PHARMACOLOGY - RESEARCH, SAFETY TESTING AND REGULATION

STATINS

MEDICAL USES, MECHANISMS OF ACTION AND CLINICAL OUTCOMES

PHARMACOLOGY - RESEARCH, SAFETY TESTING AND REGULATION

Additional books in this series can be found on Nova's website under the Series tab.

Additional e-books in this series can be found on Nova's website under the e-book tab.

PHARMACOLOGY - RESEARCH, SAFETY TESTING AND REGULATION

STATINS

MEDICAL USES, MECHANISMS OF ACTION AND CLINICAL OUTCOMES

ERIC R. TRAVERS
EDITOR

NOVA BIOMEDICAL

New York

Library of Congress Cataloging-in-Publication Data

ISBN: 978-1-63463-057-3

Library of Congress Control Number: 2014950599

Published by Nova Science Publishers, Inc. † New York

CONTENTS

PREFACE

Statins are well-known drugs to lower cholesterol levels and play an important role in the prevention of cardiovascular diseases. They inhibit hydroxymethylglutaryl–coenzyme A (HMGCoA) reductase, an enzyme that plays a central role in the production of cholesterol in the liver. Despite the growing experience in the use of statins, it is still difficult to predict the individual patient response in term of efficacy and possible adverse effects. This book discusses several medical uses for statins. It also discusses the mechanisms of action and clinical outcomes of using statins.

Chapter 1 - Statins, HMG-CoA reductase inhibitors, are well-known drugs to lower cholesterol levels and play an important role in the prevention of cardiovascular diseases [associated with increased levels of primarily low-density-lipoprotein (LDL)-cholesterol], especially in the early stages of disease. The effect of statins has been studied in different animal models, including small rodents (rats and mice), but rodents have somewhat different pathways for lipid metabolism and different serum lipoprotein profiles compared to humans (high levels of HDL, no CETP, somewhat refractory to atherogenesis, etc.). It would appear important to focus on the similarities and differences of the effects of hypolipidemic drugs (e.g., statins) in humans and small laboratory animals, since the latter are extensively utilized in pre-clinical studies to screen the potency and efficacy of new hypolipidemic drugs In this regard, it might be useful to better understand the mechanism of action of statins in mice (the most widely-used animal model in pre-clinical hypolipidemic drug testing), because it has been reported that about 50% of all published studies which evaluated the effects of statins in rodents do not demonstrate any hypolipidemic effect, since rodents carry approximately 80% of their cholesterol as HDL. In fact, almost all mouse models of atherogenesis do not mimic the most important event in human atherosclerosis, that is, plaque rupture leading to vessel occlusion. However, the poloxamer 407-induced mouse model of hyperlipidemia is a dose-dependent mouse model that produces an atherogenic plasma lipid profile somewhat similar to humans (including formation of ox-LDL), although it must be emphasized that serum triglyceride concentrations are more sensitive to the effects of poloxamer 407 due to its general lipase inhibitory effects. This model previously evaluated the hypolipidemic efficacy of commercially-available, FDA-approved statins in mice, which mirrored the trend (rank-order) in efficacy observed in humans. Additionally, this model was utilized previously to induce fibrofatty aortic lesions in mice after 4 months, and subsequently mediate regression of established plaque following an additional 4 months of treatment with atorvastatin. In this study, atorvastatin was tested in mice with atherosclerotic lesions produced by either long-term (4 mo) treatment with poloxamer 407, or mice which consumed a classic high-fat, cholate-containing diet for 4 months. In general, one needs to use higher doses of statin drugs in mice to produce a therapeutic effect. Acute lipemia induced by poloxamer 407 can be effectively treated only by high doses of statins (e.g., atorvastatin). The difficulties associated with recapitulating the phenotypic signatures associated with human atherogenic serum lipid profiles and development of atherosclerotic lesions are discussed. Lastly, some side effects of statins in humans and experimental animal models (e.g., resistance to statin therapy) are discussed, as well as the advantages and disadvantages of various alternative mouse models of atherogenesis resulting from genetic modification.

Chapter 2 - The aim of this chapter is to assess the experimental and clinical evidence regarding potential neuroprotective effects of statins and their possible perioperative benefit. Statins are drugs used to control cholesterol disorders and prevent cardiovascular diseases by four mechanisms: improvement of endothelial function, modulation of inflammatory responses, maintenance of plaque stability, and prevention of thrombus formation. It is possible that these various effects may also be neuroprotective. The anti-inflammatory effects of statins on endothelial cell mechanisms are better understood than their role in neuroprotection or tumoral apoptosis and evidence is only just emerging that statins may be beneficial. Data regarding perioperative use of statins in neurosurgery is scarce, controversial and inconclusive since there is a lack of convincing randomized, prospective clinical trials. More trials in humans are needed to determine whether statins could contribute to the current management of neurosurgical diseases. Not much is known about utilizing statins as a prophylactic treatment and some would probably advocate that we should be treating ‘at risk’ patients with statins perioperatively or at least it is important to try to put this into a clinical perspective.

Chapter 3 - The use of statins has recently attracted the attention of clinicians. Indeed, statins are probably the most common chronic treatment used for cardiovascular disease (18 million prescription purchase in France and 173.7 million in United States, per year). Moreover, their so-called pleiotropic effects open the gates to much larger medical applications. However, it is still difficult to predict the individual's response to statin therapy. Recent research has shown that variants of candidate genes affect statin efficacy and safety. Clinicians often assume that symptoms occurring with statins are caused by statins, encouraging discontinuation. But so far, only asymptomatic liver enzymes, muscle aches and development of new-onset diabetes mellitus has been proven to be related to statin therapy. To lower cholesterol levels, clinicians could prescribe statin monotherapy or a statin in combination with another agent. There are potential benefits to treating with multiple agents, such as the different mechanisms of action of other lipid-modifying agents, may be a solution against the adverse effects of statins and their intolerance. Given their pleiotropic effects, statins could be used in non-dyslipidemic diseases.

In this chapter, the authors will first examine the properties of statins including their structure, metabolism, and potency. The authors will also look at the pharmacogenomics of statins as well their mechanisms of action from their lipid-lowering effects to the more complex anti-inflammatory, immunomodulatory, anti-thrombotic, and anti-oxidant properties found independently of the lipid-lowering properties. Following this, the authors will review the potential adverse effects of statins including the mechanisms leading to myopathy and new-onset diabetes mellitus. In this regard, they will assess the benefits and harmful intensification of statin monotherapy compared to the combination of statins and other lipid-modifying medications. Then, the authors will discuss the guidelines regarding the use of statins in the well-established scope of cardiovascular diseases. Finally, the authors will review the potential benefits of statins in non-dyslipdemic disorders in chronic diseases such as rheumatoid arthritis, venous thromboembolism, and polycystic ovary syndrome, as well as in critical illnesses such as sepsis, acute lung injury/acute respiratory distress syndrome or after subarachnoidal hemorrhage. The authors will particularly focus on the latter.

Chapter 4 - Statins are widely used drugs that reduce mortality associated with cardiovascular disease. Despite an extensive evidence base for both their efficacy and adverse effects, the effect of statins on the brain and behaviour remains controversial, with some types of data suggesting harmful effects from statins but with other types of data suggesting beneficial effects. This article reviews these diverse sources of evidence, combining information from randomised clinical trials, case studies and adverse reaction monitoring programs, preclinical research, and epidemiological studies. Statins are discussed for potential psychiatric effects, effects on learning and memory, neuroprotective effects, effects on Alzheimer's disease, and on cerebral blood flow. The authors conclude that although there is some evidence that high doses of statins may have adverse psychiatric effects in some people, these are rare and can be managed through dose alteration or change in statin, and should not impact on current practice for the use of statins management of cardiovascular disease.

Chapter 5 - Cardiac surgery is associated with excellent results for patients treated for acquired cardiac disease such as coronary artery or valve disease. However, the constantly ageing patient population presents with a rising prevalence of relevant co-morbidities leading to a significant risk for postoperative major adverse cardiovascular events. This trend implies the importance of an optimal perioperative medical treatment. In this context, statins have shown to be linked with beneficial effects after on-pump coronary artery bypass graft procedures while less evidence is available for patients referred to valve surgery. This chapter aims to summarize the current evidence for perioperative statin therapy for various kinds of surgery.

Chapter 6 - Atherosclerosis is a disease that begins in childhood. Evidence of fatty streaks, the earliest precursor of atherosclerotic lesions, has been found in the coronary arteries of children as young as two years of age. Hypercholesterolemia is a risk factor for coronary artery disease. Hypercholesterolemia can be either primary, when it is characteristic of the main disease, or secondary when it occurs as a result of either a disease process or drug treatment.

Given the risk of vascular disease, including myocardial infarction (MI), cerebrovascular accidents (CVA, also known as strokes), peripheral vascular disease (PVD), and ruptured aortic aneurysm, any or all of which may follow atherosclerosis, it is important to prevent or slow the early development of atherosclerotic lesions. This prevention necessitates the control of key risk factors such hypercholesterolemia, dyslipidemia, hypertension etc. However, at what point this prevention ought to occur, and in what form, is uncertain.

This uncertainty stems from the fact that using pharmacological primary prevention in the paediatric population is controversial. In an adult patient the course of action is clear. Hypercholesterolemia warrants the initiation of a statin. Statins, also known as hydroxymethylglutaryl Co-enzyme A inhibitors (or HMG-CoA inhibitors) act by altering cholesterol metabolism. In considering the paediatric population, the clinical course of vascular disease and the effect of altering this clinical course,are less certain. Questions of safety, efficacy and ethics abound.The use of statins in the paediatric population will be examined in this chapter.

Chapter 7 - Portal hypertension is a common clinical consequence of chronic liver disease that is associated with significant morbidity and mortality. Newly described pathophysiological mechanisms has opened new perspectives for therapeutic approaches, where statins may represent an attractive option to reduce portal pressure by targeting multiple molecular pathways such as endothelial dysfunction, oxidative stress, prostanoids production, angiogenesis and HSC activation. In this work the authors described how statins may correct hemodynamic abnormalities in portal circulation of cirrhotic patients and also summarize some promising results humans and animals in studies.

Chapter 8 - Worldwide, epithelial ovarian cancer constitutes the most lethal gynecological malignancy. Annually, about 240.000 women are newly diagnosed and 150.000 die of this disease. Its lethality is mainly explained by a late diagnosis, at advanced stages, and by a transient response to available therapies. Thus, despite optimal surgical cytoreduction and a complete response to platinum-based chemotherapy, the majority of cases eventually relapses and dies of their disease determining a 5-year survival not exceeding 40%.

Current hypothesis for ovarian carcinogenesis establishes as a major determinant for malignant transformation of ovarian surface epithelium the chronic exposure to an inflammatory environment. Several conditions predispose to chronic inflammation, one of them the obesity. More importantly, recent studies confer a prognosis even worse to those ovarian cancer patients that are obese. A possible explanation for a more deleterious outcome in this subpopulation can be found in the presence of metabolic abnormalities and higher levels circulating of pro-inflammatory mediators. In fact, studies by the author's group and others show that alterations in lipid metabolism and the presence of higher levels of leptin, both conditions commonly found in the obese population, favor a pro-inflammatory environment that promotes cell growth, invasion, metastasis, and resistance to chemotherapeutic agents by the cancer cells.

Interestingly, some retrospective evidence suggests that patients receiving statins during their ovarian cancer treatment experience a better outcome than those not receiving them. Statins, HMGCoA reductase inhibitors, are usually prescribed to reduce cholesterol levels but they also possess pleiotropic effects that negatively influence ovarian carcinogenesis. By inhibiting the mevalonate pathway, statins would have a systemic effect, similar to that observed in atherosclerosis, reducing the inflammatory stimuli present in the tumor microenvironment and inhibiting the activation of multiple intracellular signaling cascades critical for metabolism, proliferation, cell death, migration, invasion, metastasis, and drug sensitivity of the ovarian cancer cell.

In the present chapter the authors summarize the current evidence on molecular mechanisms supporting the beneficial effect of statins in ovarian cancer. In particular, reasons to maintain statin use among those newly diagnosed ovarian cancer patients already taking this medication. Furthermore, reasons to consider this drug in the design of future clinical trials in the treatment of epithelial ovarian cancer.

Chapter 9 - Inhibitors of 3-hydroxy- 3-methylglutaryl-coenzyme A reductase (HMG-CoA) or statins are important drugs used in the treatment of dyslipidemia by reducing the biosynthesis of cholesterol. In addition to the main effect of lowering blood cholesterol levels, they have pleiotropic effects of which can be highlighted: i) improvement of endothelial function through modulation of endothelial nitric oxide synthase (eNOS) activity and inhibition of endothelin; ii) anti-inflammatory effects resulting from the reduction of proinflammatory cell signaling, oxidative stress, interaction of leukocytes to endothelial cells, and platelet and tissue factor activation; iii) stabilization of atherosclerotic plaque; iv) reduction of osteoclast formation and stimulation of osteoblasts (antiosteoporotic effect); and v) immunomodulation. It is known that these effects are variable and are not common to all statins. Even so, given the potential of these drugs, statins are currently the most prescribed medicines worldwide, and generally are extremely well tolerated by patients. However, adverse effects with different magnitudes can be observed in muscles, with occurrences ranging from a mild myalgia to rhabdomyolysis, progressing to acute renal failure and even death. The statin-induced rhabdomyolysis is a rare event, and is estimated to occur in 0.3 per 100,000 patient years of exposure, with a mortality rate of 9%. Regarding muscular symptoms, myalgia is characterized by pain with or without muscle weakness, not accompanied by an increased in creatine phosphokinase (CPK) enzyme, contrasting to myositis, that leads to an increase of this enzyme associated with muscle symptoms. Conversely, rhabdomyolysis, in generally, is characterized by muscle symptoms and significant increases in CPK levels (generally greater than 10 times the normal upper limit), and elevated levels of creatinine, renal dysfunction, dark urine, and myoglobinuria. Therefore, monitoring CPK levels is recommended during treatment with statins, since it is known the occurrence of an increase in their levels with potential severe effects on muscles even in the absence of muscular symptomatology. On the other hand, the opposite also occurs with muscle manifestations even in the absence of elevated CPK. The mechanisms by which statins develops miotoxicity remains not fully understood. Among the hypotheses proposed, the blocked in cholesterol biosynthesis induced by statins can be a myotoxicity determinant since the reduction in cholesterol content of cell membranes of skeletal muscle could make them unstable. Another hypothesis considers the farnesyl pyrophosphate and geranylgeranyl pirosfofate decrease, which normally activate regulatory proteins binding to guanosine triphosphate (GTP), which promotes cell maintenance and growth while decreasing apoptosis. Lastly, the hypothesis of myopathy occurrence across the depletion of coenzyme Q10 (CoQ10) in mitochondria is also considered. In association with drug therapy in clinical practice, it is often recommended to dyslipidemic patients the practice of regular physical exercises, which are known to be the most effective and cheapest intervention in reducing morbidity and mortality from cardiovascular diseases. However, miotoxicity can negatively interfere with the exercise or, in the opposite direction, the exercises may, itself, potentiate the statin myotoxic effect.

Chapter 10 - Hyperlipidemia is one of the major risk factors of cardiovascular disease (CVD). Hydroxymethylglutaryl coenzyme-A (HMG-CoA) reductase inhibitors, or statins, have now become the most commonly prescribed drugs to intended lower serum low-density lipoprotein cholesterol levels, which eventually prevent primary or secondary CVD events. However, it has also been argued that statin therapy may associate with new onset diabetes mellitus (DM) in clinical trials and metaanalyses. This association is universally observed across different statins –the homologous class effect– in some studies, while there could be varying levels of risk or gradient risk increases depending on the individual statins or their doses in some studies. Although the strength of association is weak and heterogeneous, the consistency cannot be denied. Therefore, it is critical that clinicians be aware of this presumed risk of developing DM because DM *per se* is a risk factor for CVD. This minireview presents current knowledge on the association between statins and developing DM and discusses the benefit-risk balance, i.e., the balance between numbers needed to treat and the numbers needed to harm, as well as potential confounding factors that could play a role in the statin-DM association. This comprehensive evaluation draws the conclusion that the benefits of statin therapy outweigh the new onset DM and reinforces the importance of continued statin therapy, –though the statin-DM association continues to be considered a risk among a certain segment of patients with specific characteristics. This motivates more further, more in-depth research to realize treatment optimization through identifying the most beneficial patient population while minimizing the risk of new onset DM.

In: Statins
Editor: Eric R. Travers
ISBN: 978-1-63463-057-3

Chapter 1

STATIN TREATMENT IN EXPERIMENTAL LIPEMIA AND ATHEROSCLEROSIS: THE SIMILARITIES AND DIFFERENCES WITH HUMANS

Thomas P. Johnston[1*] and Tatyana A. Korolenko[2]
[1]Division of Pharmaceutical Sciences,
University of Missouri-Kansas City, Kansas City, Missouri, US
[2]Institute of Physiology and Fundamental Medicine,
Siberian Branch of the Russian
Academy of Medical Sciences, Novosibirsk, Russia

ABSTRACT

Statins, HMG-CoA reductase inhibitors, are well-known drugs to lower cholesterol levels and play an important role in the prevention of cardiovascular diseases [associated with increased levels of primarily low-density-lipoprotein (LDL)-cholesterol], especially in the early stages of disease. The effect of statins has been studied in different animal models, including small rodents (rats and mice), but rodents have somewhat different pathways for lipid metabolism and different serum lipoprotein profiles compared to humans (high levels of HDL, no CETP, somewhat refractory to atherogenesis, *etc.*). It would appear important to focus on the similarities and differences of the effects of hypolipidemic drugs (e.g., statins) in humans and small laboratory animals, since the latter are extensively utilized in pre-clinical studies to screen the potency and efficacy of new hypolipidemic drugs In this regard, it might be useful to better understand the mechanism of action of statins in mice (the most widely-used animal model in pre-clinical hypolipidemic drug testing), because it has been reported that about 50% of all published studies which evaluated the effects of statins in rodents do not demonstrate any hypolipidemic effect, since rodents carry approximately 80% of their cholesterol as HDL. In fact, almost all mouse models of atherogenesis do not mimic the most important event in human atherosclerosis, that is, plaque rupture leading to vessel occlusion. However,

* Thomas P. Johnston, Ph.D., R.Ph. Professor, Division of Pharmaceutical Sciences, School of Pharmacy, University of Missouri-Kansas City, Health Sciences Research Building, Room 4243, 2464 Charlotte Street, Kansas City, MO 64108, P 816-235-1624, F 816-235-5779Email: johnstont@umkc.edu.

the poloxamer 407-induced mouse model of hyperlipidemia is a dose-dependent mouse model that produces an atherogenic plasma lipid profile somewhat similar to humans (including formation of ox-LDL), although it must be emphasized that serum triglyceride concentrations are more sensitive to the effects of poloxamer 407 due to its general lipase inhibitory effects. This model previously evaluated the hypolipidemic efficacy of commercially-available, FDA-approved statins in mice, which mirrored the trend (rank-order) in efficacy observed in humans. Additionally, this model was utilized previously to induce fibrofatty aortic lesions in mice after 4 months, and subsequently mediate regression of established plaque following an additional 4 months of treatment with atorvastatin. In this study, atorvastatin was tested in mice with atherosclerotic lesions produced by either long-term (4 mo) treatment with poloxamer 407, or mice which consumed a classic high-fat, cholate-containing diet for 4 months. In general, one needs to use higher doses of statin drugs in mice to produce a therapeutic effect. Acute lipemia induced by poloxamer 407 can be effectively treated only by high doses of statins (e.g., atorvastatin). The difficulties associated with recapitulating the phenotypic signatures associated with human atherogenic serum lipid profiles and development of atherosclerotic lesions are discussed. Lastly, some side effects of statins in humans and experimental animal models (e.g., resistance to statin therapy) are discussed, as well as the advantages and disadvantages of various alternative mouse models of atherogenesis resulting from genetic modification.

Keywords: Animal Models, Atherosclerosis, Hyperlipidemia, Statin

1. Cardiovascular Diseases: Atherosclerosis

Cardiovascular disease is the leading cause of death and morbidity in developed countries. Because cardiac and vascular complications are complex multifactorial pathologies, in which both genetic and environmental factors are implicated, it makes them very difficult to prevent [1]. One cardiovascular disease in particular; namely, atherosclerosis, still presents a challenge as to the exact underlying mechanisms involved with the atherogenic cascade. However, clinical and experimental evidence acquired to date has allowed the biomedical and scientific research communities to formulate, or suggest, putative mechanisms involved with atheroma formation. In general, atherosclerosis may be described as a clinical condition in which an artery wall thickens due to the slow accumulation of macrophages and fatty substances such as cholesterol, cellular waste products, and calcium (in advanced disease), which ultimately cause restricted blood flow through the artery. In the worst case scenario, the artery becomes totally occluded such that there is either negligible, or no blood flow, through the vessel. Atherosclerosis contributes to the most frequent underlying cause of coronary artery disease (CAD), carotid artery disease, and peripheral vascular disease, which, when taken together, constitutes the leading cause of mortality worldwide [2]. Many reviews have been written on the pathogenesis of atherosclerosis [3,4], so only a brief review will be provided here.

It is thought that high plasma concentrations of low-density lipoprotein (LDL) cholesterol, and especially oxidized LDL (oxLDL), initiate the progression of atherosclerotic lesion formation. Following this initiation step, endothelial cells express various adhesion molecules, which cause leukocytes to attach to the endothelium. Some of the primary adhesion molecules which play a pivotal role in leucocyte attachment are vascular cell adhesion molecule-1 (VCAM-1), intercellular adhesion molecule-1 (ICAM-1), and E-selectin. These adhesion molecules specifically recruit monocytes and T-lymphocytes, which are the predominant cell types found in early atherosclerotic lesions. Following adhesion to the vessel wall, monocytes migrate to the sub-endothelial space, where they differentiate into macrophages. These macrophages up-regulate the expression of scavenger receptors, which then incorporate cholesterol and oxLDL to form lipid-laden foam cells. The continued production and accumulation of foam cells ultimately leads to the development of fatty streaks within the vessel wall. Inflammation also plays a critical role in atheroma formation, because the foam cells manufacture cytokines and reactive oxygen species (ROS), which augment the inflammatory process.

The process continues as smooth muscle cells migrate from the medial layer into the intimal or sub-endothelial space where they begin to proliferate, engulf modified lipoproteins, and subsequently contribute to the formation of more complex lesions. These smooth muscle cells also secrete extracellular matrix proteins, which serve as a precursor to the development of fibrous plaque [5]. Narrowing of the vessel lumen begins to occur due to a chronic inflammatory state, which is influenced by a broad range of cellular and humoral responses [6,7]. When plaque rupture occurs in advanced lesions, blood components are brought in contact with lipids, as well as tissue factors, comprising the plaque, which ultimately results in formation of a thrombus and accompanying ischemia. Ischemia then leads to conditions such as myocardial infarction and stroke [8,9].

While atherosclerosis is a multifactorial disease involving numerous genetic and environmental variables, the most common risk factor for the development of this disease is the alteration of cholesterol levels in the blood [3,4]. For this reason, the statin class of drugs has been used for the last 20 years to effectively lower cholesterol, and, in particular, LDL cholesterol, in the blood. In fact, statin drugs are considered a first-line therapeutic intervention for the treatment of hypercholesterolemia that cannot be controlled with lifestyle modifications (regular exercise, diet, etc.) [10,11]. However, despite the great success of statin drugs, approximately 70% of statin-treated patients still experience adverse coronary events [12]. Thus, there is a continued push toward the development of new therapeutics that specifically target risk factors other than hypercholesterolemia, which can be used either alone, or in combination with, a statin drug [2]. Animal models that assist with the elucidation of the pathogenesis and causes of atherosclerosis are needed in the current search for new therapeutics. Therefore, a brief overview of statin therapy, as well as their use in both humans and experimental animal models, the latter, of which, attempt to recapitulate the phenotypic signatures of atherosclerosis in humans, will be presented below.

2. Overview of Statins in Hyperlipidemia and Atherosclerosis

Statins are widely prescribed cholesterol-lowering drugs with proven efficacy in humans. Statins partially exert their effect by inhibiting 3-hydroxy-3-methylglutaryl (HMG) coenzyme A (CoA) reductase, a rate-limiting enzyme involved with cholesterol neosynthesis. It is worthwhile to note that the plasma cholesterol-lowering effect of statins derives primarily from an enhanced uptake of LDL by upregulation of LDL receptor (LDLr) expression on the surface of the hepatocyte membrane and, to a lesser extent, from reduced endogenous cholesterol biosynthesis. The clinically-relevant members of the statin family of drugs include atorvastatin, cerivastatin, fluvastatin, lovastatin, pravastatin, pitavastatin, rosuvastatin, and simvastatin. Data to date clearly demonstrate a linear relationship between the degree of LDL-cholesterol lowering achieved by statins and benefits, with a 10% and a 21% reduction in all-cause mortality and major vascular events, respectively, per every 38.7 mg/dl decrease in LDL-cholesterol [13]. This is further supported by data demonstrating superiority of more, compared to less, intensive LDL-cholesterol lowering [13].

It is interesting to note that benefits from statins have been observed in people with coronary heart disease, stroke, and diabetes, as well as those who are apparently healthy. Meta-analyses have also re-confirmed the overall safety of statins, with neither a significant increase in non-vascular mortality, nor in incident or fatal cancer [13]. In fact, statins are well tolerated apart from myalgia, although its frequency is greater in clinical use than found in randomized clinical trials (RCTs). Observational data in over 2 million individuals have also shown that acute renal failure may be a dose-related side effect of statins, although it has a very low incidence [14]. Treatment of approximately 1,700 persons over 3 months with high-dose, compared to low-dose, statin therapy was associated with one hospitalization [15]. Previous meta-analysis of RCTs has revealed that one incident case of new type-2 diabetes may occur for every 255 individuals treated for 2 years with statins [16]. There have also been studies that have postulated impairment of cognition with statin use, but this was based on less robust observational data. One important analysis compared coronary heart disease (CHD) risk reduction with statin therapy in subjects with genotypes that impact LDL-cholesterol concentrations throughout their life and in RCTs with follow-up at approximately 4-5 years [14]. There was an approximate 3-fold greater reduction in CVD death, non-fatal myocardial infarction, and coronary revascularization (when the latter could be assessed) per every 38.7 mg/dl reduction in LDL-cholesterol concentrations with lifetime exposure compared to that seen in RCTs.

One current dilemma with the use of statins involves when to initiate statin therapy in apparently healthy adults. The early stages of atherosclerosis are preset in many asymptomatic younger adults in the second and third decades of life [17]. One of the potential indicators in apparently healthy, asymptomatic adults that could possibly be utilized to determine when statin therapy should be commenced in this target population are those with a family history of premature CHD, which is currently supported by guidelines [18]. Quantification of coronary artery calcification in intermediate-risk patients is already used by many clinicians [19].

Despite the extremely strong evidence base supporting the use of statins, other LDL-cholesterol lowering therapies are needed, and this is why experimental animal models, which are able to reliably recapitulate the pathophysiologic features of CHD and subsequent atherosclerosis are desperately needed. The reason that additional LDL-cholesterol lowering therapies are needed is because the LDL-cholesterol target suggested by guidelines, currently about 70 to 77 mg/dl for high-risk patients, are often not achieved with statin monotherapy. Patients may become 'statin intolerant'. The phrase 'statin intolerance' refers to an inability to use statins because of muscle symptoms or elevated creatine kinase (CK), and the major diagnostic challenge is to unambiguously link these to statin use [20]. Roughly, about 5% to 10% of statin users develop statin intolerance [20].

Finally, in addition to the high "residual risk" despite attainment of the recommended LDL-cholesterol target, more aggressive statin therapy may be warranted in special situations. Some of these special conditions include familial hypercholesterolemia (FH), when LDL-cholesterol concentrations are routinely greater than about 100 mg/dl despite statin therapy, and those patients with a genetic elevation in lipoprotein(a). In fact, FH is thought to affect about 1 in 200 individuals, making it the most common genetically transmitted disease [21]. The potential use of combination LDL-cholesterol lowering therapy is supported by greater reductions in serum LDL-cholesterol concentrations when a statin is used in combination with another LDL-cholesterol lowering intervention (drug, sequestrant, proprotein convertase subtilisin/kexin type 9 (PCSK9) inhibitor, microsomal triglyceride transfer protein (MTP) inhibitor, antisense oligonucleotide, etc.) compared to simply an increase in the statin dose when used as monotherapy [14,22].

While this chapter's focus is on the lipid-lowering effects of statins in both humans and experimental animal models of hyperlipidemia, nevertheless, it must be mentioned that statins also produce additional health benefits independent of their lipid-lowering effects. These additional pharmacological advantages to statin therapy are generally referred to as 'pleiotropic effects' [23]. Several pleiotropic effects will be mentioned below, but this does not represent an exhaustive list of all of the beneficial effects that have been observed with statins to date. Some of the nonlipid-related therapeutic effects of statins include, but are not limited to, improved endothelial function and decreased LDL oxidation, foam cell formation, smooth muscle cell proliferation, plaque rupture, and thrombus formation [23-27]. Furthermore, statins have also been found to exert both anti-inflammatory and anti-angiogenic effects, both of which are relevant to vascular disease, as well as the pathogenesis of age-related macular degeneration (AMD) [28-30]. In fact, as it relates to vision, mice administered simvastatin for 6 weeks showed significantly improved retinal structure and function [31]. Due to the fact that antioxidants are beneficial for the treatment of AMD, some investigators have evaluated the effects of statins on the development and progression of AMD and have suggested that the clinically-observed protective effects of statins in patients with AMD was due to their antioxidant activity [32]. In fact, it has been shown that statins lead to promoter activation of the antioxidative defense protein heme oxygenase-1 (HO-1), which might explain their pleiotropic antioxidative, anti-inflammatory effects [33].

3. Animal Models of Atherosclerosis

Animal models have been tremendously useful in helping to understand the pathogenetic steps and causes of atherosclerosis in humans. The first study which investigated the deliberate induction of atherogenesis in an animal model occurred when a Russian scientist, Ignatowski, demonstrated in 1908 that atherosclerosis could be consistently and reliably produced in rabbits by feeding them milk and egg yolks [34]. Since this initial study, animal models involving mice, rats, guinea pigs, hamsters, birds, swine, and non-human primates have provided valuable information regarding diagnostic and therapeutic strategies for atherosclerosis, with extensive investigation of the sequence of events occurring in the artery wall during the course of the disease process [2]. Of all of the animal models of atherosclerosis utilized to date, rodents and rabbits are still the most commonly used animal models involved with preclinical atherosclerosis research [2]. With the advent of genetic manipulation and the genesis of gene-knockout models, mice have now surpassed rabbits as the most widely used animal model with which to investigate the pathogenesis of atherosclerosis. Mouse models used to induce hyperlipidemia and atherosclerosis can loosely be categorized as those based on manipulation of diet (e.g., a high-fat, cholate-containing diet), modification of genes (e.g., various gene-knockout models; apoE, LDLr, etc.), and those models in which an exogenous compound is administered. Each of these mouse models has its unique set of advantages and disadvantages, and no one mouse model is ideal for investigating every aspect of this multifactorial disease process. Mouse models of hyperlipidemia and atherosclerosis based on dietary or genetic manipulation have been reviewed on numerous occasions [35,36], so the present authors will not provide a review of those models here. However, a model that was developed by one of the authors (T.P. Johnston) [37-49] using an exogenously-administered compound called poloxamer 407 (P-407) will be reviewed in this chapter, since it has proven useful to screen the therapeutic efficacy of statins.

4. The P-407-Induced Mouse Model of Hyperlipidemia and Atherosclerosis

The P-407-induced animal model of hyperlipidemia and atherosclerosis was initially developed by Johnston et al., in 1992 using rats [50], although these investigators switched to C57BL/6 mice once the same pharmacological effects to P-407 observed in Sprague-Dawley rats could be reliably reproduced in mice [51]. The P-407 mouse model of hyperlipidemia is a dose-controlled animal model that utilizes P-407 (a block copolymer and surfactant) to titrate the serum levels of cholesterol and triglycerides to any desired concentration. Since 1992, Johnston et al., has continued to use the P-407-induced mouse model of atherosclerosis to identify and characterize alterations in atherogenic plasma lipids, changes in the activity of key enzymes involved with lipid metabolism, and numerous other aspects involved in the pathogenesis of atherosclerosis [37-49]. In fact, as will be discussed below, this mouse model of hyperlipidemia and atherosclerosis has been shown to be useful for assessing the efficacy and potency of antihyperlipidemic agents in several drug classes (including statins) and mirrors the clinical efficacy observed with these drugs in humans [52]. The P-407-induced mouse model of hyperlipidemia and atherosclerosis will now be briefly described.

Poloxamer 407 (P-407) is a block copolymer that is used primarily as a surface-active-agent. When 5-6 week-old C57BL/6 male or female mice weighing approximately 15 g are administered a single 0.5 g/kg dose of P-407 in 0.5 mL by intraperitoneal injection, plasma concentrations of total cholesterol, and especially triglycerides (TG), are elevated for about 96 hours [50,51,53,54]. Maximum plasma concentrations of total cholesterol and TG are observed 24 hours after dosing, with a return to baseline values approximately 72 hours after maximum plasma lipid concentrations were attained (i.e., 96 h). The authors have previously demonstrated that the rise in plasma TGs occurs as a result of P-407's inactivation of capillary-bound lipoprotein lipase (LPL) [53], while the rise in plasma total cholesterol occurs due to P-407-mediated inactivation of cholesterol 7α-hydroxylase, which is the rate-limiting enzyme responsible for elimination of cholesterol into bile [52]. It is important to note that P-407 appears to be a general lipase inhibitor, hence, the enzymatic activity of LPL, hepatic lipase (HL), endothelial lipase (EL), and pancreatic lipase (PL) are all inhibited with similar log dose-activity profiles and IC_{50} values [45]. Administration of P-407 to mice also affects the distribution of lipoprotein fractions, which will be described below.

In addition to research investigating the effect that P-407-induced hyperlipidemia has on the activity of several lipases and other key enzymes involved in lipid metabolism, the authors have also reported changes in the activity of several classes of proteases in heart, liver, and the serum of P-407-treated mice [47-49]. Specifically, the authors have investigated the activity of matrix metalloproteases (MMPs) and both cysteine proteases (i.e., cathepsins B and L) and aspartate proteases (i.e., cathepsin D) following P-407 administration to mice. How proteases of different classes participate in the early stages of atherosclerosis is still unknown; in particular, their role in damage/injury to the coronary vessels and the heart. Prior to describing our results concerning hyperlipidemia and protease activity, a very brief discussion will be provided below concerning the role of MMPs and cysteine and aspartate proteases (cathepsins B, L, D) in atherosclerosis.

MMPs represent the main group of molecules regulating and processing adhesion molecules, proteases, and protease inhibitors [55]. Importantly, MMPs are responsible for the degradation and turnover of extracellular matrix [56,57]. As such, MMPs are suggested to be involved in the later stages of atherosclerosis (i.e., stability and rupture of atherosclerotic plaques) [58].

Cysteine proteases have been identified as major elastolytic and collagenolytic enzymes, causing arterial wall atherosclerotic changes [59]. Expressed by macrophages and smooth muscle cells, cysteine proteases can participate not only in protein degradation inside lysosomes, but also the degradation of the extracellular environment following their release from lysosomes [60,61]. As just mentioned, cysteine proteases have a central role in extracellular matrix (ECM) remodeling and have been implicated in the development and progression of cardiovascular diseases, e.g., atherosclerosis [62]. In particular, cathepsins have the capacity to degrade low-density lipoprotein and reduce cholesterol efflux from macrophages, aggravating foam cell formation. Oxidized LDL-cholesterol (oxLDL) (formed in the P-407 model) damages the lysosomal membrane and cause the release of cathepsins B and L into the cytosol, which may then act as cleavage enzymes during apoptosis and subsequently contribute to the formation of the necrotic core [63-65]. The action of oxLDL on the translocation of cathepsins B and L from the lysosome to the cytosol can be considered an atherosclerosis-stimulating role for cathepsins B and L. Not surprisingly, both mRNA and protein levels of cathepsins B and L are increased in murine and human atherosclerotic lesions [66,67]. Cathepsin B has been implicated in the genesis and development of heart failure, since an increase in myocardial expression of cathepsin B was found in patients suffering from heart failure [68]. Serum cathepsin L has been shown to be an accurate and independent biomarker for coronary heart disease. Importantly, cathepsin L has been suggested to be a distinguishing feature of unstable atherosclerotic plaque and myocardial ischemic injury [69]. Lastly, it has been found that the aspartate protease, cathepsin D, is increased in both plasma and monocytes of patients with acute coronary artery disease [70]. In addition, the extracellular regions of macrophage-rich intima contained in atherosclerotic lesions test positive for cathepsin D, whereas normal arteries do not reveal the presence of cathepsin D [71].

Korolenko et al., [47-49] have demonstrated that protease activity was modulated during sustained hyperlipidemia induced by the administration of P-407 to mice. Specifically, mice were administered either P-407 (500 mg/kg), or normal saline, by intraperitoneal injection two times per week for four months. As assessed using fluorescent spectroscopy, P-407-induced hyperlipidemic mice had a significant ($p < 0.01$) increase in both the specific activity of cysteine proteases (cathepsins B & L) and the aspartate protease (cathepsin D), as well as the activity of MMP, in heart tissue. However, only cathepsin B and MMP activity were significantly ($p < 0.01$) increased in the liver of P-407 hyperlipidemic mice. Interestingly, treatment with a statin (atorvastatin) in acute P-407-induced lipemia resulted in an increase in serum MMP activity in both control and P-407 hyperlipidemic mice. These results demonstrate that sustained hyperlipidemia induced in P-407-treated mice modulates protease activity, which potentially plays a key role in atheroma formation in this mouse model of atherogenesis.

In addition to determining the activity of select proteases in P-407 hyperlipidemic mice, we have also extensively characterized the lipoprotein fractions associated with the resulting atherogenic plasma lipid profile. Previously, we reported that long-term administration of P-407 (0.5 g/kg every third day for 4 mo) to C57BL/6 mice resulted in an average plasma TG concentration of 2,800 ± 460 mg/dl compared with 86 ± 7 mg/dl for controls [51]. Plasma samples evaluated chromatographically for the distribution of TG among the lipoproteins VLDL, IDL/LDL, and HDL resulted in virtually all of the TG being associated with the VLDL fraction [54]. In contrast to the TG lipoprotein distribution for saline-treated control mice, plasma from P-407-treated mice revealed a complete absence of TG associated with the IDL/LDL fraction. Additionally, agarose gel analysis indicated the presence of chylomicrons and very-large, TG-rich VLDL in P-407-treated mice. Evaluation of the apolipoprotein content of high-density lipoprotein (HDL) obtained from the plasma of P-407-treated mice by using Western blots, centrifugation, and SDS-PAGE demonstrated that there was more apolipoprotein-E (apoE) relative to apolipoprotein-A1 (apoA1) in the HDL fraction when compared to controls [54]. A reduction in apoA1 content of the HDL lipoprotein fraction would be expected to enhance atherosclerotic lesion formation, since it has been demonstrated that it is primarily the particles with apoA1 only that confer the protective effect of HDL [72]. This is just one of the many factors that contribute to the formation of fibrofatty aortic lesions in mice starting at about one month after initiating repetitive dosing of P-407 at a dose of 0.5 g/kg every third day for four months [37,47,51,73,74]. The atherosclerotic lesions thus formed are similar in number, density, and morphology to human atheromas and also parallel the time course observed for lesion development in mice fed a high-fat, cholate-containing diet for 4 months [37,47,51,73,74]. Because this model significantly increases plasma levels of non-HDL cholesterol, it is most beneficial for the evaluation and assessment of Type IV hyperlipoproteinemias in humans, which are characterized by an abnormal increase in VLDL. The major lipid elevated in a Type IV hyperlipoproteinemia is TG with, or without, a moderate increase in plasma total cholesterol. As we have shown previously, long-term administration (> 4 mo) of P-407 to mice results in a shift from HDL cholesterol (~80% in rodents) to primarily VLDL cholesterol [54].

Formation of atherosclerotic lesions in the P-407-induced mouse model of hyperlipidemia also results from the formation of oxidized LDL cholesterol. In contrast to cupric sulfate, we have previously shown that P-407 has no intrinsic capacity to oxidize human LDL *in vitro* [75,76]. However, when P-407 was administered to mice and subsequently caused an elevation in plasma concentrations of LDL cholesterol, we detected antibodies to oxidized LDL containing malondialdehyde (MDA-modified oxLDL) [75,76].

Disturbances in triglyceride metabolism also promotes atherogenesis by increasing the expression of vascular cell adhesion molecules (CAMs). Patients with markedly elevated triglyceride levels have decreased HDL cholesterol concentrations and abnormalities in fatty acid metabolism. *In vitro* studies have demonstrated that low levels of HDL cholesterol and oxidized fatty acids increase the endothelial expression of CAMs in response to cytokines. Adhesion of leukocytes to the vascular endothelium and their subsequent transmigration into the intima are key events in atherogenesis as mentioned above in the section entitled, "*Cardiovascular Diseases: Atherosclerosis*". The soluble shed forms of cellular adhesion molecules (sCAMs) found in the plasma are considered surrogate markers for the cellular expression of CAMs. The presence of oxLDL cholesterol and fatty acids in the plasma, hypertriglyceridemia, and reduced plasma concentrations of HDL cholesterol are all thought to stimulate an increase in the cellular expression of CAMs, such as VCAM-1, ICAM-1, and E-selectin. We have previously demonstrated that the plasma levels of sVCAM-1, sICAM-1, and sE-selectin were all significantly elevated following a single dose of P-407 in mice, although the temporal relationship between the plasma sCAM concentration-time profiles and the plasma lipid concentration-time profiles were not coincident [44]. The sCAMs all attained a maximum plasma concentration at approximately 48 h after a single dose of P-407, whereas plasma HDL cholesterol, non-HDL cholesterol, and triglycerides all attained a maximum concentration at about 24 h after P-407 administration [44]. Thus, this is one more factor which contributes to the formation of atherosclerotic lesions in the P-407-induced mouse model of hyperlipidemia.

Lastly, we have previously demonstrated that human macrophages cultured with P-407 exhibited a concentration-dependent reduction in cholesterol efflux to apolipoprotein A1 (apoA1) linked to down-regulation of the ATP-binding cassette transporter A1 (ABCA1) [40]. Since activation of peroxisome proliferator-activated receptor gamma (PPARγ), as well as PPARα, increase the expression of liver X receptor alpha (LXRα) in macrophages and promote the expression of ABCA1, which, in turn, mediates cholesterol efflux to apoA1, we investigated whether P-407 interfered with this signaling pathway. An *in vitro* transactivation assay was used to evaluate whether P-407 could either activate, or inhibit, the transcriptional activity of PPARγ [42]. We found that P-407 was unable to modulate PPARγ activity in cell-based transactivation assays. Furthermore, P-407 did not perturb plasma insulin and blood glucose concentrations following administration to mice. However, P-407 did cause a significant increase in the serum concentration of circulating free fatty acids in mice beginning 3 h after administration and lasting greater than 24 h post-dosing by, as yet, an unknown mechanism [42].

5. Statin Drug Therapy

5.1. Genetically-Modified Mouse Models of Atherosclerosis

With the introduction of hyperlipidemia mouse models suitable for the study of atherosclerosis, it is now possible to evaluate and compare the efficacy of clinically-established statins with respect to their antiatherosclerotic activity. We first examine genetically-modified mouse models of hyperlipidemia and atherosclerosis and their ability to predict the effect of statins in humans. Subsequently, we will address the potential of classic diet-induced mouse models of hyperlipidemia, as well as the P-407-induced mouse model of hyperlipidemia and atherosclerosis (discussed above) to evaluate statin efficacy.

To begin, some of the currently accepted mouse models of hyperlipidemia and atherosclerosis that have resulted from gene manipulation are the apolipoprotein-E deficient (apoE$^{-/-}$), LDL receptor deficient (LDLr$^{-/-}$), combination LDLr$^{-/-}$ and apoB editing efficiency deficient (LDLr$^{-/-}$/apoBEC$^{-/-}$), combination of LDLr$^{-/-}$ and apoB100 deficient (LDLr$^{-/-}$/apoB$^{-/-}$), combination of LDLr$^{-/-}$ and apoE$^{-/-}$ (LDLr$^{-/-}$/apoE$^{-/-}$), and the apoE*3-Leiden (E3L) models. The apoE*3-Leiden mutation is a rare dominant-negative mutation in the human *apoE3* gene. The E3L transgenic mouse, in which a mutated form of the human *apoE3* gene has been introduced, displays a hyperlipidemic phenotype and develops atherosclerosis while being fed a cholesterol-rich diet.

In general, statins that are efficacious in lowering cholesterol in man do not necessarily do so in the established apoE$^{-/-}$ and LDLr$^{-/-}$ models. However, in contrast to both the apoE$^{-/-}$ and LDLr$^{-/-}$ models, the E3L model appears to respond well to statins. Treatment of apoE$^{-/-}$ mice with pravastatin, fluvastatin, cerivastatin, pitavastatin, or simvastatin did not lower plasma cholesterol [77-84], and, in some cases, even increased plasma cholesterol [85-89]. Any cholesterol-lowering effects of statins in apoE$^{-/-}$ mice were only observed when the cholesterol concentration in the experimental diet was relatively low (0.15% w/w) [90-92], or when more potent, third-generation statins (e.g., atorvastatin and rosuvastatin) were used [93-95].

Despite the absence of a hypocholesterolemic response, cerivastatin [83], pitavastatin [83], fluvastatin [79,83], pravastatin [78], and simvastatin [84] reduced aortic lipid deposition in statin-treated apoE$^{-/-}$ mice. However, subsequent analysis of the resulting atherosclerotic plaques was not without question. Several studies reported antiatherogenic effects, such as a reduction in intraplaque hemorrhage and calcification [88], as well as an increased thickness of the fibrous cap [78]. However, a different study with fluvastatin in apoE$^{-/-}$ mice documented an absence of any effect on lesion size and number, despite a very pronounced reduction in plasma total cholesterol together with a concomitant increase in plasma HDL cholesterol [90].

The LDLr$^{-/-}$ model (or the combined LDLr$^{-/-}$/apoE$^{-/-}$ model) is used very seldom to evaluate antiatherogenic properties of statins. In the few papers that have been published using this model, statins appeared to exert a variable effect on the plasma cholesterol levels and resultant atherosclerosis. Low-dose pravastatin did not significantly decrease atherosclerosis in LDLr$^{-/-}$ mice [96,97], despite a lowering of plasma cholesterol [97]. In a different study, atorvastatin was reported to decrease plasma cholesterol in LDLr$^{-/-}$ mice, but neither lesion scores, nor lesion sizes, were reported [91]. Lastly, simvastatin has been shown to cause a reduction in atherosclerosis in LDLr$^{-/-}$ mice, albeit sometimes with a simultaneous lowering of plasma cholesterol [89] and other times without an effect on plasma cholesterol concentrations [98].

In contrast to the apoE$^{-/-}$ and LDLr$^{-/-}$ mouse models, the effects of statins have been evaluated in the E3L model with much more consistent results. The effects of statins in the E3L model are more uniform and predictive of the human condition, and the results reported to date consistently demonstrate both hypolipidemic and antiatherosclerotic effects. Statins evaluated in the E3L model include atorvastatin [99-103], lovastatin [104], and rosuvastatin [105,106]. This model has also been utilized to investigate antiatherosclerotic effects of statins which are independent of their cholesterol-lowering properties [99,102,105]. Comparison of a statin-treated group *versus* a cholesterol-matched control group revealed that statins can reduce atherosclerosis beyond and independent of the reduction achieved by lowering plasma cholesterol alone. Pleiotropic (including anti-inflammatory) statin effects in the vasculature and the liver may at least partly explain these additional beneficial effects of statins [107].

5.2. Diet-Induced Mouse Models of Atherosclerosis

Prior to the development and characterization of genetically-modified animal models of hyperlipidemia and atherosclerosis, scientists utilized a variety of animal species, which were fed an atherogenic diet, in an attempt to evaluate the efficacy of various anti-hyperlipidemic agents, including statins. The most widely utilized animal model for this purpose was the C57BL/6 mouse that was intentionally fed a high-fat, high-cholesterol, cholic acid-containing diet to produce hypercholesterolemia. The cholic acid was generally included in the mouse chow at a concentration of 0.25% to 0.5%, which promotes fat and cholesterol absorption from the intestine [108]. When 5-6 week old mice were maintained on this diet for an extended time period, predictable elevations in serum lipids occurred. In fact, if mice were maintained on this specialized diet for approximately 4 months, aortic fibrofatty lesions began to develop. However, while induction of an atherogenic plasma lipid profile was easy to attain, it was suggested that cholic acid may also promote inflammation of liver and vascular endothelial tissue, decrease bile acid production, and alter circulating HDL-cholesterol concentrations and, hence, may independently affect the development of atherosclerosis [109]. Therefore, it has been suggested that inflammation resulting from inclusion of cholic acid in the diet may contribute to tissue injury and independently initiate the atherogenic cascade, since one hypothesis for the pathogenesis of atheroma formation is the "Response-to-Injury" theory [109]. It must be noted, however, that no animal model that attempts to replicate hyperlipidemia and subsequent atherosclerotic lesion formation is perfect. As an example, mice typically do not develop hypertriglyceridemia when ingesting a high-fat atherogenic diet [74,110]. Nevertheless, despite the limitations inherent with all animal models, they still have proven useful for screening the therapeutic efficacy of existing, as well as new anti-hyperlipidemic drugs and non-drug therapies. An example of a limitation associated with an existing experimental animal model of hyperlipidemia is the New Zealand white rabbit. This classic diet-induced animal model of hyperlipidemia was extensively utilized for many years to evaluate the effectiveness of a variety of anti-hyperlipidemic drugs. However, the limitation with this model was feeding a high-fat, cholesterol-rich diet to an animal that is an herbivore and would not normally ingest cholesterol in its diet. Nevertheless, the high-fat fed New Zealand white rabbit model is still utilized to determine the efficacy of anti-hyperlipidemic therapies.

A recent example of the advantages of mouse models for screening anti-hyperlipidemic agents, including statins, is provided by the work of Paraskevas et al., [111]. This group examined the effect of a number of anti-hyperlipidemic drugs, including a fibrate, ezetimibe, and both low-dose (10 mg/kg/day) and high-dose (40 mg/kg/day) atorvastatin to treat dyslipidemia associated with the metabolic syndrome in C57BL/6 mice fed a high-fat, high cholesterol, cholate-containing diet for up to 22 weeks [111]. High-dose atorvastatin treatment achieved the greatest reductions in total cholesterol and LDL-cholesterol levels compared with low-dose atorvastatin, a fibrate, or ezetimibe therapy [111]. Interestingly, mice that received the high-fat diet plus high-dose atorvastatin treatment had a similar lipid profile with those mice that received a standard non-atherogenic diet, which seems to suggest that high-dose atorvastatin treatment could abolish and fully reverse the lipid changes induced by the high-fat diet [111]. Thus, the work described above by Paraskevas et al., [111] merely serves as only one current example of the usefulness of mouse models, in which dietary intervention is used to create a hyperlipidemic state, to screen the effectiveness of statin drugs. In summary, the literature is replete with examples of high-fat, diet-induced hyperlipidemic mouse models in which a statin was evaluated for its ability to favorably modulate the lipid and lipoprotein fractions associated with cholesterol and, therefore, will not be further discussed.

5.3. The P-407-Induced Mouse Model of Atherosclerosis

Previously, we investigated the usefulness of the P-407-induced mouse model of hyperlipidemia to rank-order the clinical efficacy (lipid-lowering potential) of several HMG-CoA reductase inhibitors. Briefly, thirty C57BL/6 mice were administered P-407 (0.5 g/kg every third day) for four months by intraperitoneal injection and attained a steady-state plasma TG concentration of $2,800 \pm 460$ mg/dl. The statin drugs evaluated were pravastatin sodium, atorvastatin calcium, simvastatin, lovastatin, and fluvastatin sodium.

The effect of statin therapy on the percent reduction in plasma TG in C57BL/6 mice is shown in Figure 1. As may be noted from Figure 1, the relative rank order of effectiveness (potency) of the 5 statins tested in this model of hyperlipidemia was pravastatin > atorvastatin > simvastatin > lovastatin > fluvastatin. All post-statin treatment plasma TG concentrations were significantly ($p < 0.05$) less than the steady-state value of $2,800 \pm 460$ mg/dl for this model.

The potency of the 5 statin drugs evaluated in our model appears to be in close agreement with the rank order observed in humans with one exception. Pravastatin exhibited the greatest plasma TG-lowering effect in our mouse model of hyperlipidemia. It is of interest to note that pravastatin demonstrates the greatest aqueous solubility (>300 mg/mL) of the 5 statins evaluated. However, it should be noted that fluvastatin sodium is also water soluble, but its administration did not result in a plasma TG-lowering effect similar to pravastatin. Clinically, fluvastatin sodium has been found to be the least potent of the 5 statin drugs [112] and that finding was corroborated in our model as well.

Use of plasma TG-lowering data in mice following statin therapy would appear to be a reasonable parameter with which to assess statin efficacy in humans because: (1) the P-407-induced hyperlipidemic mouse model elevates plasma TG much more profoundly than cholesterol, and (2) it is now well established that inhibitors of HMG-CoA reductase primarily lower plasma TG and, to a lesser extent, LDL-cholesterol in normal chow-fed rats by inhibiting hepatic triglyceride secretion [113-117]. The exact mechanism(s) responsible for the TG-lowering action of the statin drugs is still being studied, but probably reflects the decrease in VLDL levels, since the major lipid class associated with VLDL is endogenous triglycerides [72]. Regardless, statin therapy in our model most likely caused a reduction in plasma TG both by decreasing VLDL levels and by inhibiting hepatic triglyceride secretion similar to the action of these agents in rats.

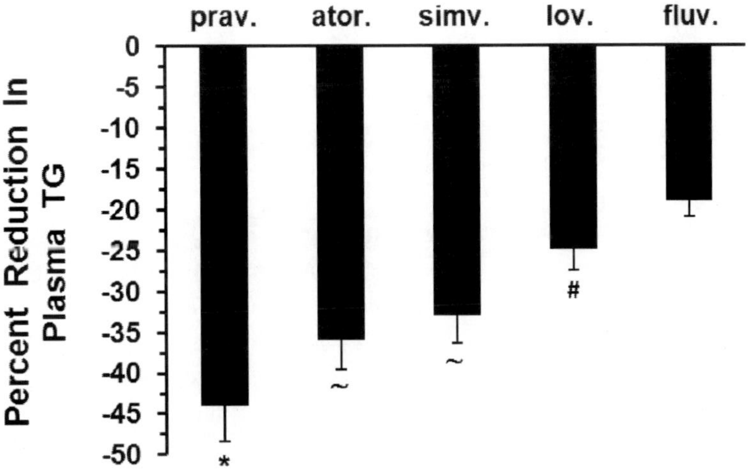

Figure 1. The effect of statin drug therapy on the percent reduction in plasma triglycerides in C57CL/6 mice. Prav., ator., simv., lov., and fluv. represent abbreviations for pravastatin sodium, atorvastatin calcium, simvastatin, lovastatin, and fluvastatin sodium, respectively. * indicates a significantly ($p < 0.05$) greater percent reduction in plasma triglycerides relative to each of the other statin drugs tested. ~ indicates a significantly ($p < 0.05$) greater percent reduction in plasma triglycerides when either ator or simv. is individually compared with either lov. or fluv., but no significant difference in the mean values between ator. and simv. # indicates a significantly ($p < 0.05$) greater percent reduction in plasma triglycerides for mice treated with lov. when compared with the same parameter for fluv. (From T.P. Johnston, *J. Cardiovasc. Pharmacol.* 2004, 43(4):595-606 with permission from Wolters Kluwer Health).

Our most recent work has again confirmed that a statin drug does affect plasma lipid concentrations following administration to mice made hyperlipidemic with P-407 [48]. However, in this investigation, we expanded our analysis of lipoproteins by using a novel small-angle X-ray scattering (SAXS) method to quantify lipoprotein *sub*fractions [118]. The effects of high-dose atorvastatin (75 mg/kg x 2 by oral gavage) on lipoprotein fractions and *sub*fractions associated with cholesterol and triglyceride were investigated in mice in the early stage of hyperlipidemia using SAXS [48]. According to Otvos [119] lipoprotein fractions can be divided into four main classes: high-density, low-density, very-low-density, and chylomicrons, or into seven *sub*fractions: $HDL_{(2)}$, $HDL_{(3)}$, $LDL_{(1-3)}$, IDL, $VLDL_{(1-2)}$, $VLDL_{(3-5)}$ and chylomicrons. Atorvastatin was administered to mice with acute lipemia induced by a single dose of P-407. The hyperlipidemia induced by P-407 alone resulted in a significant (p

< 0.01) increase in atherogenic LDL-cholesterol (IDL-cholesterol and $LDL_{(1-3)}$-cholesterol *sub*fractions) and very-low density lipoprotein-cholesterol ($VLDL_{(1-2)}$-cholesterol and $VLDL_{(3-5)}$-cholesterol *sub*fractions), as well as a slight, but statistically non-significant increase in the HDL-cholesterol fraction ($HDL_{(2)}$-cholesterol *sub*fraction). Treatment of P-407-mediated acute lipemia in mice with high-dose atorvastatin cause a reduction in total serum cholesterol, total LDL-cholesterol ($LDL_{(1-3)}$-cholesterol *sub*fraction), and the $LDL_{(1-3)}$-triglyceride *sub*fraction. Therefore, high-dose atorvastatin therapy would appear to exert its lipid-lowering effects in the early stages of acute lipemia in P-407-induced hyperlipidemic mice [48]. As an aside, it is interesting to compare the efficacy of two different statins to lower plasma cholesterol in two different rodents (mice *vs.* rats) using fairly similar total daily doses [48,120]. Korolenko et al., demonstrated an approximate 43% reduction in plasma cholesterol in P-407-induced hyperlipidemic mice using high-dose atorvastatin therapy (75 mg/kg x 2 by oral gavage) [48], whereas, Porter et al., demonstrated an approximate 28% decrease in plasma cholesterol in P-407-induced hyperlipidemic rats administered pravastatin sodium at a dose that ranged from 40 to 90 mg/kg/day [120]. In both studies, however, plasma levels of TG were more sensitive to the effects of a given statin drug when compared to reductions in plasma cholesterol [48,120].

While it was demonstrated that the P-407-induced mouse model of hyperlipidemia was able to rank-order the potency of several statin drugs [52], further studies were required to more fully characterize the effect(s) of P-407 on HMG-CoA reductase both *in vitro* and *in vivo*. Thus, we conducted a series of experiments designed to determine whether HMG-CoA reductase might be playing a role in the hypercholesterolemic response to P-407 [121]. In the first experiment, we isolated microsomes from rat livers and incubated microsomal protein with different concentrations of P-407 (0-5 mM) in a manner similar to the procedures used to evaluate the *in vitro* effects of P-407 on heparin-releasable LPL [53]. It was found that at all concentrations of P-407, microsomal HMG-CoA reductase activity was the same as that determined in hepatic samples from animals that did not receive P-407 [121]. These data indicated that P-407 did not affect HMG-CoA reductase directly.

In a second set of experiments, we previously determined the *in vivo* effect of a single dose of P-407 on hepatic HMG-CoA reductase activity. A 300-mg injection of P-407 caused microsomal HMG-CoA reductase activity to increase significantly above control values 2 hours following treatment. Activity remained elevated ($p < 0.05$) for at least 24 hours, with maximal activity (2.8-fold above control) occurring 15 hours following injection. By 48 hours, enzyme activity fell to 9.4 pmol/min/mg protein, 10% of control activity. By hour 72 following treatment, hepatic microsomal HMG-CoA reductase activity had returned to control levels. These findings are similar to those of Goldfarb [122] and Kuroda et al., [123] in that both investigators demonstrated that administering Triton WR 1339 into rats caused a stimulation of HMG-CoA reductase activity. In addition, they reported that the change in HMG-CoA reductase activity they observed was preceded by a drop in hepatic cholesterol.

Since it has been reported that the hepatic concentration of cholesterol plays a role in the regulation of HMG-CoA reductase activity [124], we measured hepatic cholesterol concentrations in P-407-treated rats. For 4 hours following P-407 administration, hepatic cholesterol content was increased ($p < 0.05$) above control levels. This increase was occurring at a time when plasma cholesterol concentrations and HMG-CoA reductase activity were increasing rapidly. At hour 15, liver cholesterol content had fallen approximately 40% below control concentrations. This was the time point at which HMG-CoA reductase activity of

P-407-treated animals was maximal. By hour 24, hepatic cholesterol content was back to the control level, a time when HMG-CoA reductase activity and plasma cholesterol concentrations were still elevated significantly above control values [121].

Following a single dose of P-407 to rats, the above findings would suggest P-407 affects plasma cholesterol, the rate-limiting enzyme in cholesterol biosynthesis, and hepatic cholesterol content. The fact that there is not a tight relationship between these variables indicates that hepatic cholesterol is not solely responsible for regulating the changes in either circulating cholesterol concentrations or enzyme activity. The data do suggest, however, that changes in cholesterol biosynthesis, due to temporary and reversible changes in HMG-CoA reductase activity, could be at least partially responsible for the elevations in plasma cholesterol we see in P-407-treated animals. The *in vitro* data indicate that the *in vivo* enzyme activation seen with a single dose of P-407 is not a direct effect of the compound on the enzyme, but rather is modulated through an indirect process. It should also be emphasized that the role of covalent modification (phosphorylation) in regulating HMG-CoA reductase activity in rodents has yet to be determined.

In contrast to single-dose studies, experiments that involve long-term, repetitive administration of P-407 to mice demonstrate no change in hepatic microsomal HMG-CoA reductase activity when compared with saline-treated controls. On 2 different occasions [52,54], we have reported that long term studies (4-6 months) did not result in a significant difference in HMG-CoA reductase activity in P-407-treated mice relative to controls. This is nicely demonstrated in Table 1, which also shows the mean value for the biologic activity of HMG-CoA reductase determined for a group of mice fed a traditional high-fat diet for comparison [52]. Also listed in Table 1 are the mean values of activity associated with two other enzymes that are involved with the catabolism of cholesterol. Specifically, microsomal cholesterol 7α-hydroxylase (C7αH) and mitochondrial sterol 27 hydroxylase (S27H) were assayed for activity in the livers of mice following 4 months of treatment with either a high-fat diet or P-407. It can be noted from Table 1 that there was a significant decrease in the activity of C7αH in P-407-treated animals when compared with controls (24 ± 3.3 *vs.* 37 ± 9.0 pmol/min/mg, respectively). With mice that were fed the high-fat diet, there was a significant decrease in the activity of HMG-CoA reductase when compared to controls (11 ± 5.1 *vs.* 165 ± 56 pmol/min/mg, respectively).

Table 1. Effects After 4 Months of Dietary/P-407 Treatment on the Activity of HMG-CoA Reductase, C7αH, and S27H in Mouse Liver

Treatment	HMG-CoA Reductase (pmol/min/mg)	C7αH (pmol/min/mg)	S27H (pmol/min/mg)
Control	165 ± 56[a]	37 ± 9.0	28 ± 8.6
High-fat diet	11 ± 5.1[b]	28 ± 7.1	38 ± 14
P-407	149 ± 12	24 ± 3.3[b]	35 ± 13

[a] Duplicate measurements on at least 4 mice per group were included for each enzyme.

[b] Significantly ($p < 0.05$) different from the mean value associated with controls.

From T.P. Johnston, *J. Cardiovasc. Pharmacol.* 2004, 43(4):595-606 with permission from Wolters Kluwer Health.

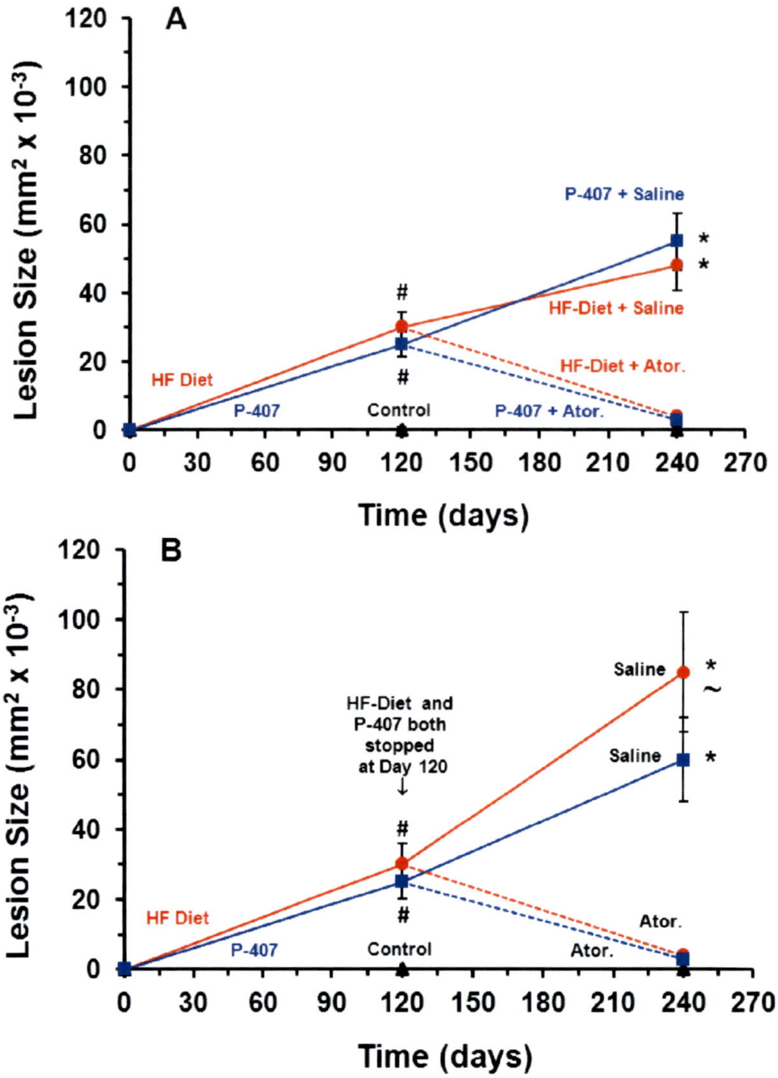

Figure 2. The effect of either atorvastatin (20 mg/kg/d) (dotted line connecting symbols) or saline (solid line connecting symbols) administration on mean aortic lesion size in C57BL/6 mice in which either-407 (filled blue squares) or a high-fat diet (filled red circles) were continued to 8 months (A) or discontinued at 4 months (B). The filled black triangles (line indistinguishable from the x-axis) represent mice in the control group that received neither P-407, nor a high-fat diet. Using the Student's *t*-test, * indicates a significant ($p < 0.05$) difference in mean values of lesion size at 8 months for saline-treated mice *versus* atorvastatin-treated mice for each atherogenic stimulus, # indicates a significant ($p < 0.05$) increase in mean lesion size for mice in either treatment group *versus* control at 4 months, and ~ indicates a significant ($p < 0.05$) increase in the mean lesion size at 8 months when saline-treated mice fed the high-fat diet for only 4 months (B) were compared with saline-treated mice in the 'progression' high-fat diet group (A). (From T.P. Johnston, *J. Cardiovasc. Pharmacol.* 2004, 43(4):595-606 with permission from Wolters Kluwer Health).

Our previous work has also demonstrated clinical significance because of the emphasis placed on the potential for regression of atherosclerotic lesions using statin drugs. We conducted an 8-month-long experiment that investigated whether the statin drug, atorvastatin, could mediate the regression of P-407-induced aortic atherosclerotic lesions in mice [74].

Briefly, female C57BL/6 mice were treated with either normal saline (controls), 0.5 g/kg of P-407, or a high-fat, high-cholesterol, cholate-containing diet for 120 days. Mice in each of the groups were then equally and randomly divided and treated with either atorvastatin or saline for an additional 120 days (Figure 2).

Aortas of mice treated with 20 mg/kg of atorvastatin in both the P-407-treated and high-fat diet groups and that were either maintained on the high-fat diet or treated with P-407 from day 120 to 240 (Figure 2A) or removed from each treatment (atherogenic stimulus) at day 120 (Figure 2B), revealed no presence of aortic atherosclerotic lesions at 8 months relative to saline-treated mice and were indistinguishable from aortas retrieved from control mice. Thus, this study demonstrated that atorvastatin at a dose of 20 mg/kg/day caused the complete regression of aortic atherosclerotic lesions induced in C57BL/6 mice by either administration of P-407, or ingestion of a high-fat diet containing cholic acid (Figure 2A,B) [74]. Interestingly, this study also demonstrated that progression of aortic lesion size still continues from day 120 onward when both atorvastatin is discontinued and each atherogenic stimulus (i.e., P-407 and HF-diet) is removed (Figure 2B). A possible, but untested, reason for the continued increase in lesion size from day 120 onward in the absence of either atherogenic stimulus may be that once atherosclerotic lesions are firmly established in this model at 4 months, the cascade of biochemical events involved with atheroma formation has been irreversibly set into motion. That is, lipids, cells, cellular components/debris, etc. may potentially continue to migrate to the lesion and add to its overall size. It may also be possible that cellular adhesion molecules, as well as macrophage (foam cell)-derived cytokines and reactive oxygen species, continue to exert their effects even after withdrawal of each atherogenic stimulus, although further testing is required to confirm this hypothesis.

Conclusion and Future Directions

Animal models have proven very beneficial for investigating the pathogenesis of hyperlipidemia and subsequent atherosclerotic heart disease in humans, but there are some very real differences. While no one animal model is ideal for evaluating the effectiveness of existing, or newer, anti-hyperlipidemic agents, nevertheless, despite their limitations, animal models have demonstrated enormous potential in predicting the therapeutic potency and efficacy of statins. Animal models of hyperlipidemia and atherosclerosis developed using dietary intervention, genetic manipulation, and those resulting from the administration of an exogenous hyperlipidemia-inducing compound have also demonstrated their usefulness with other lipid-lowering drug classes, as well as non-drug mediated therapies. Overall, due to cost, convenience, and a well-known genome, mouse models have become the most frequently used animal model for preclinical investigation of the molecular and cellular mechanisms responsible for hyperlipidemia and associated arteriosclerotic heart disease, and they continue to be the species of choice for the preclinical evaluation of therapeutic interventions aimed at reversing hyperlipidemia and the progression of coronary artery disease. Unfortunately, however, there still exists a need for mouse models of atherogenesis to mimic the most important event in human atherosclerosis, that is, plaque rupture leading to vessel occlusion. This should be a future direction, or goal, of those scientists involved with cardiovascular research focussed on hyperlipidemia and coronary artery disease.

Additionally, future research should also include identification of a mouse model that would accurately predict 'statin intolerance', since this limits the use of statins in some patients for which statin therapy is recommended as a first-line defense, for example, those patients with familial hypercholesterolemia. Mouse models must also be able to reliably replicate all of the conditions or symptoms observed clinically in specific patient populations, for instance, Type 2 diabetics that present with the metabolic syndrome secondary to morbid obesity. As an example, hypertriglyceridemia is one of the conditions exhibited by patients with the metabolic syndrome and Type 2 diabetes, but high-fat, high-cholesterol, diet-induced atherogenic mouse models do not produce hypertriglyceridemia. Nevertheless, despite this shortcoming, current and future mouse models will continue to be heavily utilized for not only investigating hyperlipidemia, disturbances in lipid metabolism, and atherosclerosis, but also for evaluating the effectiveness of both drug and non-drug mediated therapeutic interventions to either slow, or possibly reverse, this disease process.

REFERENCES

[1] Zaragoza, C; Gomez-Guerrero, C; Martin-Ventura, JL; Blanco-Colio, L; Lavin, B; Mallavia, B; Tarin, C; Mas, S; Ortiz, A; Egido, J. Animal models of cardiovascular diseases. *J. Biomed. Biotech.* 2011, Article ID 497841, doi:10.1155/2011/497841.

[2] Li, X; Liu, Y; Zhang, H; Ren, L; Li, Q; Li, N. Animal models for the atherosclerosis research: a review. *Protein Cell* 2011, 2(3):189-201.

[3] Weber, C; Noels, H. Atherosclerosis: current pathogenesis and therapeutic options. *Nat. Med.* 2011, 17:1410-1422.

[4] Steinberg, D. Thematic review series: the pathogenesis of atherosclerosis. An interpretive history of the cholesterol controversy: part II: the early evidence linking hypercholesterolemia to coronary disease in humans. *J. lipid Res.* 2005, 46:179-190.

[5] Ross, R. Atherosclerosis – an inflammatory disease. *N. Engl. J. Med.* 1999, 340:115-126.

[6] Hansson, GK. Inflammation, atherosclerosis, and coronary heart disease. *N. Engl. J. Med.* 2005, 352:1685-1695.

[7] Hansson, GK. Atherosclerosis – an immune disease: The Anitschkov Lecture 2007. *Atherosclerosis* 2009, 202:2-10.

[8] Davies, MK; Hollman, A. Atherosclerosis and myocardial infarction. *Heart* 1998, 79:218.

[9] Libby, P; Aikawa, M. Stabilization of atherosclerotic plaques; new mechanisms and clinical targets. *Nat. Med.* 2002, 8:1257-1262.

[10] Knopp, RH; Paramsothy, P. Treatment of hypercholesterolemia in patients with metabolic syndrome: how do different statins compare? *Nat. Clin. Pract. Endocrinol. Metab.* 2006, 2:136-137.

[11] Knopp, RH. Drug treatment of lipid disorders. *N. Engl. J. Med.* 1999, 341:498-511.

[12] Mohrschladt, MF; Westendorp, RGJ; Gevers-Leuven, JA; Smelt, AHM. Cardiovascular disease and mortality in statin-treated patients with familial hypercholesterolemia. *Atherosclerosis* 2004, 172:329-335.

[13] Baigent, C; Blackwell, L; Emberson, J; Holland, LE; Reith, C; Bhala, N; Peto, R; Barnes, EH; Keech, A; Simes, J; Collins, R. Efficacy and safety of more intensive lowering of LDL cholesterol: a meta-analysis of data from 170,000 participants in 26 randomized trials. *Lancet* 2010, 376:1670-1681.

[14] Tonkin, A; Byrnes, A. Treatment of dyslipidemia. *F1000Prime Reports* 2014, 6:17 doi: 10.12703/P6-17.

[15] Dormuth, CR; Hemmelgarn, BR; Paterson, JM; James, MT; Teare, GF; Raymond, CB; Lafrance, J; Levy, A; Garg, AX; Ernst, P. Use of high potency statins and rates of admission for acute kidney injury: multicenter, retrospective observational analysis of administrative databases. *BMJ* 2013, 346:f880 doi: 10.1136/bmj.f880.

[16] Sattar, N; Preiss, D; Murray, HM; Welsh, P; Buckley, BM; Craen, Ade; Seshasai, S; McMurray, JJ; Freeman, DJ; Jukema, JW; Macfarlane, PW; Packard, CJ; Stott, DJ; Westendorp, RG; Shepherd, J; Davis, BR; Pressel, SL; Marchioli, R; Marfisi, RM; Maggioni, AP; Tavazzi, L; Tognoni, G; Kjekshus, J; Pedersen, TR; Cook, TJ; Gotto, AM; Clearfield, MB; Downs, JR; Nakamura, H; Ohashi, Y; et al., Statins and risk of incident diabetes: a collaborative meta-analysis of randomized statin trials. *Lancet* 2010, 375:735-742.

[17] Strong, JP; Malcom, GT; McMahan, CA; Tracy, RE; Newman, WP; Herderick, EE; Cornhill, JF. Prevalence and extent of atherosclerosis in adolescents and young adults: implications for prevention from the Pathobiological Determinants of Atherosclerosis in Youth Study. *JAMA* 1999, 281:727-735.

[18] Greenland, P; Alpert, JS; Beller, GA; Benjamin, EJ; Budoff, MJ; Fayad, ZA; Foster, E; Hlatky, MA; Hodgson, JM; Kushner, FG; Lauer, MS; Shaw, LJ; Smith, SC; Taylor, AJ; Weintraub, WS; Wenger, NK; Jacobs, AK; Anderson, JL; Albert, N; Buller, CE; Creager, MA; Ettinger, SM; Guyton, RA; Halperin, JL; Hochman, JS; Nishimura, R; Ohman, EM; Page, RL; Stevenson, WG; Tarkington, LG; et al., 2010 ACCF/AHA guideline for assessment of cardiovascular risk in asymptomatic adults: a report of the American College of Cardiology Foundation/American Heart Association Task Force on Practice Guidelines. *J. Am. Coll. Cardiol.* 2010, 56:e50-103.

[19] Polonsky, TS; McClelland, RL; Greenland, P. Coronary artery calcium score and risk classification for coronary heart disease prediction: the multi-ethnic study of atherosclerosis. *JAMA* 2010, 303:1610-1616.

[20] Ahmad, Z. Statin intolerance. *Am. J. Cardiol.* 2014, 113:1765-1771.

[21] Nordestgaard, BG; Chapman, MJ; Humphries, SE; Ginsberg, HN; Masana, L; Descamps, OS; Wiklund, O; Hegele, RA; Raal, FJ; Defesche, JC; Wiegman, A; Santos, RD; Watts, GF; Parhofer, KG; Hovingh, GK; Kovanen, PT; Boileau, C; Averna, M; Borén, J; Bruckert, E; Catapano, AL; Kuivenhoven, JA; Pajukanta, P; Ray, K; Stalenhoef, A; Stroes, E; Taskinen, M; Tybjærg-Hansen, A. Familial hypercholesterolaemia is underdiagnosed and undertreated in the general population: guidance for clinicians to prevent coronary heart disease: consensus statement of the European atherosclerosis society. *Eur. Heart J.* 2013, 34:3478-3490.

[22] Laufs, U; Weintraub, WS; Packard, CJ. Beyond statins: what to expect from add-on lipid regulating therapy? *Eur. Heart J.* 2013, 34:2660-2665.

[23] Bellosta S, Ferri N, Arnaboldi L, Bernini F, Paoletti R, Corsini A. Pleiotropic effects of statins in atherosclerosis and diabetes. *Diabetes Care*. 2000;23(suppl 2):B72-B78.

[24] Bellosta S, Ferri N, Bernini F, Paoletti R, Corsini A. Non-lipid related effects of statins. *Ann. Med.* 2000;32:164-176.
[25] Hess DC, Fagan SC. Pharmacology and clinical experience with simvastatin. *Expert Opin. Pharmacother.* 2001;2:153-163.
[26] Kuvin JT, Karas RH. The effects of LDL reduction and HDL augmentation on physiologic and inflammatory markers. *Curr. Opin. Cardiol.* 2003;18:295-300.
[27] Takemoto M, Liao JK. Pleiotropic effects of 3-hydroxy-3- methylglutaryl coenzyme a reductase inhibitors. *Arterioscler Thromb. Vasc. Biol.* 2001;21:1712-1719.
[28] Inoue I, Goto S, Mizotani K, Awata T, Mastunaga T, Kawai S, Nakajima T, Hokari S, Komoda T, Katayama S. Lipophilic HMG-CoA reductase inhibitor has an anti-inflammatory effect: reduction of MRNA levels for interleukin-1beta, interleukin-6, cyclooxygenase-2, and p22phox by regulation of peroxisome proliferator-activated receptor alpha (PPARalpha) in primary endothelial cells. *Life Sci.* 2000;67:863-876.
[29] Jialal I, Stein D, Balis D, Grundy SM, Adams-Huet B, Devaraj S. Effect of hydroxymethylglutaryl coenzyme a reductase inhibitor therapy on high sensitive C-reactive protein levels. *Circulation.* 2001;103:1933-1935.
[30] Pruefer D, Scalia R, Lefer AM. Simvastatin inhibits leukocyte endothelial cell interactions and protects against inflammatory processes in normocholesterolemic rats. *Arterioscler Thromb. Vasc. Biol.* 1999;19:2894-2900.
[31] Barathi, VA; Yeo, SW;Guymer, RH; Wongg, TY; Luu, CD. Effects of simvastatin on retinal structure and function of a high-fat atherogenic mouse model of thickened Bruch's membrane. *Invest Ophthalmol. Vis. Sci.* 2014, 55:460-468.
[32] Simons M. Molecular multitasking: statins lead to more arteries, less plaque. *Nat. Med.*. 2000;6:965-966.
[33] Lee TS, Chang CC, Zhu Y, Shyy JY. Simvastatin induces heme oxygenase-1: a novel mechanism of vessel protection. *Circulation.* 2004;110:1296-1302.
[34] Ignatowski, AC. Influence of animal food on the organism of rabbits. *Izv. Imp. Voyenno-Med. Akad. Peter* 1908, 16:154-173.
[35] Kennedy, AJ; Ellacot, KLJ; King, VL; Hasty, AH. Mouse models of the metabolic syndrome. *Dis. Model Mech.* 2010 3:156-166.
[36] Whitman, SC. A practical approach to using mice in atherosclerosis research. *Clin. Biochem. Rev.* 2004, 25:81-93.
[37] Johnston, TP. The P-407-induced murine model of dose-controlled hyperlipidemia and atherosclerosis: A review of findings to date. *J. Cardiovasc. Pharmacol.* 2004, 43(4):595-606.
[38] Wasan, KM; Subramanian, R; Kwong, M; Goldberg, IJ; Wright, T; Johnston, TP. Poloxamer 407-mediated alterations in the activities of enzymes regulating lipid metabolism in rats. *J. Pharm. Pharm. Sci.* 2003, 6(2):189-197.
[39] Leon, C; Wasan, KM; Sachs-Barrable, K; Johnston, TP. Acute P-407 administration to mice causes hypercholesterolemia by inducing cholesterolgenesis and down-regulating low-density lipoprotein receptor expression. *Pharm. Res.* 2006, 23(7):1597-1607.
[40] Johnston, TP; Jaye, M; Webb, CL; Krawiec, JA; Alom-Ruiz, SP; Sachs-Barrable, K; Wasan, KM. Poloxamer 407-mediated reduction in the gene expression of ATP-binding-cassette transporter A1 may contribute to increased cholesterol in peripheral tissues of P-407-treated rats. *Eur. J. Pharmacol.* 2006, 536(3):232-240.

[41] Johnston, TP; Waxman, DJ. The induction of atherogenic dyslipidemia in poloxamer 407-treated mice is not mediated through PPARalpha. *J. Pharm. Pharmacol.* 2008, 60(6):753-759.

[42] Johnston, TP; Waxman, DJ. Circulating free fatty acids are increased independently of PPARgamma activity after administration of poloxamer 407 to mice. *Can. J. Physiol. Pharmacol.* 2008, 86(9):643-649.

[43] Tanaka, H; Ishida, T; Johnston, TP; Yasuda, T; Ueyama, T; Kojima, Y; Kundu, RK; Quertermous, T; Ishikawa, Y; Hirata, K. Role of endothelial lipase in plasma HDL levels in a murine model of hypertriglyceridemia. *J. Atheroscler Thromb.* 2009, 16(4):327-338.

[44] Johnston, TP. Poloxamer 407 increases soluble adhesion molecules, ICAM-1, VCAM-1, and E-selectin, in C57BL/6 mice. *J. Pharm. Pharmacol* 2009, 61(12):1681-1688.

[45] Johnston, TP. Poloxamer 407 as a general lipase inhibitor: its implications in lipid metabolism and atheroma formation in C57BL/6 mice. *J. Pharm. Pharmacol.* 2010, 62(12):1807-1812.

[46] Yasuda, T; Johnston, TP; Shinohara, M; Inoue, M; Ishida, T. The effect of poloxamer 407 on the functional properties of HDL in mice. *J. Pharm. Pharmacol.* 2012, 64(5):677-687.

[47] Korolenko, TA; Tuzikov, FV; Johnston, TP; Tuzikova, NA; Kisarova, YA; Zhanaeva, SY; Alexeenko, TV; Zhukova, NA; Brak, IV; Spiridonov, VK; Filjushina, EE; Cherkanova, MS; Monoszon, AA. The influence of repeated administration of poloxamer 407 on serum lipoproteins and protease activity in mouse liver and heart. *Can. J. Physiol. Pharmacol.* 2012, 90(11):1456-1468.

[48] Korolenko, TA; Tuzikov, FV; Cherkanova, MS; Johnston, TP; Tuzikova, NA; Loginova, VM; Filjushina, EE; Kaledin, VI. Influence of atorvastatin and carboxymethylated glucan on the serum lipoprotein profile and MMP activity of mice with lipemia induced by poloxamer 407. Can *J. Physiol. Pharmacol.* 2012, 90(2):141-153.

[49] Korolenko, TA; Johnston, TP; Dubrovina, NI; Kisarova, YA; Zhanaeva, SY; Cherkanova, MS; Filjushina, EE; Alexeenko, TV; Machova, E; Zhukova, NA. Effect of poloxamer 407 administration on the serum lipid profile, anxiety level, and protease activity in the heart and liver of mice. *Interdiscip Toxicol.* 2013, 6(1):18-25.

[50] Wout, ZG; Pec, EA; Maggiore, JA, Williams, RH; Palicharla, P; Johnston, TP. Poloxamer 407-mediated changes in plasma cholesterol and triglycerides following intraperitoneal injection to rats. *J. Parenter. Sci. Technol.* 1992, 46(6):192-200.

[51] Palmer, WK; Emeson, EE; Johnston, TP. Poloxamer 407-induced atherogenesis in the C57BL/6 mouse. *Atherosclerosis* 1998, 136(1):115-123.

[52] Johnston, TP; Nguyen, LB; Chu, WA; Shefer, S. Potency of select statin drugs in a new mouse model of hyperlipidemia and atherosclerosis. *Int. J. Pharm.* 2001, 229(1-2):75-86.

[53] Johnston, TP; Palmer, WK. Mechanism of poloxamer 407-induced hypertriglyceridemia in the rat. *Biochem. Pharmacol.* 1993, 46:1037-1042.

[54] Johnston, TP; Baker, JC; Jamal, AS; Hall, D; Emeson, EE; Palmer, WK. Potential downregulation of HMG-CoA reductase after prolonged administration of P-407 in C57BL/6 mice. *J. Cardiovasc. Pharmacol.* 1999, 34(6):831-842.

[55] Knäuper, V; Will, H; López-Otin, C; Smith, B; Atkinson, SJ; Stanton, H; Hembry, RM; Murphy, G. Cellular mechanisms for human procollagenase-3 (MMP-13) activation. Evidence that MT1-MMP (MMP-14) and gelatinase A (MMP-2) are able to generate active enzyme. *J. Biol. Chem.* 1996, 271:17124-17131.
[56] Chow, AK; Cena, J; Schulz, R. Acute actions and novel targets of matrix metalloproteases in the heart and vasculature. *Br. J. Pharmacol.* 2007, 152:189-205.
[57] Cudic, M; Fields, GB. Extracellular proteases as targets for drug development. *Curr. Protein. Pept. Sci.* 2009, 10:297-307.
[58] Thrailkill, KM; Clay Bunn, R; Fowlkes, JL. Matrix metalloproteinases: their potential role in the pathogenesis of diabetic nephropathy. *Endocrine* 2009, 35:1-10.
[59] Sjöberg, S; Shi, GP. Cysteine protease cathepsins in atherosclerosis and abdominal aortic aneurysm. *Clin. Rev. Bone Miner Metab* 2011, 9:138-147.
[60] Peterson, JT. The importance of estimating the therapeutic index in the development of matrix metalloproteinase inhibitors. *Cardiovasc Res* 2006, 69: 677-687.
[61] Qin, Y; Shi, GP. Cysteinyl cathepsins and mast cell proteases in the pathogenesis and therapeutics of cardiovascular diseases. *Pharmacol. Ther.* 2011, 131:338-350.
[62] Lutgens, SPM; Cleutjens, KBJM; Daemen, MJAP; Heeneman, S. Cathepsin cysteine proteases in cardiovascular disease. *FASEB J.* 2007, 21:3029-3041.
[63] Li, W; Yuan, XM. Increased expression and translocation of lysosomal cathepsins contribute to macrophage apoptosis in atherogenesis. *Ann. NY Acad. Sci.* 2004, 1030:427-433.
[64] Li, W; Dalen, H; Eaton, JW; Yuan, XM. Apoptotic death of inflammatory cells in human atheroma. *Arterioscler Thromb. Vasc. Biol.* 2001, 21:1124-1130.
[65] Li, W; Yuan, XM; Olsson, AG; Brunk, UT. Uptake of oxidized LDL by macrophages results in partial lysosomal enzyme inactivation and relocation. *Arterioscler Thromb. Vasc. Biol.* 1998, 18:177-184.
[66] Jormsjo, S; Wuttge, DM; Sirsjo, A; Whatling, C; Hamsten, A; Stemme, S; Eriksson, P. Differential expression of cysteine and aspartic proteases during progression of atherosclerosis in apolipoprotein E-deficient mice. *Am. J. Pathol.* 2002, 161:939-945.
[67] Liu, J; Sukhova, GK; Yang, JT; Sun, J; Ma, L; Ren, A; Xu, WH; Fu, H; Dolganov, GM; Hu, C; Libby, P; Shi, GP. Cathepsin L expression and regulation in human abdominal aortic aneurysm, atherosclerosis, and vascular cells. *Atherosclerosis* 2006, 184:302-311.
[68] Ge, J; Zhao, G; Chen, R; Li, S; Wang, S; Zhang, X; Zhuang, Y; Du, J; Yu, X; Li, G; Yang, Y. Enhanced myocardial cathepsin B expression in patients with dilated cardiomyopathy. *Eur. J. Heart Failure* 2006, 8:284-289.
[69] Liu, Y; Li, X; Peng, D; Tan, Z; Liu, H; Qing, Y; Xue, Y; Shi, G-P. Usefulness of serum cathepsin L as an independent biomarker in patients with coronary heart disease. *Am. J. Cardiol.* 2009, 103:476-481.
[70] Vivanco, F; Mas, S; Darde, VM; De la Cuesta, F; Alvarez-Llamas, G; Barderas, MG. Vascular proteomics. *Proteomics Clin. Appl.* 2007, 1:1102-1122.
[71] Hakala, JK; Oksjoki, R; Laine, P; Du, H; Grabowski, GA; Kovanen, PT; Pentikainen, MO. Lysosomal enzymes are released from cultured human macrophages, hydrolyze LDL *in vitro*, and are present extracellularly in human atherosclerotic lesions. *Arterioscler Thromb Vasc. Biol.* 2003, 23:1430-1436.

[72] Witzium, JL. Drugs used in the treatment of hyperlipoproteinemias. In J.G. Hardman, L.E. Limbird, P.B. Molinoff, R.W. Rudden (Eds.), *The Pharmacological Basis of Therapeutics*, 9th ed. New York:McGraw-Hill; 1996; 875-897.

[73] Johnston, TP; Coker, JW; Paigen, BJ; Tawfik, O. Sex does not seem to influence the formation of aortic lesions in the P-407-induced mouse model of hyperlipidemia and atherosclerosis. *J. Cardiovasc. Pharmacol.* 2002, 39:404-411.

[74] Johnston, TP; Baker, JC; Hall, D; Jamal, S; Palmer, WK; Emeson, EE. Regression of poloxamer 407-induced atherosclerotic lesions in C57BL/6 mice using atorvastatin. *Atherosclerosis* 2000, 149(2):303-313.

[75] Johnston, TP; Zhou, X. Oxidation of low-density lipoprotein cholesterol following administration of poloxamer 407 to mice results from an indirect effect. *J. Cardiovasc. Pharmacol.* 2007, 49(4):246-252.

[76] Zhou, X; Johnston, TP; Johansson, D; Parini, P; Funa, K; Svensson, J; Hansson, GK. Hypercholesterolemia leads to elevated TGF-beta1 activity and T helper 3-dependent autoimmune responses in atherosclerotic mice. *Atherosclerosis* 2009, 204(2):381-387.

[77] Grothusen, C; Bley, S; Selle, T; Luchtefeld, M; Grote, K; Tietge, UJ; Drexler, H; Schieffer, B. Combined effects of HMG-CoA-reductase inhibition and renin-angiotensin system blockade on experimental atherosclerosis. *Atherosclerosis* 2005, 182:57-69.

[78] Johnson, J; Carson, K; Williams, H; Karanam, S; Newby, A; Angelini, G; George, S; Jackson, C. Plaque rupture after short periods of fat feeding in the apolipoprotein E-knockout mouse: model characterization and effects of pravastatin treatment. *Circulation* 2005, 111:1422-1430.

[79] Li, Z; Iwai, M; Wu, L; Liu, HW; Chen, R; Jinno, T; Suzuki, J; Tsuda, M; Gao, XY; Okumura, M; Cui, TX; Horiuchi, M. Fluvastatin enhances the inhibitory effects of a selective AT1 receptor blocker, valsartan, on atherosclerosis. *Hypertension* 2004, 44:758-763.

[80] Nachtigal, P; Pospisilova, N; Pospechova, K; Jamborova, G; Kopecky, M; Jaynes, R; Briestensky, J; Santar, I; Smahelova, A; Solichova, D; Zdansky, P; Semecky, V. MDOC and atorvastatin have potential antiinflammatory effects in vascular endothelium of $apoE^{-/-}$ mouse model of atherosclerosis. *Life Sci.* 2006, 78:1983-1989.

[81] Naoum, JJ; Zhang, S; Woodside, KJ; Song, W; Guo, Q; Belalcazar, LM; Hunter, GC. Aortic eNOS expression and phosphorylation in Apo-E knockout mice: differing effects of rapamycin and simvastatin. *Surgery* 2004, 136:323-328.

[82] Navab, M; Anantharamaiah, GM; Hama, S; Hough, G; Reddy, ST; Frank, JS; Garber, DW; Handattu, S; Fogelman, AM. D-4F and statins synergize to render HDL antiinflammatory in mice and monkeys and cause lesion regression in old apolipoprotein E-null mice. *Arterioscler Thromb. Vasc. Biol.* 2005, 25:1426-1432.

[83] Sata, M; Nishimatsu, H; Osuga, J; Tanaka, K; Ishizaka, N; Ishibashi, S; Hirata, Y; Nagai, R. Statins augment collateral growth in response to ischemia but they do not promote cancer and atherosclerosis. *Hypertension* 2004, 43:1214-1220.

[84] Sparrow, CP; Burton, CA; Hernandez, M; Mundt, S; Hassing, H; Patel, S; Rosa, R; Hermanowski-Vosatka, A; Wang, PR; Zhang, D; Peterson, L; Detmers, PA; Chao, YS; Wright, SD. Simvastatin has anti-inflammatory and antiatherosclerotic activities independent of plasma cholesterol lowering. *Arterioscler Thromb. Vasc. Biol.* 2001, 21:115-121.

[85] Quarfordt, SH; Oswald, B; Landis, B; Xu, HS; Zhang, SH; Maeda, N. *In vivo* cholesterol kinetics in apolipoprotein E-deficient and control mice. *J. lipid Res.* 1995, 36:1227-1235.

[86] Fu, T; Borensztajn, J. Simvastatin causes the formation of cholesterol-rich remnants in mice lacking apoE. *Biochem. Biophys. Res. Commun.* 2006, 341:1172-1176.

[87] Choudhury, RP; Carrelli, AL; Stern, JD; Chereshnev, I; Soccio, R; Elmalem, VI; Fallon, JT; Fisher, EA; Reis, ED. Effects of simvastatin on plasma lipoproteins and response to arterial injury in wild-type and apolipoprotein-E-deficient mice. *J. Vasc. Res.* 2004, 41:75-83.

[88] Bea, F; Blessing, E; Bennett, B; Levitz, M; Wallace, EP; Rosenfeld, ME. Simvastatin promotes atherosclerotic plaque stability in apoE-deficient mice independently of lipid lowering. *Arterioscler Thromb. Vasc. Biol.* 2002, 22:1832-1837.

[89] Bea, F; Blessing, E; Shelley, MI; Shultz, JM; Rosenfeld, ME. Simvastatin inhibits expression of tissue factor in advanced atherosclerotic lesions of apolipoprotein E deficient mice independently of lipid lowering: potential role of simvastatin-mediated inhibition of Egr-1 expression and activation. *Atherosclerosis* 2003, 167:187-194.

[90] Gervais, M; Pons, S; Nicoletti, A; Cosson, C; Giudicelli, JF; Richer, C. Fluvastatin prevents renal dysfunction and vascular NO deficit in apolipoprotein E-deficient mice. *Arterioscler Thromb. Vasc. Biol.* 2003, 23:183-189.

[91] Galman, C; Ostlund-Lindqvist, AM; Bjorquist, A; Schreyer, S; Svensson, L; Angelin, B; Rudling, M. Pharmacological interference with intestinal bile acid transport reduces plasma cholesterol in LDL receptor/apoE deficiency. *FASEB J.* 2003, 17:265-267.

[92] Wang, YX; Martin-McNulty, B; Huw, LY; da Cunha, V; Post, J; Hinchman, J; Vergona, R; Sullivan, ME; Dole, W; Kauser, K. Anti-atherosclerotic effect of simvastatin depends on the presence of apolipoprotein E. *Atherosclerosis* 2002, 162:23-31.

[93] Chen, J; Li, D; Schaefer, R; Mehta, JL. Cross-talk between dyslipidemia and renin-angiotensin system and the role of LOX-1 and MAPK in atherogenesis studies with the combined use of rosuvastatin and candesartan. *Atherosclerosis* 2006, 184:295-301.

[94] Chen, J; Li, D; Schaefer, RF; Mehta, JL. Inhibitory effect of candesartan and rosuvastatin on CD40 and MMPs expression in apo-E knockout mice: novel insights into the role of RAS and dyslipidemia in atherogenesis. *J. Cardiovasc. Pharmacol.* 2004, 44:446-452.

[95] Bisgaier, CL; Essenburg, AD; Auerbach, BJ; Pape, ME; Sekerke, CS; Gee, A; Wolle, S; Newton, RS. Attenuation of plasma low density lipoprotein cholesterol by select 3-hydroxy-3-methylglutaryl coenzyme A reductase inhibitors in mice devoid of low density lipoprotein receptors. *J. lipid Res.* 1997, 38:2502-2515.

[96] Kwak, BR; Veillard, N; Pelli, G; Mulhaupt, F; James, RW; Chanson, M; Mach, F. Reduced connexin43 expression inhibits atherosclerotic lesion formation in low-density lipoprotein receptor-deficient mice. *Circulation* 2003, 107:1033-1039.

[97] Dunoyer-Geindre, S; Kwak, BR; Pelli, G; Roth, I; Satta, N; Fish, RJ; Reber, G; Mach, F; Kruithof, EK; de Moerloose, P. Immunization of LDL receptor-deficient mice with beta2-glycoprotein 1 or human serum albumin induces a more inflammatory phenotype in atherosclerotic plaques. *Thromb Haemost* 2007, 97:129-138.

[98] Chen, Z; Fukutomi, T; Zago, AC; Ehlers, R; Detmers, PA; Wright, SD; Rogers, C; Simon, DI. Simvastatin reduces neointimal thickening in low-density lipoprotein

receptor-deficient mice after experimental angioplasty without changing plasma lipids. *Circulation* 2002, 106:20-23.

[99] Verschuren, L; Kleemann, R; Offerman, EH; Szalai, AJ; Emeis, SJ; Princen, HM; Kooistra, T. Effect of low dose atorvastatin versus diet-induced cholesterol lowering on atherosclerotic lesion progression and inflammation in apolipoprotein E*3-Leiden transgenic mice. *Arterioscler Thromb. Vasc. Biol.* 2005, 25:161-167.

[100] van De Poll, SW; Romer, TJ; Volger, OL; Delsing, DJ; Bakker Schut, TC; Princen, HM; Havekes, LM; Jukema, JW; van Der Laarse, A; Puppels, GJ. Raman spectroscopic evaluation of the effects of diet and lipid-lowering therapy on atherosclerotic plaque development in mice. *Arterioscler Thromb. Vasc. Biol.* 2001, 21:1630-1635.

[101] Delsing, DJ; Jukema, JW; van de Wiel, MA; Emeis, JJ; van Der Laarse, A; Havekes, LM; Princen, HM. Differential effects of amlodipine and atorvastatin treatment and their combination on atherosclerosis in ApoE*3-Leiden transgenic mice. *J. Cardiovasc. Pharmacol.* 2003, 42:63-70.

[102] Trion, A; de Maat, M; Jukema, W; Maas, A; Offerman, E; Havekes, L; Szalai, A; van Der Laarse, A; Princen, H; Emeis, J. Anti-atherosclerotic effect of amlodipine, alone and in combination with atorvastatin, in APOE*3-Leiden/hCRP transgenic mice. *J. Cardiovasc. Pharmacol.* 2006, 47:89-95.

[103] van De Poll, SW; Delsing, DJ; Jukema, JW; Princen, HM; Havekes, LM; Puppels, GJ, van Der Laarse, A. Raman spectroscopic investigation of atorvastatin, amlodipine, and both on atherosclerotic plaque development in APOE*3 Leiden transgenic mice. *Atherosclerosis* 2002, 164:65-71.

[104] van Vlijmen, BJ; Pearce, NJ; Bergo, M; Staels, B; Yates, JW; Gribble, AD; Bond, BC; Hofker, MH; Havekes, LM; Groot, PH. Apolipoprotein E*3-Leiden transgenic mice as a test model for hypolipidaemic drugs. *Arzneimittelforschung* 1998, 48:396-402.

[105] Kleemann, R; Princen, HM; Emeis, JJ; Jukema, JW; Fontijn, RD; Horrevoets, AJ; Kooistra, T; Havekes, LM. Rosuvastatin reduces atherosclerosis development beyond and independent of its plasma cholesterol-lowering effect in APOE*3-Leiden transgenic mice: Evidence for antiinflammatory effects of rosuvastatin. *Circulation* 2003, 108:1368-1374.

[106] Delsing, DJ; Post, SM; Groenendijk, M; Solaas, K; van Der Boom, H; van Duyvenvoorde, W; de Wit, EC; Bloks, VW; Kuipers, F; Havekes, LM; Princen, HM. Rosuvastatin reduces plasma lipids by inhibiting VLDL production and enhancing hepatobiliary lipid excretion in ApoE*3-leiden mice. *J. Cardiovasc. Pharmacol.* 2005, 45:53-60.

[107] Kleemann, R; Verschuren, L; De Rooij, BJ; Lindeman, J; De Maat, MM; Szalai, AJ; Princen, HM; Kooistra, T. Evidence for anti-inflammatory activity of statins and PPARalpha activators in human C-reactive protein transgenic mice *in vivo* and in cultured human hepatocytes *in vitro*. *Blood* 2004, 103:4188-4194.

[108] Nishina, PM; Lowe, S; Verstuyft, J; Naggert, JK; Kuypers, FA; Paigen, B. Effects of dietary fats from animal and plant sources on diet-induced fatty streak lesions in C57BL/6 mice. *J. lipid Res.* 1993, 34:1413-1422.

[109] Getz, GS; Reardon, CA. Diet and murine atherosclerosis. *Arterioscler Thromb. Vasc. Biol.* 2006, 26:242-249.

[110] Gao, S; He, L; Ding, Y; Liu, G. Mechanisms underlying different responses of plasma triglyceride to high-fat diets in hamsters and mice: role of hepatic MTP and triglyceride secretion. *Biochem. Biophys. Res. Commun.* 2010, 398:619-626.

[111] Paraskevas, KI; Pantopoulou, A; Vlachos, IS; Agrogiannis, G; Iliopoulos, DG; Karatzas, G; Tzivras, D; Mikhailidis, DP; Perrea, DN. Comparison of fibrate, ezetimibe, low- and high-dose statin therapy for the dyslipidemia of the metabolic syndrome in a mouse model. *Angiology* 2011, 62:144-154.

[112] Jones, P; Kafonek, S; Laurora, I; Hunninghake, D. Comparative dose efficacy study of atorvastatin *versus* simvastatin, pravastatin, lovastatin, and fluvastatin in patients with hypercholesterolemia. *Am. J. Cardiol.* 1998, 81(5):582-587.

[113] Yoshino, G; Matsushita, M; Iwai, M; Morita, M; Matsuba, K; Hirano, T; Furukawa, S; Kazumi, T; Baba, S. Effect of pravastatin on newly-secreted very low density lipoprotein composition in rats. *Horm. Metab. Res.* 1991, 23(4):193-195.

[114] Khan, BV; Wilcox, HG; Heimberg, M. Cholesterol is required for secretion of very-low-density lipoprotein by rat liver. *Biochem. J.* 1989, 259:807-814.

[115] Kasim, SE; LeBoeuf, RC; Khilnani, S; Tallapaka, L; Dayananda, D; Jen, KL. Mechanisms of triglyceride-lowering effect of an HMG-CoA reductase inhibitor in a hypertriglyceridemic animal model, the Zucker obese rat. *J. lipid Res.* 1992, 33(1):1-7.

[116] Khan, BV; Fungwe, TV; Wilcox, HG; Heimberg, M. Cholesterol is required for the secretion of the very-low-density lipoprotein: *in vivo* studies. *Biochim. Biophys. Acta* 1990, 1044(3):297-304.

[117] Yoshino, G; Kazumi, T; Kasama, T; Iwai, M; Iwatani, I; Matsuba, K; Matsushita, M; Baba, S. Effect of CS-514 (pravastatin) on VLDL-triglyceride kinetics in rats. *Atherosclerosis* 1988, 73(2-3):191-195.

[118] Tuzikov, FV; Tuzikova, NA; Galimov, RV; Panin, LE; Nevinsky, GA. General model to describe the structure and dynamic balance between different human serum lipoproteins and its practical application. *Med. Sci. Monit.* 2002, 8(6):MT79-MT88.

[119] Otvos, JD. Measurement of lipoprotein subclass profiles by nuclear magnetic resonance spectroscopy. *Clin. Lab.* 2002, 48(3-4):171-180.

[120] Porter, JA; Carter, BL; Johnston, TP; Palmer, WK. Effects of pravastatin on plasma lipid concentrations in poloxamer 407-induced hyperlipidemic rats. *Pharmacotherapy* 1995, 15:92-98.

[121] Johnston, TP; Palmer, WK. Effect of poloxamer 407 on the activity of microsomal 3-hydoxy-3-methylglutaryl CoA reductase in rats. *J. Cardiovasc. Pharmacol.* 1997, 29:580-585.

[122] Goldfarb, S. Rapid increase in hepatic HMG-CoA reductase activity and *in vivo* cholesterol synthesis after Triton WR 1339 injection. *J. lipid Res.* 1978, 19:489-494.

[123] Kuroda, M; Tanzawa, K; Tsujita, Y; Endo,A. Mechanism for elevation of hepatic cholesterol synthesis and serum cholesterol levels in Triton WR-1339-induced hyperlipidemia. *Biochim. Biophys. Acta* 1977, 489(1):119-125.

[124] Shefer, S; Nguyen, LB; Salen, G; Ness, GC; Chowdhary, IR; Lerner, S; Batta, AK; Tint, GS. Differing effects of cholesterol and taurocholate on steady state hepatic HMG-CoA reductase and cholesterol 7 alpha-hydroxylase activities and mRNA levels in the rat. *J. lipid Res.* 1992, 33(8):1193-1200.

In: Statins
Editor: Eric R. Travers

ISBN: 978-1-63463-057-3

Chapter 2

STATINS: POTENTIALLY NEUROPROTECTIVE AGENTS

***Sergey V. Pisklakov*[1*] *and Anuradha Patel*[2†]**

[1]Neuroanesthesia Service, Clinical Competence Committee,
Department of Anesthesiology and Perioperative Care,
New Jersey School of Medicine, Newark, New Jersey, US
[2]Pediatric Anesthesia, Department of Anesthesiology and Perioperative Care,
New Jersey School of Medicine, Newark, New Jersey, US

ABSTRACT

The aim of this chapter is to assess the experimental and clinical evidence regarding potential neuroprotective effects of statins and their possible perioperative benefit. Statins are drugs used to control cholesterol disorders and prevent cardiovascular diseases by four mechanisms: improvement of endothelial function, modulation of inflammatory responses, maintenance of plaque stability, and prevention of thrombus formation. It is possible that these various effects may also be neuroprotective. The anti-inflammatory effects of statins on endothelial cell mechanisms are better understood than their role in neuroprotection or tumoral apoptosis and evidence is only just emerging that statins may be beneficial. Data regarding perioperative use of statins in neurosurgery is scarce, controversial and inconclusive since there is a lack of convincing randomized, prospective clinical trials. More trials in humans are needed to determine whether statins could contribute to the current management of neurosurgical diseases. Not much is known about utilizing statins as a prophylactic treatment and some would probably advocate that we should be treating 'at risk' patients with statins perioperatively or at least it is important to try to put this into a clinical perspective.

* Director of Neuroanesthesia Service, Chairman of Clinical Competence Committee; 185 S Orange Ave. MSB E-552, Newark, NJ 07101, USA; Tel: 9739725255; Fax: 9739724172; E-mail: pisklase@rutgers.edu.

† Associate Professor, Section Chief; 185 S Orange Ave; MSB E-552, Newark, NJ 07101, USA; Tel: 9739725255; Fax: 9739724172.

The aim of this literature chapter is to assess the experimental and clinical evidence regarding potential neuroprotective effects of statins and their possible perioperative benefit. Statins are drugs primarily used to control cholesterol disorders and prevent cardiovascular disease. They inhibit hydroxymethylglutaryl–coenzyme A (HMGCoA) reductase, an enzyme that plays a central role in the production of cholesterol in the liver (Figure 1). Since elevated serum cholesterol levels have been associated with cardiovascular diseases [1], statins are known to be effective in decreasing mortality and morbidity in patients with cardiovascular disease. Statins are currently recommended for patients at high risk of developing heart disease and they are known to lower cholesterol, decrease the number of cardiac events, and reduce the risk of stroke [2]. Improvement of endothelial function, modulation of inflammatory responses, maintenance of plaque stability, and prevention of thrombus formation are other actions of statins beyond their lipid-lowering activity in the prevention of atherosclerosis [3]. The anti-inflammatory effects of statins on endothelial cell mechanisms are better understood than their role in neuroprotection or tumoral apoptosis and evidence is only just emerging that statins may be beneficial in the neurosurgical patient.

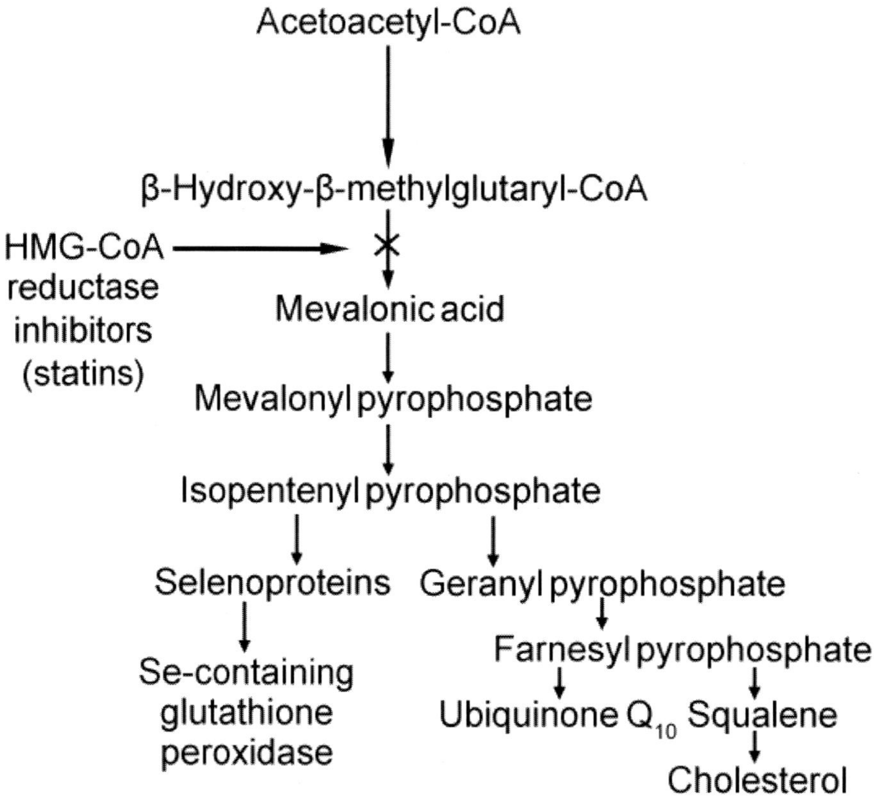

Figure 1. The mevalonate pathway. Statins inhibit production of HMG-CoA reductase, which is responsible for the conversion of HMG-CoA to mevalonate and thus prevent downstream cholesterol, ubiquinone-, and dolichol - dependent effects. (Adopted from: Hothersall E, Mc Sharry C, Thomson NC (2006) Potential therapeutic role for statins in respiratory disease. Thorax 61: 729-734).

Statins as Anti-Inflammatory Agents

A brief review of the anti-inflammatory properties of statins is necessary to understand their possible role in neuroprotection. The anti-inflammatory properties of statins are exemplified by reduced plasma concentrations of the inflammatory cytokines like Tissue Necrosis Factor (TNF) and InterLeukin (IL)-6 in patients receiving pravastatin [4]. Inflammatory processes play a pivotal role in the pathogenesis of atherosclerosis, and elevated plasma levels of markers of inflammation such as high sensitivity C- Reactive Protein (hs-CRP), serum amyloid A, IL-6 and soluble intercellular adhesion molecule-1 have been shown to predict cardiovascular events. Mechanism by which statins may reduce vascular event rates is related to potential anti-inflammatory effects of these agents [5-8]. There is data that preoperative statin therapy attenuates the release of pro-inflammatory IL-6 and up-regulates anti-inflammatory IL-10 after cardiac surgery with cardioplegia [9].

Cell-contact-dependent interactions between T cells and macrophages are now recognized to be of fundamental importance in promoting chronic inflammation in several autoimmune diseases [10]. There is evidence that statins affect macrophage function. Macrophages are capable of degrading the extracellular matrix and, by secreting Matrix MetalloProteinase (MMP), may weaken the fibrous cap and thus predispose an atheromatous plaque to rupture. Statins as Fluvastatin and Simvastatin have recently been shown to inhibit MMP-9 (gelatinase B) activity and secretion by macrophages [11]. Statins cause decreased macrophage expression of soluble intercellular adhesion molecule-1 and lipopolysaccharide-induced secretion of IL-6 and TNF by monocytes and macrophages [12-14]. Simvastatin therapy for 8 weeks reduces monocyte expression of TNF and IL-1 [15]. Statins are known to inhibit T-cell activation [16,17]. This effect is reversed by mevalonic acid, directly implicating HydroxyMethylGlutaryl- Coenzyme A (HMG-CoA) reductase in this activity. Lovastatin and simvastatin suppress critical T-cell co stimulatory events [18]. Overall, clinical data regarding the anti-inflammatory role of statins has until recently been limited and it is difficult to say if all statins have clinically relevant anti-inflammatory effects or whether any one agent is more powerful than another in this regard.

Statins in the Perioperative Care of Patients

What is the role of statins in perioperative care? The use of statins in the general population is widespread. Many patients presenting for surgery are regularly taking them but the evidence for the prophylactic use of statins perioperatively is weak and lacks prospective controlled studies. Statins have beneficial effects beyond those of lipid lowering, including reducing the perioperative risk of cardiac complications and sepsis [19]. It was shown that patients hospitalized with an acute coronary syndrome, ischemic stroke, or revascularization and prescribed a statin demonstrated a lower incidence of sepsis compared with controls [20]. One retrospective cohort analysis determined that statin used before hospital admission, and continued after sepsis, correlated with decreased mortality rates from septicemia [21]. Some studies have been performed in animals with death as the endpoint. For example, in mice, pretreatment with simvastatin before induction of sepsis using the cecal ligation puncture model increased survival rate four-fold [22]. In a subsequent study of treatment with a number of different statins given after the onset of sepsis, statins also improved survival [23].

The 2007 American Heart Association guidelines [24] indicate that there is evidence that supports the use of statins perioperatively to prevent cardiac complications during non-cardiac surgery. The guidelines state that it is unclear how we would identify those patients in whom to initiate statin therapy and for what duration. Abrupt stopping of statins is associated with an increased morbidity and mortality [25] as measured by an increase in troponins and cardiac events. Some authors suggest that statins are effective in lipid-independent conditions like sepsis [20], nephropathy, decreasing the rate of renal damage in diabetics [26], Alzheimer's disease and dementia, decreasing incidence and progression of autoimmune disease [27,28], rheumatoid arthritis [29], organ transplantation, decreasing rejection rates [30], gastrointestinal disease, possibly decreasing the incidence of colon cancer [31], inflammatory bowel disease [32], osteoporosis and macular degeneration [33]. Although the proposed benefits of statin therapy seem to be as widespread as their use, their use is associated with significant adverse effects. Most common are hepatic dysfunction and muscle problems like myalgia and rhabdomyolysis [12,34]. Myalgia is possibly related to mitochondrial dysfunction. Statins inhibit synthesis of mevalonate, a precursor of ubiquinone that is a central compound of the mitochondrial respiratory chain. Statin therapy can be associated with high blood lactate/pyruvate ratio. All this is suggestive of mitochondrial dysfunction [35].

Trials of statin therapy have had conflicting findings on the risk of development of diabetes mellitus in patients given statins. Statin therapy is associated with a slightly increased risk of development of diabetes, but the risk is low both in absolute terms and when compared with the reduction in coronary events [36]. The mechanism underlying the increase in type II Diabetes in patients undergoing statin therapy has not been fully identified. It is possible that statins may influence muscle or liver insulin sensitivity directly, but there is no specific experimental evidence to support any feasible hypothesis [37,38]. Other possible adverse effects include cognitive loss, neuropathy, pancreatic and sexual dysfunction [39]. The question remains, should we use statins perioperatively for neurosurgical patient? To elucidate this it would be important to know if statins provide neuroprotection.

Neuroprotective Effects of Statins

Modern concept of providing cerebral protection focuses on blocking the cascade of events that occur during ischemia. Cytokines are prominent mediators of inflammatory and immunologic responses in the brain and are produced by neurons, glial cells, and endothelium. Although, the precise mechanism of cerebral ischemic damage by cytokines needs to be further elucidated, their importance has been shown by studies demonstrating a reduction in cerebral infarct size in animals treated with cytokine receptor antagonists. Surgical stress triggers an inflammatory response and releases mediators into human plasma such as interleukins. Craniotomy performed under general anesthesia may be associated with different levels of stress and plasma IL-6 level is significantly increased [40]. Aspirin has shown laboratory evidence of neuronal protection due to its anti-inflammatory action [41]. Possibly statins as agents with anti-inflammatory properties could do same. Cytokines have a major role in ischemic neuronal damage primarily during reperfusion which is followed by leukocyte infiltration, primarily neutrophils. Cytokines are necessary for the optimal function of leukocytes, and they are considered the key mediators of acute phase responses to tissue injury. The adhesion of leukocytes to the walls of cerebral blood vessels is induced by cytokines. Tumor necrosis factor alpha and interleukin 1-beta seem to play a significant role in ischemic brain injury. This cytokine-induced leukocyte infiltration into ischemic brain tissue activates an inflammatory reaction, which results in the release of oxygen free radicals (Figure 2). Statins are known to attenuate the inflammatory cytokine response to ischemia [42].

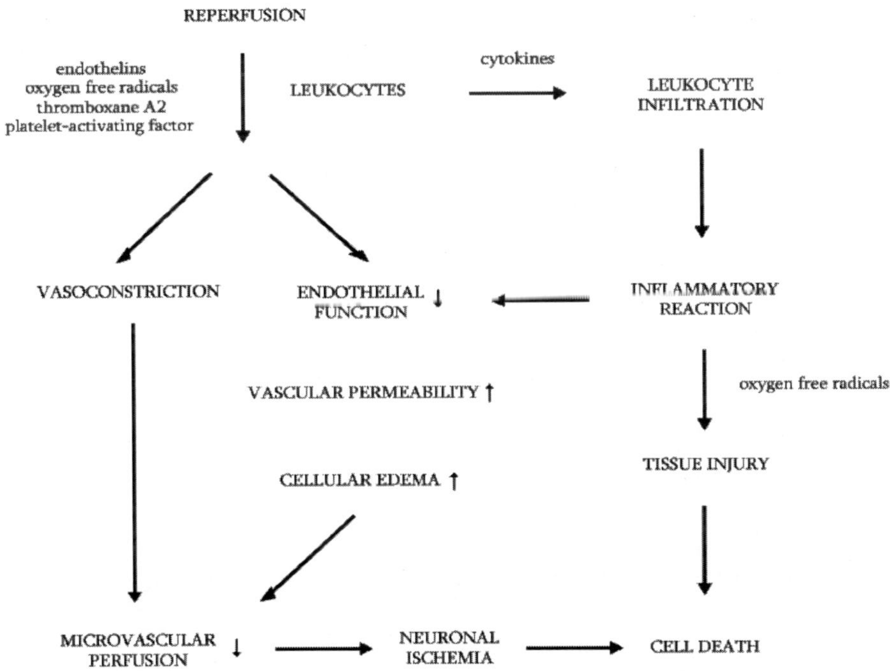

Figure 2. Cytokines and their role in ischemic neuronal damage during reperfusion. (Based on adaptation from Barone FC, Feuerstein GZ (1999) Feuerstein Journal of Cerebral Blood Flow and Metabolism 19: 819-834).

Endothelial glycocalyx plays one of the pivotal roles in ischemic damage. Drugs that can specifically increase the synthesis of glycocalyx components, refurbish it, or selectively prevent its enzymatic degradation could be very beneficial but do not seem to be available. Pharmacological blockers of radical production may be useful to diminish the oxygen radical stress on the glycocalyx; statins inhibitory effect on the cytokine tumor necrosis factor and inflammatory mediators release can be one of the tenable therapeutic options to improve glycocalyx layer [43].

The effect of simvastatin on the development of cerebral aneurysms and vasospasm was studied in rats. Treatment with simvastatin decreased induced aneurysm development [44]. If statins decrease the progression of cerebral aneurysms then the incidence of SAH may be lower in patients treated with statins. There are no long enough followup studies to answer this question now. Initiating simvastatin at the time of SAH also decreased vasospasm and improved neurobehavioral outcomes [45]. Retrospective clinical studies are conflicting with some reporting decreased vasospasm, improved short-term clinical outcome and decreased mortality with statins, and others finding no effect or an increased risk of vasospasm in patients on statins [46].

Three randomized clinical trials revealed controversial results [47-49]. In those studies statins had no effect on mortality and did not significantly decrease symptomatic vasospasm, but the numbers of patients treated were small. In other studies statins have exhibited some promise in the setting of SubArachnoid Hemorrhage (SAH): significantly reduced incidence of vasospasm and rebleeds, delayed ischemic deficits and mortality [49,50] and worse outcome if statins were discontinued [51]. This means statins may provide cerebrovascular protection which is lost if therapy is discontinued.

As the major regulator of homeostasis, the vascular endothelium exerts a number of vasoprotective effects, such as vasodilatation, suppression of smooth muscle cell growth, and inhibition of inflammatory responses. These effects are largely mediated by nitric oxide. Nitric oxide opposes the effects of endothelium-derived vasoconstrictors and inhibits oxidation of low-density lipoprotein. Poor production or activity of nitric oxide leads to impaired endotheliumdependent vasodilatation. A number of clinical trials have shown that statins improve endothelial dysfunction in patients with coronary risk factors beyond what could be attributed to their impact on plasma lipids. Several possible mechanisms by which statin therapy may improve endothelial dysfunction may include upregulation of nitric oxide production or activity and reduction of oxidative stress. One important pathway appears to be the effects of statins on NO production via increased availability of nitric oxide synthase [52]. This means statins possess beneficial effects during ischemic stroke and reperfusion. Statins can ameliorate ischemic damage by improving blood flow to the ischemic brain and by making the brain parenchyma intrinsically more resistant to the effects of ischemia. The proposed mechanisms includes upregulation of endothelial nitric oxide synthase (which promotes vasodilation) while inhibiting inducible nitric oxide synthase (which increases ischemic damage) [42].

Statins can be beneficial in Traumatic Brain Injury (TBI) [53]. After the initial insult to the brain, the delayed secondary effects of TBI often cause long-term severe injury. The secondary events are neurochemically mediated resulting in brain ischemia and hypoxia. The various effects of statins, especially anti-inflammatory and vasoactive effects, have been found to counter some of the secondary damage from traumatic brain injury and restore neural function. Therefore, statins may offer a potential novel therapeutic strategy for TBI [54,55].

Statins showed significant benefit in models of TBI [56]. Simvastatin promotes functional recovery after Traumatic Brain Injury (TBI) in rat; however, the underlying mechanisms remain poorly understood. TBI causes inflammatory reaction, including increased levels of IL-1β, IL-6 and TNF-α, as well as activated microglia. Simvastatin selectively reduces IL-1β expression and inhibits the activation of microglia and astrocytes after TBI, which may be one of the mechanisms underlying the therapeutic benefits of simvastatin treatment of TBI [57]. Simvastatin decreases post-TBI polymorphonuclear neutrophil infiltration and prevents release of proinflammatory mediators leading to blood-brain barrier disruption. Simvastatin does not stop the full insult of brain edema and restore BBB permeability but, it is able to limit the extravasation of large molecules in the pericontusional areas of TBI [58]. Animal TBI models showed functional and histological improvement after administration of statins [59,60]. Mice that were pretreated with atorvastatin and simvastatin, and then subjected to controlled head injury displayed recovery in vestibulomotor function, decreased degeneration of neurons within the hippocampus, and a decreased reduction in cerebral blood flow following the trauma. These results of neurocognitive improvements were reproduced in animals that were given atorvastatin post-injury as well. The mechanism by which atorvastatin attenuates this neuroinflammatory cytokinemediated response seems to be by diminishing microglial activation which contributes to the development of cerebral edema and neuronal injury. Atorvastatin significantly lowered post-injury TNFα and IL-6 levels as compared to control mice [59]. Simvastatin, similarly attenuated inflammatory mediator, IL-1β, and decreased reactive astrogliosis, thereby rescuing neuronal cells and increasing survival in the hippocampus and dentate gyrus post-injury [57,61]. Lovastatin also showed anti-inflammatory protective mechanisms in pretreated rats by reducing TNFα and IL-1β mRNA levels and enhancing motor and somatosensory function [62]. Statins promote angiogenesis and neurogenesis which are keys to recovery from traumatic brain injury [63]. Lu et al. administered atorvastatin to rats on day 1 and for 14 consecutive days after TBI and found a significant improvement in motor and spatial function [64]. Lu et al. found comparable outcomes with simvastatin [53]. Animal models had significant improvement in functional recovery after administration of atorvastatin which was quantitatively identified by an increase of angiogenesis [65].

Statins are drugs known to improve endothelial function, modulate inflammatory responses, and maintain plaque stability and prevention of thrombus formation. Based on laboratory evidence statins could offer substantial benefit in the perioperative management of neurosurgical diseases. The origin of neuroprotective effects of statins has not been well explained and the available data regarding perioperative use of statins in neurosurgery is inconclusive. There is certainly a lack of convincing randomized double-blind prospective clinical trials. Further studies in humans are needed to determine whether statins could contribute to the current management of neurosurgical diseases. An important question remains about utilizing statins as a prophylactic treatment as opposed to perioperative use.

REFERENCES

[1] Lewington S, Whitlock G, Clarke R, Sherliker P, Emberson J, et al. (2007) Blood cholesterol and vascular mortality by age, sex, and blood pressure: a meta-analysis of individual data from 61 prospective studies with 55,000 vascular deaths. *Lancet* 370: 1829-1839.

[2] National Institute for Health and Clinical Excellence - Quick reference guide (2010) Lipid modification - Cardiovascular risk assessment and the modification of blood lipids for the primary and secondary prevention of cardiovascular disease.

[3] Nissen SE, Nicholls SJ, Sipahi I, Libby P, Raichlen JS, et al. (2006) Effect of very high-intensity statin therapy on regression of coronary atherosclerosis: the ASTEROID trial. *JAMA* 295:1556-1565.

[4] Node K, Fujita M, Kitakaze M, Hori M, Liao JK (2003) Short-term statin therapy improves cardiac function and symptoms in patients with idiopathic dilated cardiomyopathy. *Circulation* 108: 839-843.

[5] Ridker PM, Cushman M, Stampfer MJ, Tracy RP, Hennekens CH (1997) Inflammation, aspirin, and the risk of cardiovascular disease in apparently healthy men. *N Engl J Med* 336: 973-979.

[6] Ridker PM, Hennekens CH, Buring JE, Rifai N (2000) C-Reactive protein and other markers of inflammation in the prediction of cardiovascular disease in women. *N Engl J Med* 342: 836-843.

[7] Ridker PM, Rifai N, Stampfer MJ, Hennekens CH (2000) Plasma concentration of interleukin-6 and the risk of future myocardial infarction among apparently healthy men. *Circulation* 101: 1767-1772.

[8] Harris TB, Ferrucci L, Tracy RP, Corti MC, Wacholder S, et al. (1999) Associations of elevated interleukin-6 and C-reactive protein levels with mortality in the elderly. *Am J Med* 106: 506-512.

[9] Liakopoulos OJ, Dörge H, Schmitto JD, Nagorsnik U, Grabedunkel J, et al. (2006) Effects of preoperative statin therapy on cytokines after cardiac surgery. *Thor Card Surg* 54: 250-254.

[10] McInnes IB, Leung BP, Sturrock RD, Field M, Liew FY (1997) Interleukin-15 mediates T cell-dependent regulation of tumor necrosis factor-alpha production in rheumatoid arthritis. *Nat Med* 3: 189-195.

[11] Bellosta S, Via D, Canavesi M, Pfister P, Fumagalli R, et al. (1998) HMG-CoA reductase inhibitors reduce MMP-9 secretion by macrophages. *Arterioscler Thromb Vasc Biol* 18:1671-1678.

[12] Ikeda U, Shimada K (1999) Statins and monocytes. *Lancet* 353: 2070.

[13] Niwa S, Totsuka T, Hayashi S (1996) Inhibitory effect of fluvastatin, an HMG-CoA reductase inhibitor, on the expression of adhesion molecules on human monocyte cell line. *Int J Immunopharmacol* 18: 669-675.

[14] Rosenson RS, Tangney CC, Casey LC (1999) Inhibition of proinflammatory cytokine production by pravastatin. *Lancet* 353: 983-984.

[15] Ferro D, Parrotto S, Basili S, Alessandri C, Violi F (2000) Simvastatin inhibits the monocyte expression of proinflammatory cytokines in patients with hypercholesterolemia. *J Am Coll Cardiol* 36: 427-431.

[16] Munford RS (2001) Statins and the acute-phase response. *N Engl J Med* 344: 2016-2018.

[17] Kwak B, Mulhaupt F, Myit S, Mach F (2000) Statins as a newly recognized type of immunomodulator. *Nat Med* 6: 1399-1402.

[18] Weitz-Schmidt G, Welzenbach K, Brinkmann V, Kamata T, Kallen J, et al. (2001) Statins selectively inhibit leukocyte function antigen-1 by binding to a novel regulatory integrin site. *Nat Med* 7: 687-692.

[19] Brookes ZL, McGown CC, Reilly CS (2009) Statins for all: the new premed? *Br J Anaesth* 103: 99-107.

[20] Hackam DG, Mamdani M, Li P, Redelmeier DA (2006) Statins and sepsis in patients with cardiovascular disease: a population-based cohort analysis. *Lancet* 367: 413-418.

[21] Kruger P, Fitzsimmons K, Cook D, Jones M, Nimmo G (2006) Statin therapy is associated with fewer deaths in patients with bacteraemia. *Intensive Care Med* 32: 75-79.

[22] Merx MW, Liehn EA, Janssens U, Lutticken R, Schrader J, et al. (2004) HMG-CoA reductase inhibitor simvastatin profoundly improves survival in a murine model of sepsis. *Circulation* 109: 2560-2565.

[23] Merx MW, Liehn EA, Graf J, van de Sandt A, Schaltenbrand M, et al. (2005) Statin treatment after onset of sepsis in a murine model improves survival. *Circulation* 112: 117-124.

[24] Fleisher LA, Beckman JA, Brown KA, Calkins H, Chaikof E, et al. (2007) ACC/AHA 2007 guidelines on perioperative cardiovascular evaluation and care for noncardiac surgery. *Circulation* 116: 418-499.

[25] Durazzo AE, Machado FS, Ikeoka DT, De Bernoche C, Monachini MC, et al. (2004) Reduction in cardiovascular events after vascular surgery with atorvastatin: a randomized trial. *J Vasc Surg* 39: 967-975.

[26] Usui H, Shikata K, Matsuda M, Okada S, Ogawa D, et al. (2003) HMG-CoA reductase inhibitor ameliorates diabetic nephropathy by its pleiotropic effects in rats. *Nephrol Dial Transplant* 18: 265-272.

[27] Jick H, Zornberg GL, Jick SS, Seshadri S, Drachman DA (2002) Statins and the risk of dementia. *Lancet* 356: 1627-1631.

[28] Simons M, Schwarzler F, Lutjohann D, von Bergmann K, Beyreuther K, et al. (2002)Treatment with simvastatin in normocholesterolemic patients with Alzheimer's disease: a 26-week randomized, placebo-controlled, double-blind trial. *Ann Neurol* 52: 346-350.

[29] Leung BP, Sattar N, Crilly A, Prach M, McCarey DW, et al. (2003) A novel anti-inflammatory role for simvastatin in inflammatory arthritis. *J Immunol* 170: 1524-1530.

[30] Mehra MR, Uber PA, Vivekananthan K, Solis S, Scott RL, et al. (2002) Comparative beneficial effects of simvastatin and pravastatin on cardiac allograft rejection and survival. *J Am Coll Cardiol* 40: 1609-1614.

[31] Pedersen TR, Berg K, Cook TJ, Faergeman O, Haghfelt T, et al. (1996) Safety and tolerability of cholesterol lowering with simvastatin during 5 years in Scandinavian simvastatin survival study. *Arch Intern Med* 156: 2085-2092.

[32] Sasaki M, Bharwani S, Jordan P, Joh T, Manas K, et al. (2003) The 3-hydroxy-3-methylglutaryl-CoA reductase inhibitor pravastatin reduces disease activity and inflammation in dextran-sulfate induced colitis. *J Pharmacol Exp Ther* 305: 78-85.

[33] Laufs U, Liao JK (1998) Post-transcriptional regulation of endothelial nitric oxide synthase mRNA stability by Rho GTPase. *J Biol Chem* 273: 24266-24271.

[34] Sweetman S (2009) Cardiovascular drugs. In: Martindale: the complete drug reference. *Pharmaceutical Press,* London 1155-1434.

[35] De Pinieux G, Chariot P, Ammi-Saïd M, Louarn F, Lejonc JL, et al. (1996) Lipid-lowering drugs and mitochondrial function: effects of HMG-CoA reductase inhibitors on serum ubiquinone and blood lactate/pyruvate ratio. *Br J Clin Pharmacol* 42: 333-337.

[36] Sattar N, Preiss D, Murray HM, Welsh P, Buckley BM, et al. (2010) Statins and risk of incident diabetes: a collaborative meta-analysis of randomised statin trials. *Lancet* 375: 735-742.

[37] Waters DD, Ho JE, DeMicco DA, Breazna A, Arsenault BJ, et al. (2011) Predictors of new-onset diabetes in patients treated with atorvastatin: results from 3 large randomized clinical trials. *J Am Coll Cardiol* 57: 1535-1545.

[38] Preiss D, Seshasai SR, Welsh P, Murphy SA, Ho JE, et al. (2011) Risk of incident diabetes with intensive-dose compared with moderate-dose statin therapy: a meta-analysis. *JAMA* 305: 2556-2564.

[39] Doing Things Differently (2008) *Pfizer Annual Review.*

[40] Klimek M, Hol JW, Wens S, Antonissen CH, Niehof N, et al. (2009) Inflammatory profile of awake function-controlled craniotomy and craniotomy under general anesthesia. *Mediators Inflamm.*

[41] Riepe MW, Kasischke K, Raupach A (1997) Acetylsalicylic acid increases tolerance against hypoxic and chemical hypoxia. *Stroke* 28: 2006-2011.

[42] Vaughan CJ, Delanty N (1999) Neuroprotective properties of statins in cerebral ischemia and stroke. *Stroke* 30: 1969-1973.

[43] Becker BF, Chappell D, Bruegger D, Annecke T, Jacob M (2010) Therapeutic strategies targeting the endothelial glycocalyx: acute deficits, but great potential. *Cardiovasc Res* 87: 300-310.

[44] Aoki T, Kataoka H, Ishibashi R, Nozaki K, Hashimoto N (2008) Simvastatin suppresses the progression of experimentally induced cerebral aneurysms in rats. *Stroke* 39: 1276-1285.

[45] McGirt MJ, Pradilla G, Legnani FG, Thai QA, Recinos PF, et al. (2006) Systemic administration of simvastatin after the onset of experimental subarachnoid hemorrhage attenuates cerebral vasospasm. *Neurosurgery* 58: 945-951.

[46] Sabri M, Macdonald R (2010) Statins: A Potential Therapeutic Addition to Treatment for Aneurysmal Subarachnoid Hemorrhage? *World Neurosurg* 73: 646-653.

[47] Bulsara KR, Coates JR, Agrawal VK, Eifler DM, Wagner-Mann CC, et al. (2006) Effect of combined simvastatin and cyclosporine compared with simvastatin alone on cerebral vasospasm after subarachnoid hemorrhage in a canine model. *Neurosurg Focus* 21: E11.

[48] Kramer AH (2009) Statins in the management of aneurysmal subarachnoid hemorrhage--not (yet) a standard of care. *Stroke* 40: 80-81.

[49] Sillberg VA, Wells GA, Perry JJ (2008) Do statins improve outcomes and reduce the incidence of vasospasm after aneurysmal subarachnoid hemorrhage: a meta-analysis. *Stroke* 39: 2622-2626.

[50] Moskowitz SI, Ahrens C, Provencio JJ, Chow M, Rasmussen PA (2009) Prehemorrhage statin use and the risk of vasospasm after aneurysmal subarachnoid hemorrhage. *Surg Neurol* 71: 311-317.

[51] Tapia-Pérez JH, Sanchez-Aguilar M, Schneider T (2010) The role of statins in neurosurgery. *Neurosurg Rev* 33:259-70.

[52] Davignon J, Ganz P (2004) Role of Endothelial Dysfunction in Atherosclerosis. *Circulation.* 109: 27-32.

[53] Lu D, Qu C, Goussev A, Jiang H, Lu C, et al. (2007) Statins increase neurogenesis in the dentate gyrus, reduce delayed neuronal death in the hippocampal CA3 region, and improve spatial learning in rat after traumatic brain injury. *J Neurotrauma* 24: 1132-1146.

[54] Xiong Y, Mahmood A, Chopp M (2009) Emerging treatments for traumatic brain injury. *Expert Opin Emerg Drugs* 14: 67-84.

[55] Lu D, Mahmood A, Goussev A, Schallert T, Qu C, et al. (2004) Atorvastatin reduction of intravascular thrombosis, increase in cerebral microvascular patency and integrity, and enhancement of spatial learning in rats subjected to traumatic brain injury. *J Neurosurg* 101: 813-821.

[56] Wible EF, Laskowitz DT (2010) Statins in traumatic brain injury. *Neurotherapeutics* 7: 62-73.

[57] Li B, Mahmood A, Lu D, Wu H, Xiong Y, et al. (2009) Simvastatin attenuates microglial cells and astrocyte activation and decreases interleukin-1beta level after traumatic brain injury. *Neurosurgery* 65: 179-185.

[58] Beziaud T, Ru Chen X, El Shafey N, Frechou M, Teng F, et al. (2011) Simvastatin in traumatic brain injury: Effect on brain edema mechanisms. *Crit Care Med* 39: 2300-2307.

[59] Wang H, Lynch JR, Song P, Yang HJ, Yates RB, et al. (2007) Simvastatin and atorvastatin improve behavioral outcome, reduce hippocampal degeneration, and improve cerebral blood flow after experimental traumatic brain injury. *Exp Neurol* 206: 59-69.

[60] Qu C, Lu D, Goussev A, Schallert T, Mahmood A, et al. (2005) Effect of atorvastatin on spatial memory, neuronal survival, and vascular density in female rats after traumatic brain injury. *J Neurosurg* 103: 695-701.

[61] Wu H, Mahmood A, Lu D, Jiang H, Xiong Y, et al. (2010) Simvastatin attenuates astrogliosis after traumatic brain injury through the modulation of EGFR in lipid rafts. *J Neurosurg* 113: 591-597.

[62] Chen SF, Hung TH, Chen CC, Lin KH, Huang YN, et al. (2007) Lovastatin improves histological and functional outcomes and reduces inflammation after experimental traumatic brain injury. *Life Sci* 81: 288-298.

[63] Wu H, Lu D, Jiang H, Xiong Y, Qu C, et al. (2008) Simvastatin-mediated upregulation of VEGF and BDNF, activation of PI3K/Akt Pathway, and increase of neurogenesis are associated with therapeutic improvement after traumatic brain injury. *J Neurotrauma* 25: 130-139.

[64] Lu D, Goussev A, Chen J, Pannu P, Li Y, et al. (2004) Atorvastatin reduces neurological deficit and increases synaptogenesis, angiogenesis, and neuronal survival in rats subjected to traumatic brain injury. *J Neurotrauma* 21: 21-32.

[65] Wu H, Jiang H, Lu D, Qu C, Xiong Y, et al. (2011) Induction of angiogenesis and modulation of vascular endothelial growth factor receptor-2 by simvastatin after traumatic brain injury. *Neurosurgery* 68: 1363-1371.

In: Statins
Editor: Eric R. Travers

ISBN: 978-1-63463-057-3

Chapter 3

STATINS: PHARMACOLOGY, MEDICAL USES AND CLINICAL OUTCOMES

Dr. Isabelle De Loecker
Erasme Hospital, Brussels, Belgium

ABSTRACT

The use of statins has recently attracted the attention of clinicians. Indeed, statins are probably the most common chronic treatment used for cardiovascular disease (18 million prescription purchase in France and 173.7 million in United States, per year). Moreover, their so-called pleiotropic effects open the gates to much larger medical applications. However, it is still difficult to predict the individual's response to statin therapy. Recent research has shown that variants of candidate genes affect statin efficacy and safety. Clinicians often assume that symptoms occurring with statins are caused by statins, encouraging discontinuation. But so far, only asymptomatic liver enzymes, muscle aches and development of new-onset diabetes mellitus has been proven to be related to statin therapy. To lower cholesterol levels, clinicians could prescribe statin monotherapy or a statin in combination with another agent. There are potential benefits to treating with multiple agents, such as the different mechanisms of action of other lipid-modifying agents, may be a solution against the adverse effects of statins and their intolerance. Given their pleiotropic effects, statins could be used in non-dyslipidemic diseases.

In this chapter, we will first examine the properties of statins including their structure, metabolism, and potency. We will also look at the pharmacogenomics of statins as well their mechanisms of action from their lipid-lowering effects to the more complex anti-inflammatory, immunomodulatory, anti-thrombotic, and anti-oxidant properties found independently of the lipid-lowering properties. Following this, we will review the potential adverse effects of statins including the mechanisms leading to myopathy and new-onset diabetes mellitus. In this regard, we will assess the benefits and harmful intensification of statin monotherapy compared to the combination of statins and other lipid-modifying medications. Then, we will discuss the guidelines regarding the use of statins in the well-established scope of cardiovascular diseases. Finally, we will review the potential benefits of statins in non-dyslipdemic disorders in chronic diseases such as rheumatoid arthritis, venous thromboembolism, and polycystic ovary syndrome, as well as in critical illnesses such as sepsis, acute lung injury / acute respiratory distress syndrome or after subarachnoidal hemorrhage. We will particularly focus on the latter.

Introduction

The use of statins recently attracted the attention of clinicians. Indeed, statins are probably the most common chronic treatment in cardiovascular disease (18 million prescription purchases in France and 173.7 million in the United States, per year) but moreover; their so-called pleiotropic effects open the gates to much larger medical applications. However, it is still difficult to predict the individual's response to statin therapy. Recent research has shown that variants of candidate genes affect statin efficacy and safety. Clinicians often assume symptoms occurring with statins are caused by statins, encouraging discontinuation. But so far, only asymptomatic liver enzymes, muscle aches and development of new-onset diabetes mellitus has been proven to be related to statin therapy. To lower cholesterol levels, clinicians could prescribe statin monotherapy or statins combined with another agent. There are potential benefits to treating with multiple agents, since the different mechanisms of action of the other lipid-modifying agents may be a solution against the adverse effects of statin adverse and their intolerance. Given their pleiotropic effects, statins could be used in non-dyslipidemic diseases. They open a new field in the treatment of chronic disease such as rheumatoid arthritis, venous thromboembolism, and polycystic ovary syndrome, as well as in critical illnesses such as sepsis, acute lung injury / acute respiratory distress syndrome or after subarachnoidal hemorrage.

1. Pharmacology

Different Statins, Different Properties

In 1976, a microbiological research on a new target of antibacterial activity led to the discovery of a molecule affecting bacterial growth by inhibiting a key enzyme in cholesterol biosynthesis, the HMG CoA reductase [1]. Subsequently, lovastatin was developed and provided a remarkable improvement in the therapy of dyslipidemias. However, this drug was not efficient enough for large clinical prevention studies. This urged the need for new semisynthetic molecules, of which simvastatin, which is more lipophilic and more potent thanks to an additional methyl group, was the greatest advance [2].

Structure

Lovastatin and simvastatin both have a closed ring configuration that needs to be converted, presumably in the liver, to a molecule with a structure resembling HMGCoA. This property makes them inactive pro-drugs.

Development of newer agents led to a preference for open-ring structures. Indeed, the first open-ring statin to be synthetized, pravastatin, appeared to be active on in vitro cholesterol levels with the highest activity in the liver and reduced activity in other tissues [3], which presumed to decrease the amount of adverse affects. Following this, all second and third generation statins, from pravastatin to fluvastatin, atorvastatin, rosuvastatin or the newest, pitavastatin, show open ring structure in the classical position of the HMG CoA-analog moiety.

For some time, this difference led to a number of controversies on whether the open ring molecules would have liver selectivity whereas closed ring molecules wouldn't have any particular selectivity. This issue never came to a real end [4] although, in comparative trials, the open ring pravastatin seems to be less associated with generalized, and in particular muscle, toxicity [5].

Absorption and Metabolism

The intestinal absorption of statins is variable, ranging from 30% to 85%. With the exception of hydrophilic agents, statins undergo a first pass metabolism in the liver declining the systemic bioavailability to 5-30% of the oral dose. Statins are predominantly metabolized by the cytochrome P-450 (CYP450) system and most metabolites are active. A number of variant CYP450 genes might explain, to a minimal extent, the variability in cholesterol lowering activity [6].

The hydrophilic agents, pravastatin and rosuvastatin, undergo minimal metabolic handling. They enter cells via carrier proteins whereas the other agents, lipophilic, interact directly with the membrane (Table 1).

Table 1. Properties of statins

	Structure	Solubility	Bioavailability	Metabolization CYP450	Elimination half-life	Active Metabolites
Simvastatin	Closed ring	Lipophilic	5%	3A4, 3A5	2 - 3 hours	Yes
Pravastatin	Open ring	Hydrophilic	18%	-	1.3-2.8 hours	No
Fluvastatin	Open ring	Lipophilic	19 -29 %	2C9	0.5-2.3 hours	No
Atorvastatin	Open ring	Lipophilic	12 %	3A4	15 -30 hours	Yes
Rosuvastatin	Open ring	Hydrophilic	20%	2C9	19 hours	No
Pitavastatin	Open ring	Lipophilic	51%	2C9, 2C8	12 hours	Yes

Kinetics

Regarding their mechanism of action, the kinetics of statins doesn't influence the hypolipidemic activity. Indeed, the HMG-CoA reductase inhibition leads to a blockade of an enzyme with a rapid turnover, far shorter than that influenced by drugs levels.

HMG-CoA reductase has a $t1/2\beta$ of about 4 hours whereas for instance, simvastatin has a half-life of about 12h. Atorvastatin and rosuvastatin have the longest half-life, around 20h. A prolonged half-life may have two advantages: firstly, it could improve lipid-lowering activity in non-compliant patients and secondly, the permanence of blood levels may have to do with the so-called "pleiotropic effects". These may not be active in the case of low or absent blood levels of a statin.

Potency

The different statins show different potencies on LDL-C level lowering. At maximal prescribed doses, rosuvastatin and atorvastatin are the more potent statin, reaching a reduction of around 60 percent of the LDL-C level [7,8]. They are followed by simvastatin, lovastatin, pravastatin and finally, fluvastatin [9], which is the least potent statin but also the least likely to produce muscle toxicity or drug interactions (Table 2).

Table 2. Statins potency equivalence

Approximate reduction in LDL-C level.					
	20%	30%	40%	50%	60%
Rosuvastatin	-	-	-	5 -10 mg	20 - 40 mg
Atorvastatin	-	-	10 mg	40 mg	80 mg
Simvastatin	-	10 mg	20 mg	80 mg	-
Pravastatin	10 mg	20 - 40 mg	80 mg	-	-
Fluvastatin	20 mg	80 mg	-	-	-

Regarding the effect on HDL-C, rosuvastatin is again the most effective with an increase up to 10 percent [10]. The efficacy of rosuvastatin on HDL-C level increase is followed by simvastatin, which in turn appears to be more effective than atorvastatin [11].

Rosuvastatin and atorvastatin are the most effective in decreasing triglycerides with a reduction between 14 and 33 percent [12,13]. Their effect on triglycerides are dose-dependent. Atorvastatin, for instance, produces reductions in triglycerides ranging from 27 percent at a dose of 5 mg/day to 46 percent at a dose of 80mg/day [14].

Pharmacogenomics

Despite the growing experience in the use of statins, it is still difficult to predict the individual patient response in terms of efficacy and possible adverse effects. Plasma concentrations can vary greatly, as much as 45-fold, amongst patients receiving the same dose of statins [15]. Recent advances in pharmagenomics have allowed the identification of genes that could affect the pharmacokinetic and pharmacodynamic of statins. Overall, more than 40 genes are implicated in affecting statin efficacy and safety, which reflects both the complexity of cholesterol homeostasis as well as the variability of individual's response. Some genetic variants have been linked to more serious adverse effects leading to recommendations toward these particular population subgroups.

SLCO1B1

In 2008, the SEARCH study [15] found an association between myopathy induced by high dose (80 mg) simvastatin and a polymorphism in the SLCO1B1 gene, which encodes for the OATP1B1 importer, a membrane transporter that facilitates the hepatic uptake of statins. At the rs4149056 locus, the wild-type T allele encodes valine while the minor C allele encodes alanine. The association between the C allele and statin-induced myopathy has been independently replicated by subsequent studies [16 - 19].

The frequency of the C allele is less than 3% in some African populations, 10%-20% in European and Middle Eastern populations, 10%-15% in East Asian populations, 5%-10% in South/West Asian populations, and over 20% in some populations from South and Central America [20, 21].

The rs4149056 polymorphism has been shown to influence statin pharmacokinetics in the different haplotypes: in studies on simvastatin, CC homozygotes (0%-6% of patients), with the lowest OATP1B1 activity, had higher plasma exposure to active simvastatin acid than TT homozygotes (55%-88% of patients); TC heterozygotes (11%-36% of patients) had intermediate exposure [20, 22]. Despite the observed effect on statin pharmacokinetics, there is no evidence for an effect of SLCO1B1 polymorphisms on the efficacy of statin therapy [23 - 27]. Results from the very large Heart Protection Study suggested at most a small effect of the SLCO1B1 genotype (approximately 1% per C allele) on LDL-c reduction and no significant effect on vascular outcomes [28]. However, it is clear that the higher plasma exposure to simvastatin in the C allele variant is responsible for myopathy, but the mechanism remains unknown. Overall, the SEARCH and Heart Protection Study (HPS) [15, 28] studies provide support for an association between the C allele at rs4149056 and increased susceptibility to simvastatin-induced myopathy, with odds ratios between 2.1 and 4.7 per copy of the allele [29].

The evidence for an association between the SLCO1B1 rs4149056 variant and simvastatin-induced myopathy has led to suggest that SLCO1B1 genotyping might be used clinically to guide the choice and/or dose of statin therapy, with the aim of reducing the risk of myopathy and improving adherence to therapy [30, 31]. Given the modest positive predictive value of the CC genotype but the much higher negative predictive value, the test might have greater clinical utility for selecting patients (TT homozygotes) who are able to tolerate higher-dose simvastatin, especially if they are at high risk of major coronary events. CC homozygotes have an increased risk of myopathy, so a statin therapy that has slightly lower efficacy may nevertheless result in a net clinical benefit if it lowers the risk of non-adherence as well as the risk of rare, but serious, rhabdomyolysis. It has been suggested that knowledge of the SLCO1B1 genotype may be particularly useful to inform prescribing and on-therapy safety monitoring if statins are to be used in conjunction with other drugs, and during the first year of therapy when the absolute risk of myopathy is the highest [32].

HMG-CoA Reductase Gene

Different studies have identified variations in the HMG-CoA reductase (HMGCR) gene that affect the efficacy of statins to lower cholesterol [33 - 35]. One of these variants, known as rs3846662 and found in the H7 haplotype of the HMGCR gene, is known to lower statin responsiveness [36, 37]. This variation causes alternative splicing of the mRNA, which generates a variation in enzyme expression. In the rs3846662 variant, the alternative splicing of the exon 13 leads to the expression of a non-functional protein isoform, referred to as HMGCRv_1. This protein isoform lacks amino acids in the catalytic domain where statins bind [36, 38]. Therefore, the expression of this variant significantly lowers the efficacy of statins and is inversely correlated with percentage reductions of plasma total cholesterol, low-density lipoprotein cholesterol, apolipoprotein B, and triglycerides.

According to a recent study, HMGCRv_1 expression explains only a fraction of the variation in LDL-C, apoB, and triglyceride response to statins (9%, 15%, and 6%, respectively); but when age, race, smoking status, and body mass index were added to the model, the combination of these parameters accounted for 24% of the variation in LDL-C response, 29% of the variation in apoB response, and 8% of the variation in triglycerides, with HMGCRv_1 gene expression being the most significant predictor of response in all three [36].

Apolipoprotein E

The apolipoprotein E (APOE) is secreted by the liver and plays a role in the hepatic uptake of lipoproteins. There are three isoforms of APOE in the general population, known as ε2, ε3, and ε4. Patients expressing the ε2 isoform were shown to have significantly higher LDL reductions after pravastatin and atorvastatin compared to subjects expressing the ε4 isoform [39].

KIF6

KIF6 codes for a kinesin-like protein, which is responsible for the intracellular transport of messenger ribonucleotides (mRNA‘s). The kinesin-like family 6 (*KIF6*) is potentially both a prognostic marker for coronary heart disease risk and a predictive marker of statin efficacy. Indeed, one of the KIF 6 variant, the rs20455, was initially described as an independent risk factor for coronary heart disease [40, 41]. Following this, retrospective genetic association studies were conducted to investigate whether patients carrying the rs20455 variant experience a greater coronary risk reduction from statin therapy than the others. Four studies (CARE, WOSCOPS, TIMI-22 and PROSPER) [41- 43] indicated that while rs20455 carriers experience a significantly lower coronary event risk, non-carriers show no statistically significant decrease in their baseline event rate with statin therapy. Interestingly, although carriers experienced a reduction in clinical events on therapy, they did not have a statistically significant difference in reductions of low-density lipoprotein cholesterol or inflammatory markers during statin treatment [44]. This result implies that while carriers are selected for response to statin therapy, their improved outcomes are not derived from decreased levels of LDL, but possibly from pleiotropic effects. However, four subsequent studies (HPS, TNT, IDEAL and JUPITER) [45- 47] failed to replicate the differences between carriers and non-carriers observed in earlier trials.

These latter data don't encourage the use of KIF6 genetic testing before the initiation of statin therapy, even if a test for KIF6 genotyping is now available. The only benefit could be regarding medication adherence, which is one of the major problems facing prescribers. Indeed, a recent study showed better statin therapy adherence in patients screened before the initiation of statin therapy compared to others [48]

Mechanisms of Action

The action of statins goes far beyond their lipid lowering properties since they can influence the intracellular signaling. Indeed, mevalonate is the precursor of many sterol and non-sterol products. By inhibiting the HMG CoA reductase and thus reducing the intracellular mevalonate, statins do not only reduce the cholesterol levels but also the non-sterol end products: farnesylpyrophosphate and geranylgeranylpyrophospahte, which provide the post-translational modification, or isoprenylation, of small GTP-binding proteins (Roc, Rho and Ras) (Figure 1) [49]. These anti-inflammatory, immunomodulatory, and antithrombotic effects are grouped under the name of "pleiotropic" effects and are the basis for the use of statins in non-lipid related disorders.

Lipid Lowering

Statins are competitive inhibitors of the HMGCoA reductase, the rate-limiting enzyme in cholesterol synthesis. They occupy a portion of the binding site of HMG CoA, blocking access of this substrate to the active site on the enzyme [50]. Inhibition of this enzyme results in a decrease in intrahepatic cholesterol concentration. This decrease in cholesterol concentration activates a cellular signaling cascade culminating in the activation of sterol regulatory element binding protein (SREBP), a transcription factor that up-regulates expression of the gene encoding the LDL receptor. Increased LDL receptor expression causes increased uptake of plasma LDL, and consequently decreases plasma LDL-cholesterol concentration.

Statins also reduce triglycerides plasma level through a decrease in VLDL synthesis associated with an increase of VLDL remnant particles by the LDL receptors [51].

Anti-Inflammatory

Small GTP-binding proteins have crucial roles in intracellular inflammatory signaling by acting as molecular on/off switches for various protein kinase, which regulate Nuclear Factor kappa B, Mitogen Activated Protein Kinase (MAPK), and Phosphatidyinositol-3 kinase (PI3K) systems. By inhibiting protein isoprenylation, statins reduce, without abolishing, the response of the inflammatory intracellular signaling pathway. The reduction in intensity affects the expression of cytokines, acute phase proteins, chemokines, adhesion molecules, and enzymes, and modulates leucocyte function and the coagulation system (Figure 2) [52].

Immunomodulatory

Beyond the effects over cytokines, chemokines and adhesion molecules, statins directly influence leucocyte function by a direct inhibition of the major histocompatibility complex type II (MHC II) gene of antigen presenter cells [53], and an allosteric block site of the lymphocyte function-associated antigen (LFA-1) [54, 55], which has a significant role in lymphocyte adhesion and activation.

Statins also decrease the expression of Toll-like receptor 4 (TLR4) [56 - 58], possibly by an alteration in cholesterol rich membrane domains as observed in brain plasma membranes [59].

Antithrombotic

Statins modulate coagulation through a number of mechanisms, including the increased expression and functional activity of thrombomodulin, an essential cofactor for protein C activation [60]. Statins might thus enhance protein C function. This may be relevant since recombinant activated protein C is the only pharmacological treatment shown to reduce mortality in patients with severe sepsis [61].

Endothelial Function

Whereas physiological concentrations of nitric oxide preserve microcirculatory flow, pathological levels of inducible nitric oxide synthase (NOS) contribute to excessive vasodilatation, loss of systemic vascular resistance, and vascular leaks.

Statins reduce inducible NOS expression, while maintaining constitutive NOS production [62-64]. This may be clinically important since unselected NOS blockade is associated with increased mortality [65].

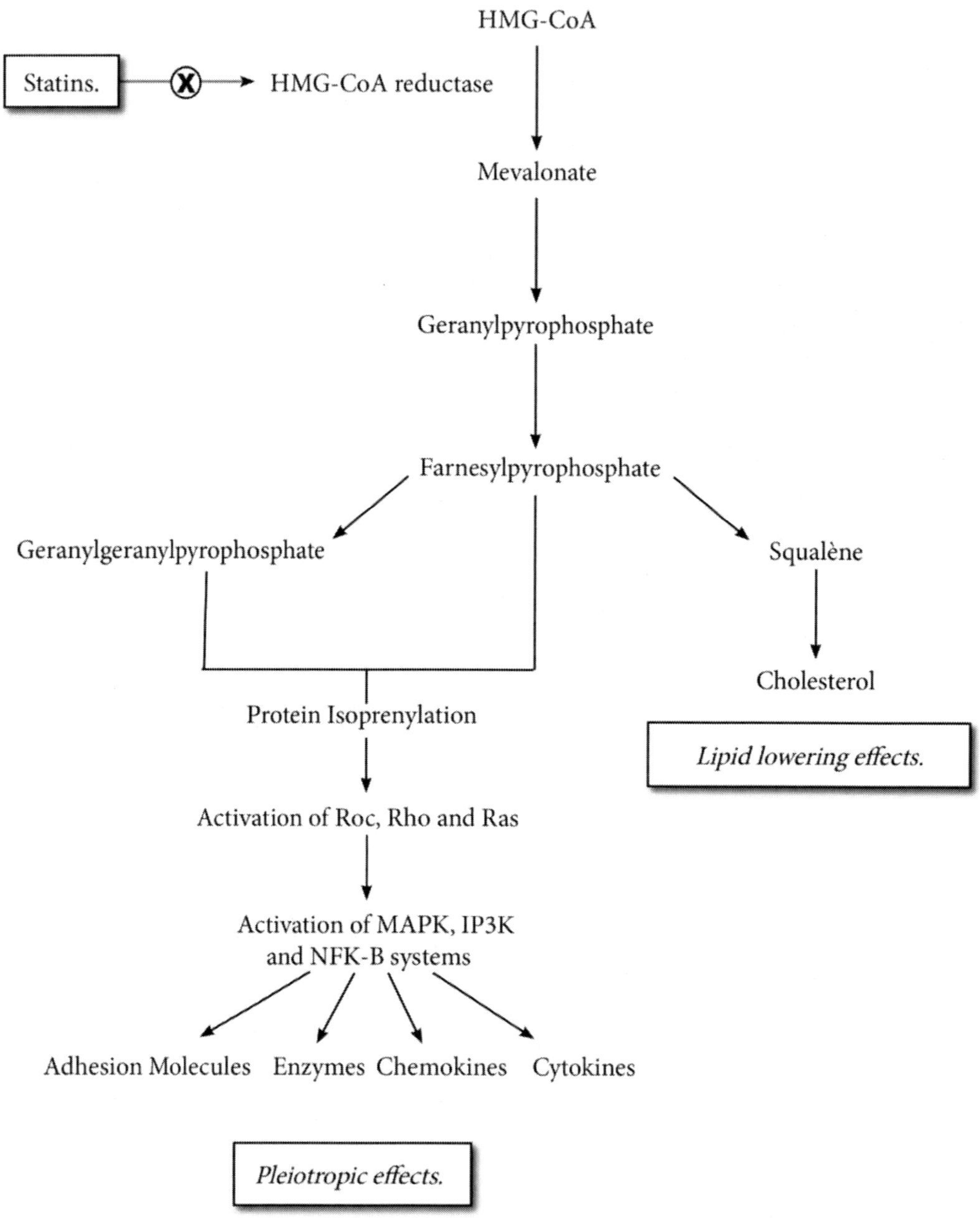

Figure 1. Mechanism of action.

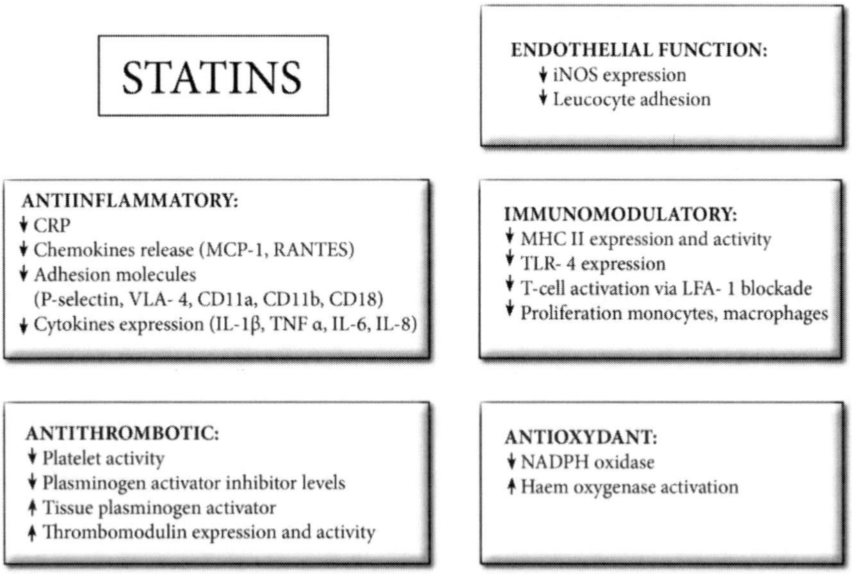

Figure 2. Pleitropic effects of statins.

Anti-Oxidant

Oxidative stress is an important factor associated with morbidity and mortality in patients with sepsis and multiorgan failure [66-68]

Stains have anti-oxidant effects by NADPH oxidase inactivation [69] and heme oxygenase activation [70 - 73].

Vitamin D

Cells of the innate and adaptative immune system express the vitamin D receptor and respond to stimulation by vitamin D's active form, 1,25-dihydroxyvitmin D [1,25(OH)$_2$D] [74]. Moreover, 1,25(OH)$_2$D leads to enhanced expression of human cathelicidin, which is an endogenous antimicrobial peptide active against a broad spectrum of infectious agents [75].

Statin therapy increases the major circulating form of vitamin D, 25-hydroxyvitamin D [25(OH)D] [76, 77], by a mechanism which is still unclear but could have beneficial effects on infection control [78, 79].

Adverse Effects

Statins are well-tolerated by most patients, but they can produce some adverse effects of which muscle injury and new-onset type 2 diabetes mellitus are the most relevant.

Muscle Injury

Myopathic syndromes associated with statin therapy range from myalgias to rhabdomyolysis. Most of the patients experience mild muscle symptoms, however severe muscle damage with renal failure may occur [80, 81].

The mechanism by which statins cause muscle toxicity remains unclear but several mechanisms have been proposed.

Firstly, statins inhibit the synthesis of coenzyme Q10 [82], also known as ubiquinone, which plays an important role in the production of muscle cell energy. This reduction in intracellular CoQ10 level may at least partially explain statin-induced muscle injury. However, studies have come to different conclusions about whether statin treatment decreases CoQ10 levels in skeletal muscle [83- 86].

Another proposed mechanism involves β oxidation. A study showed that statin-intolerant patients demonstrate increased β oxidation in response to lovastatin, implicating an intrinsic β oxidation abnormality [87]. Indeed, statins increase the expression of mitochondrial carnitine acylcarnitine transferase, which may contribute to the alteration in β oxidation [88].

Finally, atrogin-1, a muscle-specific ubiquitin protein ligase, may also play an important role in statin toxicity as it has been shown that lovastatin induces its expression in humans with statin myopathy. Myopathy can be prevented by knockdown of this protein [89].

There are no standard definitions or terminology for statin-associated muscle symptoms, which is an issue that complicates attempts to establish the incidence of the condition. An expert panel proposed these following definitions: a "mild" serum creatinine kinase (CK) increase as CK above the upper limit of normal (ULN) but less than 10 times; a "moderate" CK increase as CK 10 times above the upper limit of normal but less than 50 times and a "marked" CK increase as CK above 50 times the upper limit of normal (Table 3) [90]. Despite these clear definitions, uncertainty remains about the relationship between clinical symptoms and levels of biochemical markers of muscle toxicity such as CK. Most myopathy reported by statin users takes the form of myalgia: muscle ache, tenderness, or weakness without elevated CK. Despite the inclusion of CK levels in most diagnostic criteria for myopathy, there is some evidence that clinically significant muscle toxicity can occur without an increase in CK levels [91].

Table 3. Statin induced-myopathy proposed definitions

	Serum Creatinine Kinase level
Mild CK increase	Less than 10 times the upper limit of normal
Moderate CK increase	Between 10 and 50 times the upper limit of normal
Marked CK increase	Over 50 times the upper limit of normal

The onset of muscle symptoms is usually within 6 months of starting therapy [92]. Statin-induced myalgia typically presents as a proximal, symmetric muscle weakness and soreness. Patients often describe their symptoms as fatigue or tiredness. Some of them may complain about cramping (including nocturnal cramping) and tendon pain [93].

As previously mentioned, an elevation in serum CK is not always present and there are many other causes of muscle pain and weakness. Moreover, large clinical trials showed no difference in myalgia between statin-treated groups and placebo-controls groups, ranging from 2 to 11 percent [94 - 96]. The diagnosis of statin-induced myalgia must then be careful, and based on a precise patient history and trials of cessation and reintroduction of the drug. After discontinuation of the drug, myalgia and muscle weakness usually resolve within 2 months on average, with a maximum of 6 months [92].

Muscle toxicity is primarily induced by high doses regimen. With simvastatin for instance, the incidence of muscle injury varies from 0.02 percent at 20 mg/day to 0.3 percent at 80 mg/day [97]. Besides, the risk to induce muscle injury seems to vary among the different statins. Indeed, the more hydrophilic statins may have less muscle penetration than lipophilic statins. Moreover, some statins are less likely to be involved with drug interactions since they are not extensively metabolized by CYP4503A4. Regarding this issue, pravastatin and fluvastatin appear to be the safest [98, 99].

Another important factor, which is related to patient characteristics, includes genetics, which plays a major role in muscle sensibility. For example, variants of the SLCO1B1 gene, which encodes a transporter that mediates the hepatic uptake of statins, increase or decrease the risk of muscle injury in patients treated with statins (see Pharmacogenomics above).

Other characteristics predisposing patients to muscle injury include preexisting neuromuscular disorders [100, 101], hypothyroidism, acute or chronic renal failure, and obstructive liver disease.

Finally, concurrent drug therapy may increase the susceptibility to muscle toxicity, particularly drugs that inhibit the CYPP4503A [102] and fibrates [103]. Moreover, some drugs are independently related to the risk of statin-induced myopathy: glucocorticoids, cyclosporine [104, 105].

Patients experiencing muscle toxicity or showing serum CK 10 times above the upper limit should discontinue statin therapy. Once the symptoms have resolved and the CK returns to baseline levels, statin therapy could be switched to pravastatin or fluvastatin with careful monitoring [106]. If it is not tolerated either, an alternate-day dosing might be established. Finally, although there is limited evidence for benefits, supplementation of CoQ10 at a dose of 150 to 200 mg daily could be given [107].

New-Onset Type 2 Diabetes Mellitus

Another statin-related effect is the increased incidence of new-onset insulin resistance and type 2 diabetes mellitus (T2DM).

The JUPITER [108] trial was the first one to report a link between statin use and diabetes. Conducted in nearly 18,000 patients over a two-years period, it showed an overall increase of 27% in T2DM in patients treated with 20 mg/day rosuvastatin compared to a placebo, as well as an increase in the median hemoglobin A1c levels.

A further evaluation of this issue has been carried out with trials and meta-analyses. From these data, it appears that statin-induced T2DM is a medication class effect, not related to potency or to an individual statin and independent of the previous history of CVD [109].

However, a recent meta-analysis [110] including 17 randomized controlled trials with a total of 113,394 patients showed that different types and doses of statins seem to have different potentials to induce T2DM. This meta-analysis compares either statin versus placebo, or high-dose versus low-dose statin therapy. When high-dose statin treatment was compared to a placebo, the risk for T2DM was greater with 20 mg/day rosuvastatin(+25%) than with 40 mg/day simvastatin (+21%), 80 mg/day atorvastatin (+15%) and 40 mg/day pravastatin (+7%). With lower statin doses versus placebo, the higher risk was with 10 mg/day rosuvastatin (+11%) followed by 10 mg/day atorvastatin (+ 4%) whereas pravastatin even resulted protective (-10%). Compared to high dose, a low-dose treatment was associated with only modest benefit in the induction of T2DM: +1% for 80 vs. 10 mg atorvastatin, +7%

for 20 vs. 10 mg pravastatin, +12 % 20 vs. 10 mg rosuvastatin. These findings illustrate a new situation that emphasizes a personalized therapeutic strategy.

Although the defined process by which statins might induce T2DM remains unknown, some mechanisms have been put forward. Statins may reduce insulin secretion both directly and indirectly. First, they may directly inhibit the ATP-dependent potassium channels and thus the depolarization of the cell and the calcium influx, which leads to insulin secretion. Secondly, they may indirectly inhibit the ATP-dependent potassium channels by reducing the ATP formation thanks to an inhibition of ubiquinone synthesis. Moreover, the increased intracellular import of LDL-C by activation of the LDL receptor may facilitate the oxidation process leading to an alteration of the B cells. Oxidation products may in turn lead to the overproduction of nitric oxide by cytokines, potentially inducing B cell apoptosis and impaired insulin secretion. At last, the inhibition of isoprenoids by reduced HMGCR activity may cause a down-regulation of glucose transporter type 4 (GLUT4) expression on adipocytes, leading to impaired glucose uptake [111].

Regarding this potential effect, it is important to assess the individual risk for each patient to develop a T2DM before the initiation of the treatment. The use of a score for stratifying the risk to develop a T2DM in the course of statin treatment is an important issue. Based on the results of three important trials (TNT, IDEAL and SPARCL) [112 - 114], four main predictors have been proposed: fasting plasma glucose > 100mg/dl, triglycerides >150mg/dl, body mass index > 30 kg/m2 and arterial hypertension [115]. These four predictors produce a score ranging from 0 to 4, which predicts the risk of developing T2DM during statin treatment. Indeed, the hazard ratio for new-onset T2DM increased in parallel with the score in all of the three previously mentioned studies, independently of the comparator chosen in each trial [116]. Additional features associated with greater risk of new-onset T2DM are familial history, female gender, older age, Asian ethnicity, and duration of statin treatment. Interestingly, a study showed an association between the concomitant use of diuretics and statins and an increased risk of new-onset T2DM. No effect of beta-blockers or calcium-channel blockers was observed [117] (Table 4).

Table 4. Statin related risk of type 2 diabetes mellitus

Main features: score calculation (0-4)
Fasting plasma glucose > 100 mg/dl Plasma triglycerides > 150 mg/dl Body mass index > 30 kg/m^2 Arterial hypertension
Additional features
Familial history of type 2 diabetes mellitus Female gender Older age Asian ethnicity Duration of statin treatment Concomitant medications: diuretics,...

According to most authors, it should be emphasized that the benefits of CVD reduction by statin therapy appears to far exceed the risk of new-onset T2DM development. However, the increased risk of incident T2DM in at least a subset of patients upon statin treatment suggests the opportunity to consider different therapeutical options that may reduce the risk of T2DM, and the importance of monitoring glycemic control.

Firstly, patients should be encouraged to follow an appropriate diet with a reduction of approximately 400 kcal/day and to practice exercise. In particular, reducing carbohydrates from 46 to 11% of total calories has been shown to reduce serum triglyceride and insulin levels in statins users. It may also favorably affect markers of inflammation and altered vascular endothelial function [118].

Secondly, physicians can reduce the drug load with an alternate-day statin use or the addition of other lipid-lowering drugs such as ezetimibe [119] or colesevelam [120].

In any case, clinical assessment for new-onset T2DM needs to be conducted periodically in patients treated with statins, especially when the previously mentioned features are present: HbA1C, FPG and oral glucose tolerance test are the three diagnostic criteria that need to be checked [121].

Administration and Association

Since the majority of cholesterol synthesis occurs at night, statins should be taken in the evening. This has been confirmed by trials, which have shown greater decrease in cholesterol levels if simvastatin was administered in the evening rather than in the morning [122, 123].

Alternative Dosing Regimens

Alternative dosing regimens have been suggested to decrease the cost and to improve patient's tolerability. Results from clinical studies suggest that to reach a similar lowering in LDL-C, the every other day dose needs to be twice of the daily dose [124 -126]. Moreover, all of the major outcomes trials have used daily statin therapy so we can't assess whether the pleiotropic effects of statins remain with this kind of regimen. The only benefit of an alternate day dosing regimen is a possible improvement in patients experiencing myalgias.

High Dosing Regimens

High dosing regimens should be avoided as they increase the susceptibility of developing statin-induced myopathy. In particular, according to a FDA announcement, high-dose simvastatin (80 mg) should be limited because of increased risk of muscle damage [127]. In patients who have already been taking this dose, an alternative statin therapy should be considered since future medication therapy or illness could increase the risk for muscle injury.

Association with Other Lipid-Modifying Drugs

Regarding limitation toward the use of high dosing regimens, the use of lipid lowering agents, other than statins, might be useful. Fibrates, bile acid sequestrants, nicotinic acid, and ezetimibe differ with respect to their mechanism of action and to the degree and type of lipid lowering. The underlying lipid abnormality will guide the prescriber's choice toward one of these molecules.

Fibrates decrease serum triglycerides by 35 to 50 percent while increase serum high-density lipoprotein cholesterol (HDL-C) by 5 to 20 percent [128-130]. Despite their favorable effects on lipids, fibrates showed little to no effects on cardiovascular outcomes in the general population [131, 132]. However, a benefit can be seen in the particular subsets of patients with triglycerides level above 200 mg/dl [133, 134], or HDL-C level below 40mg/dl combined with a borderline elevated triglycerides level [130]. If combined with a statin, attention should be paid to myopathy since some fibrates have been associated with muscle injury [135, 136]. This effect may be due to a competitive inhibition of the cytochrome P450 3A4, leading to a decrease in statin metabolism.

Bile Acid Sequestrants

Bile acid sequestrants interrupt the reabsorption of bile acids in the intestine leading to a reduction in the cholesterol pool. This reduction decreases the intrahepatic cholesterol level and promotes the synthesis of LDL-receptors, which bind LDL from the plasma, causing a further decrease in blood cholesterol. In addition, bile acid sequestrants raise HDL-C level via intestinal formation of nascent HDL [137]. Low-doses reduce LDL-C by 10 to 15 percent whereas high-doses can achieve a reduction of 24 percent. When used in combination, statins and bile acid sequestrants have a synergetic action. They can lower LDL-C down to 50 percent and raise HDL-C up to 18 percent [138 - 140]. The use of acid bile sequestrants is often limited by side effects, especially gastrointestinal. Furthermore, they can inhibit the absorption of other drugs such as digoxin and warfarin.

Nicotinic Acid

Nicotinic acid, or niacin, lowers LDL-C level and raises HDL-C levels by as much as 30 to 35 percent [141]. The HDL-C raising properties occur with low doses whereas high doses are necessary to lower LDL-C. Although some benefits can be drawn from the use of niacin [142], two large randomized trials have raised serious concerns about its safety. The first one was stopped because of an increased number of ischemic strokes in patients treated with niacin [143], whereas the second one showed an increase in serious adverse events such as myopathy, gastrointestinal side effects, rash, poor glucose control, serious infection or bleeding [144]. Given these results, niacin should be restricted to patients with very high cardiovascular risk, such as homozygous or heterozygous familial hypercholestrolemia patients. Moreover, the use of niacin is limited by its intense adverse effects such as flushing, which occurs in 80 percent of patients and pruritus, paresthesias, and nausea, each of which occurs in 20 percent of patients [145].

Ezetimibe

Ezetimibe is an intestinal cholesterol absorption inhibitor, which unlike bile acid sequestrants, does not affect the absorption of triglycerides or soluble vitamins [146]. In monotherapy, eztimibe lowers LDL-C by about 17 percent. As for bile acid sequestrants, the association of ezetimibe and statins has a synergetic action since they lower LDL-C by 14 percent more than the LDL lowering effect of simvastatin alone [147]. A similar decrease in LDL-C can be achieved simply by maximizing the doseage of statins, which given their pleiotropic effects, may have a number of benefits in addition to lipid lowering. However, ezetimibe may be used to avoid high doses of statins and the associated risk of muscle injury in patients who do not meet the cholesterol level goals with moderate doses of statin.

If combination therapy regimens have shown benefit in lowering LDL-C, they fail to demonstrate a reduction in cardiovascular clinical outcomes. The ACCORD trial compared statin alone vs. statin with fenofibrate and found no difference in myocardial infarction, stroke, and cardiovascular death between groups [148]. The AIM-HIGH study compared statin vs. statin with niacin and found no difference in coronary heart disease death, myocardial infarction, stroke, acute coronary syndrome, and symptom-driven revascularization [149]. The IMPROVE-IT trial will compare statin vs. statin with ezetimibe on cardiovascular death, myocardial infarction, stroke, unstable angina, and coronary revascularization [150]. It has enrolled 18,144 patients and the results are expected for September 2014.

2. Medical Uses and Clinical Outcomes

Dyslipidemic Disorders

At the end of 2013, the American College of Cardiology along with the American Heart Association published new guidelines on the control of blood cholesterol to reduce atherosclerotic cardiovascular disease (ACVD) [151]. These new guidelines deserve to be discussed and compared to the 2011 guidelines of the European Society of Cardiology (ESC) and the European Atherosclerosis Society (EAS) [150, 153].

Both the 2013 ACC/AHA and the 2011 ESC/EAS guidelines have systematically evaluated scientific evidence. However, if the European guidelines have considered all of the available evidence as well as the importance of all lipid profiles, the American guidelines have considered only randomized trial evidence. Indeed, the ESC/EAS guidelines have a larger scope, encompassing all available data, to cover the management of all dyslipidemias and the use of all currently available medication for the prevention of CVD. On the contrary, the ACC/AHA focuses explicitly on statins only, because they are the most widely tested lipid-reducing drugs and the have the greatest evidence base for benefit in the prevention of CVD. Hence, the ACC/AHA guidelines may appear restricted because they ignore a large area of the scientific knowledge about CVD prevention. This may raise concerns, especially for those who cannot tolerate recommended dose of statins for different reasons. However, both guidelines conclude that a high LDL-C level is the major cause for ACVD and that a change in the patient lifestyle should strongly be recommended in addition of lipid-lowering therapy.

Both guidelines define four groups who would benefit from a lipid reducing therapy: patients with defined CVD, diabetes mellitus, familial hypercholerolemia, and those with an increased CVD risk based on individual assessment. However, even in the definition of these groups, differences lie between the American and European guidelines. The 2011 ESC/EAS guidelines include pre-clinical evidence of CVD on the basis of imaging. More importantly, the ESC/EAS guidelines include patients with chronic kidney disease as being at very high-risk of CVD development, whereas the ACC/AHA guidelines do not include this particular subset of patients in any category. But the feature that will have the largest impact on statin drug prescription in the US is the inclusion, according to the ACC/AHA guidelines, of individuals with a 10-year CVD risk of 7.5% or higher requiring moderate to high-intensity statin therapy whereas this group of patients requires only lifestyle change according to the ESC/EAS guidelines. On the one hand, this inclusion will increase the number of patients treated with statins and thus, more patients complaining about side effects as well as greater public health expenditure. Moreover, practically all patients over 70 years of age will now be administered moderate to high intensity therapy. Yet, as comorbidities and tolerability of these agents along with poly-pharmacy becomes more of an issue in this age group, the potential for harm is much greater. On the other hand, this lowering of the threshold for statin initiation could benefit the younger patient with a high-lifetime risk who will be initiated with statins earlier and is therefore likely to have a greater impact on the disease process.

Surprisingly, the ACC/AHA recommendations do not use LDL-C level as a treatment target. They recommend a specific dosage of statins for each group rather than a specific LDL-C level attainment. According to these guidelines, LDL-C measurement remains only to assess patient adherence to lifestyle modifications and therapy. The LDL-C target has been abandoned because of the lack of RCT evidence. Indeed, it can be argued that treatment targets are arbitrary and often based on extrapolation from available data, but they are usually based on an evaluation of larger knowledge as done in the ESC/EAS guidelines. Moreover, goal targeted therapy gives to non-specialists a broad outline of an absolute risk and gives information about which patients should receive optimized treatment. In this regard, the ESC/EAS guidelines offer clear goals and allow more flexibility in the choice of the treatment.

Non-Dyslipidemic Disorders

In addition to cholesterol lowering, statins present the so-called "pleiotropic" effects including anti-inflammatory and immunomodulatory actions. For these reasons, meta-analyses and clinical trials, retrospective for the most part, have been conducted to investigate the clinical efficacy of statin therapy on disorders not directly linked to hypercholesterolemia.

Rheumatoid Arthritis

Rheumatoid arthritis (RA) is a chronic inflammatory disease characterized by painful swelling and stiffness of the joints, eventually resulting in bone erosion and join deformity. RA is one of the most important disabling diseases, affecting more than 2 million adults in the US and medications to control it are still needed. Since statins present anti-inflammatory and immunomodulatory effects, a number of studies have been looking at their potential benefit in the treatment of this disease.

The first evidence came from a preliminary study, which showed that the administration of atorvastatin 20 mg/day for eight patients reduced CRP levels and produced clinical improvement in five patients [154]. These results were confirmed by a randomized double blind placebo-controlled trial also studying the clinical effect of atorvastatin, which showed a significant improvement of the 28-joint Disease Activity Score (DAS28) [155]. Another study, using simvastatin, showed some effects on clinical and biological parameters of disease activity but without statistical significance [154]. It may be due to a lower anti-inflammatory effect of simvastatin compared to atorvastatin. Finally, a prospective cohort study of 7,512 patients also reported beneficial effects of statins in reducing RA activity [157]. These encouraging results must be balanced with a large epidemiological study demonstrating the absence of any benefit of statins in reducing inflammation in RA patients [158]. Nevertheless, the latter study investigated a link between statin therapy and RA improvement by using oral corticoids exposure as a proxy marker of disease activity. So, we might conclude that if statins may have a beneficial effect in controlling RA inflammation and decreasing clinical manifestation, this effect is smaller than the effect of disease modifying drugs usually used to manage this disease.

However, since RA by itself represents an independent risk factor for early atherosclerosis and development of cardiovascular disease, most of the patients should already be administered statins. Even if statins prove to be only mildly effective in reducing inflammation and/or autoimmunity in RA, their potential for reducing the inflammatory and lipid mediated processes of accelerated atherosclerosis suggests that statins may at least prove to be useful for preventing CVD in RA patients [159]. But their use must stay cautious as recent results from the DREAM registry suggest that statins may interfere with the anti-rheumatic properties of Rituximab, raising concerns about their concomitant use in patients with RA [160].

Venous Thromboembolism

Although the complete patho-physiological mechanisms of venous thromboembolism (VTE) remains unclear, the increase in blood coagulability has always been considered the main cause of VTE. Further studies also indicated that endothelial dysfunction and vascular inflammation could play a role in the formation of a thrombus [161]. If several drugs are already available for the prevention and the treatment of venous thromboembolism, these drugs also induce bleeding and very serious side effects. For these reasons, an alternative therapy is still needed.

As previously described, statins decrease tissue factor expression, the major initiator of blood clotting in vivo, and suppress inflammation. These conditions result in a reduced thrombin generation.

In a model of microvascular injury in patients with coronary artery disease, simvastatin and atorvastatin have been shown to reduce thrombin generation [162, 163]. Two meta-analyses of observational studies reported that statins decrease the risk of VTE by almost 20% [164, 165]. The JUPITER trial provided the first randomized evidence that rosuvastatin 20mg/day reduces the risk of VTE. No significant protection was seen for pulmonary embolism [166]. Subset analyses of these studies suggested that rosuvastatin does not reduce the incidence of VTE in patients over 70 years old [167]. This was confirmed by the PROSPER study ((Prospective Study of Pravastatin in the Elderly at Risk) study where statins did not prevent VTE in a selected population of elderly people at risk of vascular disease [168].

More recently, a pooled analysis of 29 randomized studies showed that VTE occurred with a similar incidence in statin users and non-users, which seems to contradict the results from the JUPITER trial [169]. Nevertheless, the JUPITER trial was the only one to investigate rosuvastatin and this difference might induce the belief that rosuvastatin is different from the other statins regarding the prevention of VTE. This conclusion is supported by an analysis suggesting a difference between rosuvastatin and the other statins with an odds ratio for rosuvastatin of 0.69 (95% CI 0.39–0.92) for all trials of statins versus no statins [169]. The reasons why rosuvastatin seems to be the only statin to have a positive effective on VTE remains to be elucidated.

Polycystic Ovary Syndrome

Polycystic ovary syndrome (POCS) is a heterogeneous disorder characterized by chronic ovulatory dysfunction and hyperandrogenism with a reported prevalence of 5–7% in women of reproductive age [170, 171]. Despite high incidence, the etiology of POCS remains unknown. However, one of the most common features of PCOS is elevated androgen levels, which is considered to be the central problem. Because cholesterol is a substrate for ovarian steroidogenesis, decreased availability of cholesterol by statin treatment may result in lower androgen production. Indeed, it is well established that statins may reduce total testosterone levels by about 10–15% [172].

There is growing evidence that statin therapy may have beneficial effects in patients with POCS. Indeed, a recent meta-analysis of 4 randomized controlled trials reported a significant effect of statins on reducing total testosterone levels, even in the absence of metformine [173]. Two trials showed that atorvastatin significantly reduce hyperandrogenemia [174, 175]. A decrease in total testosterone was also observed in two other trials using simvastatin [176, 177]. More recently, the final result of one of these trials demonstrated that the beneficial effects of simvastatin on POCS are long-lasting and that overall, simvastatin is superior to metformin as it improves menstrual regularity, reduces ovarian volume and improves biochemical and clinical features of hyperandrogenism [178]. Interestingly, a direct comparison of atorvastatin and simvastatin in POCS patients showed that both drugs reduce testosterone level with the same efficacy [179].

However, the use of statins in women at risk of conceiving is limited because of their potential teratogenicity.

Sepsis

Sepsis is a syndrome precipitated by an infection and characterized by systemic inflammation and dysregulation of the coagulation cascade [180]. Despite advances in antimicrobial therapy and medical management of patients with severe infections, sepsis remains a major source of morbidity and mortality in ICUs [181-183]. Statins possess a number of pleiotropic effects that are thought to have a beneficial effect on the cascade of detrimental events that characterize the sepsis syndrome.

Experimental Studies

Two studies on animal models evaluated the mortality effect of statins given twice before the induction of sepsis. They both show a significantly improvement in survival.

Ando et al. [184] showed that cerivastatine pre-treatment at 12 and 1 hour before lipopolysaccharide (LPS)-induced sepsis improved the rate of 7-day survival from 26.7% in the non-pretreated group to 73.3% in the cerivastatin pretreated group ($P=0.016$).

Merx et al. [185] evaluated the effects of statins given at 18 and 3 hours before polymicrobial sepsis using a cecal ligation and puncture (CLP) model and found that median survival time extended to 108 hours from 28 hours in untreated mice ($P < 0.005$). This improvement in the survival rate of simvastatin treated mice is associated with a complete preservation of cardiac function at 20 hours of (CLP) and a preserved responsiveness to dobutamine, whereas cardiac function and dobutamine stimulation were severely impaired in untreated CLP mice [200].

A study of rats receiving simvastatin 20 minutes before LPS-induced sepsis [186], confirm the property of statins to recover vascular responsiveness during an experimental endotoxic shock. In this study, pretreatment with simvastatin did not significantly change the hypotension induced by LPS but reverted the impaired pressor response to phenylephrine when compared with rats treated with saline followed by LPS (40.3 ±1.7 mmHg vs. 31.4 ± 2.6 mmHg; $P < 0.05$).

Only one animal [187] study evaluated the effect of various statins after the onset of sepsis. In this study, statin treatment was initiated at 6 hours after CLP-induced sepsis, when profound hemodynamic alterations were manifest. Compared with 23±1.2 hours of mean survival time in CLP placebo-treated mice, survival was extended by 70% to 39±3.9 hours with atorvastatin, by 74% to 40±4.2 hours with pravastatin, and by 61% to 37±3.6 hours with simvastatin treatment ($P<0.05$ versus placebo). As for Merck's previous study of simvastatin pretreatment in sepsis [200], hemodynamic and cardiac function were preserved in the statin treated group. Cardiac output measured at 20 hours after sepsis induction remained stable in CLP mice treated with atorvastatin, pravastatin, or simvastatin after sepsis induction (P = NS vs. preoperative) whereas it decreased significantly in CLP placebo-treated mice ($P< 0.005$ vs. preoperative). Here again, responsiveness to catecholamine was restored in CLP mice by treatment with atorvastatin, pravastatin, or simvastatin. Dobutamine stimulation increased CO in all groups ($P<0.001$ vs. no stimulation for simvastatin, pravastatin, and atorvastatin) except in CLP placebo-treated mice. Surprisingly, no beneficial effects were observed with fluvastatin, which showed no significant survival time increase ($P= 0.759$ vs. placebo), a decrease in cardiac output at 20 hours ($P < 0.01$ vs. preoperatively), and a dampened response to dobutamine ($P < 0.05$ vs. no stimulation).

Cohort Studies

A recent meta-analysis reviewed the effect of statins on mortality in patients with infection and/or sepsis [188]. The analysis included 20 studies, 18 being cohort studies (12 retrospective and 6 prospective), 1 matched cohort study and 1 randomized control trial. Of those 20 studies, 15 [189-203] showed a mortality decrease in patients taking statins, with adjusted ORs ranging from 0,06 to 0,75. Four studies [204 - 207] showed a trend toward a benefit from statins although not reaching statistical significance. One study [208] reported an increased mortality in patients taking statins.

The primary meta-analysis regarding mortality from any cause demonstrated a significant protective effect from statins in patients with infection and/or sepsis compared to a placebo (OR, 0.49 [95% CI, 0.37- 0.61]) [74]

To further explore the effects of statins on outcomes in infection and sepsis, the studies were grouped based on the outcome definition as well as the type of infection. All 6 subgroup analyses demonstrated a significant protective benefit from statins, with pooled odds ratios all in favor of statin use: 0.61 (95% CI, 0.48- 0.73) for 30-day mortality (n= 7), 0.38 (95% CI, 0.13- 0.64) for in-hospital mortality (n= 7), 0.63 (95% CI, 0.55-0.71) for pneumonia-related mortality (n=7), 0.33 (95% CI, 0.09-0.75) for bacteremia-related mortality (n=4), 0.40 (95% CI, 0.23-0.57) for sepsis-related mortality (n= 4) and 0.50 (95% CI, 0.18-0.83) for mixed infection-related mortality (n= 4).[30]

Only one study [198] showed a statistically significant mortality increase among septic patients that were taking statins, but the statin population was older (71.7 ± 8.3 years vs. 61.5

±18.3; p= 0.001) and had more chronic illness, as defined by the APACHE II score (42% vs. 26%; p= 0.04). Statin therapy was thus associated with a worse outcome, probably because underlying clinical conditions were insufficiently considered in mortality predictors. The same results occurred for the 4 studies [194 - 197], which showed no mortality benefit of statins. It may be that the benefits of statins are hidden by these strong risk factors.

Despite the limitations regarding the heterogeneity of studies, studies design, and exposure definition, results regarding the protective effect of statins are encouraging. However, these observational studies are all about statins' use on consecutive days prior to infection and, what will be more interesting is the effect of statins given right before the sepsis triggering a use in at-risk populations, or even after the onset of sepsis for a use as an adjuvant treatment.

Placebo Controlled Randomized Trial

Basic sciences, cohort studies, and animal studies show that there might be a rationale for the clinical use of statins in sepsis. However, until now, only one double-blind placebo controlled randomized trial [209] has tried to determine if statin therapy reduces the incidence of severe sepsis in patients with acute bacterial infection. Unfortunately, because of a very slow recruitment rate, mainly due to refusal, the study was stopped prematurely after 10 months and enrolled only 83 subjects comparing to the 1,080 planned in an estimated 24 months.

Nonetheless, several clinical trials are now underway examining the potential clinical benefit of statins in sepsis.

Simvastatin and severe sepsis trial (SIMSEPT) will be the first double-blind, randomized, placebo-controlled trial of simvastatin (40mg) in the treatment of severe sepsis in humans. It will investigate the effect of simvastatin on important inflammatory markers and monitor the safety and feasibility of administering simvastatin to patients with severe sepsis [210]. The STATInS trial is a phase II, randomized, placebo-controlled study of the safety, pharmacokinetics, and effect on inflammatory marker levels of atorvastatin in intensive care patients with severe sepsis [211]. Two other phase II trials are evaluating simvastatin in adults hospitalized with sepsis with the primary outcome being time to clinical stability in one trial [212] and time to shock reversal in the other [213].

Acute Lung Injury

Acute lung injury (ALI) and acute respiratory distress syndrome are heterogeneous diseases with a complex physiopathology that may occur in response to a direct pulmonary or indirect systemic injury [214]. As sepsis, ALI/ARDS is mediated by an intense inflammatory response. Although the pathogenesis of ALI/ARDS remains poorly understood, evidence suggests that alveolar macrophages and neutrophil-mediated injury is central. These inflammatory cells release cytokines, proteases, particularly matrix metalloproteases (MMPs), and reactive oxygen species [204] causing alveolar epithelial and capillary endothelial barrier damages with exudation of fluid into the alveolar space. Limiting lung distension by small tidal volume is the only clinically proved maneuver that decreases mortality in patients with ARDS [215]. However, it is becoming increasingly apparent that even the best ventilation strategy further damages the injured lung [216]. There is, therefore, a major need to develop a pharmacological agent to improve clinical outcome in ALI/ARDS [217].

Experimental Studies

Animal studies have demonstrated that statins attenuate lung injury in models such as ischemia-reperfusion [218], peritonitis [219], and aerosolized LPS [220, 221]. Most observational [222 - 224] studies show a benefit of prior statin use in patients with pneumonia, suggesting a potential modulation in pulmonary inflammation.

This has been confirmed by a double-blind, placebo-controlled study [225] in which thirty healthy volunteers were randomized to receive simvastatin or a placebo for 4 days before LPS inhalation. Compared to the placebo, the simvastatin pre-treated group presented a reduction in neutrophil numbers ($3x10^5$ /ml [1.8-8.1] vs. 8.5×10^5 /ml [4.4-16.2]. P = 0,05 vs. placebo) and activity in the alveolar space, partially due to an increase in neutrophil apoptosis (10.3% vs. 5%; p= 0,05 vs. placebo). This increase in alveolar neutrophil apoptosis may be related to the reduced pulmonary (P= 0.01) and systemic (P= 0.03) CRP concentrations after LPS inhalation, compared to the placebo. Interestingly, the simvastatin pre-treated group also demonstrated a reduction in broncholoalveolar lavage fluid (BALF) MMP's, particularly MMP-7 (P= 0.03 vs. placebo), which is required for neutrophil influx to the lung in animal models of ALI [226]. The tumor necrosis factor α (TNF α) in BALF was also reduced by simvastatin pretreatment (P= 0.04).

Cohort Studies

Most observational [227 - 229] studies show a benefit of prior statin use in patients with pneumonia, suggesting a potential modulation in pulmonary inflammation, as did the Shyamsundar's study [225].

Two cohort studies of patients with ALI/ARDS, one being observational [230] and the other retrospective [231], showed a trend toward a reduced mortality in patients that were receiving statins previous to hospitalization, although not reaching significance.

Placebo Controlled Randomized Trials

Recently, Craig et al. [232] reported a randomized, double blinded, placebo-controlled trial in sixty patients with ALI. Patients were receiving 80 mg of simvastatin or a placebo until cessation of mechanical ventilation or up to 14 days. Although a pulmonary anti-inflammatory effect occurs early in the course of simvastatin treatment with a 2.5-fold reduction in IL-8 BALF (P= 0.05) and a 2.9-fold reduction in IL-6 BALF (P=NS) compared to the placebo, there was no difference in extravascular lung water at day 7 (13.7 [7.1] vs. 13.4 [8.0] for placebo; p= 0.90). Nonetheless, at day 14 the simvastatin treated group showed a reduction in oxygenation index (P=0.08) as well as a reduction in plateau pressure (P=0.09) and in the lung injury score (P=0.12), without reaching statistical significance compared to the placebo.

However, the SOFA score at day 14 was significantly reduced in the simvastatin-treated group compared with placebo (P= 0.01). Analysis of SOFA score organ components at day 14 revealed that simvastatin resulted in a significant improvement in the coagulation (P= 0.04), renal (P= 0.003), and cardiovascular (P= 0.0001) organ dysfunction. Statins effects on endothelial function can explain the improvements in systemic organ dysfunction to a greater degree than respiratory dysfunction, which is likely to be mediated by alveolar epithelial dysfunction as well [228].

Interestingly, this study also shows that, although anti-inflammatory effects can occur as early as day 3, more prolonged treatment may be required for these effects to be translated into improvements in organ dysfunction.

If this study has shown that simvastatin has an effect on systemic and, to a lesser degree, pulmonary outcomes in patients with ALI, it was not designed to detect a difference in duration of ventilation or mortality. The National Institutes of Health Acute Respiratory Distress Syndrome Network was recruiting patients with sepsis-induced ALI into the Statins for Acutely Injured Lungs study (SAILS) [233], which was designed for clinical outcomes measures with an estimated enrollment of 1,000 patients. However, the study was stopped because of futility after 745 patients had been enrolled. There was no significant difference between study groups in 60-day in-hospital mortality (28.5% with rosuvastatin and 24.9% with placebo, P=0.21) or in mean (±SD) ventilator-free days (15.1±10.8 with rosuvastatin and 15.1±11.0 with placebo, P=0.96).

Aneurismal Subarachnoid Hemorrhage

Vasospasm and related delayed ischemic neurologic deficits (DINDs) remain a major cause of morbidity and mortality after an aneurysmal subarachnoid hemorrhage (aSAH). Current non-surgical treatment options are limited to triple-H therapy [234] (hypertensive, hypervolemic, hemodilution) and the calcium-channel blocker nimodipine [235], but their effects remain modest.

The interest of statins in aSAH reside in their ability to raise endothelial nitric oxide synthase expression, decrease oxidative stress, diminish inflammation, prevent platelet activation, and promote angiogenesis. These effects increase the diameter of spastic vessels, improve endothelial function, and protect against ischemia [236]

Placebo Controlled Randomized Trials

In 2008, a meta-analysis from Sillberg et al. [237] concluded that in patients with aSAH, statins reduced the incidence of vasospasm, DID, and mortality. However, this meta-analysis was criticized for its methodology and interpretation of results [238, 239]. A stronger meta-analysis was thus needed.

Recently, a meta-analysis of four randomized [240 - 244], double-blinded placebo-controlled trials investigating the effects of acute statin treatment on vasospasm, DINDs, and their outcome was performed including 190 statin-naïve patients with aSAH [245].

For the analysis of the occurrence of transcranial Doppler (TCD) vasospasm, data from 3 of the four studies were available [232, 234, 235]. The overall number of patients who had TCD vasospasm was 42 in the statin group and 46 in the placebo group (pooled RR, 0.99 [95% CI, 0.66 to 1.48]).

In the four studies, the total number of patients who developed DIND was 20 in the statin group and 39 in the placebo group, but this difference was not statistically significant (pooled RR, 0.57 [95% CI, 0.29 to 1.13]). However, a subgroup analysis for the type of statins showed that patients randomized to pravastatin (n= 40) had a significant lower risk of DCI (RR, 0.17 [95% CI, 0.04 to 0.70]) compared to a placebo.

As for TCD vasospasm and DID, definitions used for poor outcome were different in each of the studies. In 2 studies, the functional outcome was assessed with the modified Ranking Scale (mRS) [232, 234]. The Glasgow Outcome Scale scores of the latter study

[235] were transformed to a Rankin grading. Furthermore, the timing of measuring differed between groups either at discharge or at 6 months. The overall number of patients with poor outcome was 38 in the statin group and 42 in the placebo group (pooled RR, 0.92 [95% CI, 0.68 to 1.24]).

The results of this meta-analysis do not lend statistically significant support to a beneficial effect of statins in patients with aSAH.

This seems to be a contradiction with another concomittant meta-analysis [246] of six randomized control trials (RCTs), which concluded that in RCTs, statins were found to significantly reduce the occurrence of DINDs [OR 0.38 (0.23-0.65); P < 0.001]. But in comparison with Vergouwen's meta-analysis [236], this analysis included two more RCTs [247, 248] of lower quality, correspondence with the authors having revealed that they had "pseudo-randomized" designs, without being blind or placebo controlled [237]; With removal of these two non-peer-reviewed studies, heterogeneity in results regarding DINDs were more pronounced ($I^2 = 47\%$) compared to all the six RCTs combined ($I^2 = 20\%$), and if the results did not change when using a fixed-effects model, it was dampened and no longer statistically significant when a random effects model was applied [OR 0.40 (0.15-1.05), *P*= 0.06].

Cohort Studies

If RCTs are clearly the preferred study design to assess treatment efficacy, the small numbers of patients in these RCTs may unbalance the baseline characteristics and thus, influence the results. The addition of observational studies can greatly increase the sample size, thereby reducing the chance of type II errors.

In the same paper [93], Kramer analyzes six observational studies (five cohort [249 - 253], and one case-control [254]) including 1,542 patients of whom 385 received statins. Statin-use was not associated with any reduction in DINDs [OR 0.96 (0.71- 1.31); *P*= 0.80], mortality [OR 1.16 (0.78- 1.73); *P*= 0.47], or poor neurological recovery [OR 1.20 (0.84 - 1.72); *P*= 0.31].

When the results of these six observational studies were combined with those of the 6 RCTs, statins had no statistically significant effect.

Interpreting results about possible beneficial effects of immediate statin therapy in statin-naïve patients following a SAH is limited by small sample sizes and low to moderate quality of available RCTs, and very low quality for observational studies. Some of the inconsistencies of results may reflect substantial differences among study design.

Four registered clinical trials are currently assessing the efficacy of statins aSAH.

The Simvastatin in Aneurysmal Subarachnoid Hemorrhage (STASH) trial [255] is a multi-center placebo-controlled double-blinded phase III trial assessing that a Simvastatin 40 mg treatment, given within 96 hours of the ictus over 3 weeks, will reduce the incidence and duration of delayed ischemic deficits following subarachnoid hemorrhage when compared to a placebo, leading to improvements in the short and long term clinical course for these patients.

The target enrollment was 1,600 patients, with projected completion in February 2013.

Another study investigates the effect of statin therapy on cerebral blood flow in patients with aSAH, using a positron emission tomography [256]. A third study is randomizing 240 patients with 40 or 80 mg of simvastatin or placebo, with presence of DIDs listed as a primary endpoint [257]. And finally, a double-blind placebo randomized control trial with an estimated enrollment of 80 patients was conducted in Sao Paulo with clinical outcome at 6 months being the primary endpoint [258]

CONCLUSION

After more than 25 years of use of statins, these drugs have provided a huge benefit in cardiovascular prevention. Despite this large experience and while the mechanism of cholesterol reduction is well established, a number of other properties of these drugs remains unclear, such as the importance of pharmacogenomics and the potential benefit of pleiotropic effects. Until now, there have been a number of candidate genes shown to affect statin efficacy and safety. For some of those, genetic testing is available and recommendations regarding the results have been made. Whether genetic screening will become routine remains to be seen. In the meantime, the benefits of pharmacogenomic studies on statins lies in the identification of new candidate genes involved in fine-tuning cholesterol homeostasis, making them possible new therapeutic targets. The risk of muscle toxicity and new-onset type 2 diabetes mellitus related to statin treatment is not negligible, especially for specific subsets of patients. Specific attention should be paid to muscle symptoms and creatinine kinase levels, and to metabolic syndrome features and glucose levels when evaluating a patient for statin therapy as well as after the initiation of the treatment. Importantly, the benefits of cardiovascular disease reduction by statin therapy far exceed the risk of developing serious adverse effects. Some combination therapy regimen, such as bile acid sequestrants and eztimibe, may confer benefits regarding reduced adverse effects and decreased LDL-C levels. These regimens, however, lack evidence in reducing clinical outcomes such as cardiovascular death, myocardial infarction, revascularization, or stroke.

Regarding the treatment of dyslipidemias, the new ACC/AHA American guidelines differ considerably from ESC/EAS European guidelines as they require a more careful assessment of patient risk and more importantly, they lower the primary prevention threshold, which will be beneficial to younger patients but may lead to an increase in the number of patients treated. The benefit of statins goes way beyond simple lipid lowering. Anti-inflammatory, immunomodulatory, and anti-thrombotic effects have been shown, pooled under the name of pleiotropic effects. Since statins do not target individual inflammatory mediators but possibly reduce the overall magnitude of the systemic response, they are an important feature in modulating the host response to inflammatory stress in chronic diseases such as rheumatoid arthritis, as well as in acute illnesses such as sepsis, acute lung injury, and subarachnoid hemorrhage. In addition, the pleiotropic effects of statins can also be related to the fact that, by inhibiting the cholesterol biosynthesis, they can have a significant impact on steroidogenesis and thus be effective in disorders such as polycystic ovary syndrome. In conclusion, the use of statins is in constant evolution regarding both how it is prescribed and why it is prescribed. Future developments will lead to patient-tailored prescriptions and to broader indications including non-dyslipidemic disorders.

REFERENCES

[1] Endo A, Kuroda M, Tanzawa K. Competitive inhibition of 3-hydroxy-3-methylglutaryl coenzyme A reductase by ML-236a and ML_236b fungal metabolites having hypocholesterolemic activity. *FEBS Lett* 1976; 72 :323-6.

[2] Sirtori CR. Pharmacology and mechanism of action of the new HMG-CoA reductase inhibitors. *Pharmacol Res* 1990;22:555-63

[3] Gemershausen JI, Hunt VM, Bostedor RG et al. Tissue selectivity of the cholesterol lowering agents lovastatin, simvastatin and pravastatin in rats in vivo. *Biochem Biophys Res Commun* 1989; 158: 667-75

[4] Sirtori CR. Tissue selectivity of hydroxymethylglutaryl coenzyme a (HMG-CoA) reductase inhibitors. *Pharmacol Ther* 1993; 60:431-59

[5] Bruckert E, Hayem G, Dejager S et al. Mild to moderate muscular symptoms with high-dosage statin therapy in hyperlipidemic patients - the PRIMO study. *Cardiovasc Drugs Ther* 2005; 19:403-14

[6] Sirtori CR, Mombelli G, Triolo M et al. Clinical response to statins: mechanism(s) of variable activity and adverse effects. *Ann Med* 2012;44:419-32

[7] Rosenson RS. Rosuvastatin: a new inhibitor of HMG-coA reductase for the treatment of dyslipidemia. *Expert Rev Cardiovasc Ther* 2003; 1:495.

[8] Jones PH, Davidson MH, Stein EA, et al. Comparison of the efficacy and safety of rosuvastatin versus atorvastatin, simvastatin, and pravastatin across doses (STELLAR* Trial). *Am J Cardiol* 2003; 92:152.

[9] Brown AS, Bakker-Arkema RG, Yellen L, et al. Treating patients with documented atherosclerosis to National Cholesterol Education Program-recommended low-density-lipoprotein cholesterol goals with atorvastatin, fluvastatin, lovastatin and simvastatin. *J Am Coll Cardiol* 1998; 32:665.

[10] Jones PH, Davidson MH, Stein EA, et al. Comparison of the efficacy and safety of rosuvastatin versus atorvastatin, simvastatin, and pravastatin across doses (STELLAR* Trial). *Am J Cardiol* 2003; 92:152.

[11] Kastelein JJ, Isaacsohn JL, Ose L, et al. Comparison of effects of simvastatin versus atorvastatin on high-density lipoprotein cholesterol and apolipoprotein A-I levels. *Am J Cardiol* 2000; 86:221.

[12] Davidson M, McKenney J, Stein E, et al. Comparison of one-year efficacy and safety of atorvastatin versus lovastatin in primary hypercholesterolemia. Atorvastatin Study Group I. *Am J Cardiol* 1997; 79:1475.

[13] Dart A, Jerums G, Nicholson G, et al. A multicenter, double-blind, one-year study comparing safety and efficacy of atorvastatin versus simvastatin in patients with hypercholesterolemia. *Am J Cardiol* 1997; 80:39.

[14] Bakker-Arkema RG, Davidson MH, Goldstein RJ, et al. Efficacy and safety of a new HMG-CoA reductase inhibitor, atorvastatin, in patients with hypertriglyceridemia. *JAMA* 1996; 275:128.

[15] Link E, Parish S, Armitage J, Bowman L, Heath S, Matsuda F, Gut I, Lathrop M, Collins R. SLCO1B1 variants and statin-induced myopathy--a genomewide study. *N Engl J Med.* 2008 Aug 21;359(8):789-99.

[16] Voora D, Shah SH, Spasojevic I, Ali S, Reed CR, Salisbury BA, Ginsburg GS. The SLCO1B1*5 genetic variant is associated with statin-induced side effects. *J Am Coll Cardiol.* 2009 Oct 20;54(17):1609-16.

[17] Brunham LR, Lansberg PJ, Zhang L, Miao F, Carter C, Hovingh GK, Visscher H, Jukema JW, Stalenhoef AF, Ross CJ, Carleton BC, Kastelein JJ, Hayden MR. Differential effect of the rs4149056 variant in SLCO1B1 on myopathy associated with simvastatin and atorvastatin. *Pharmacogenomics J.* 2012 Jun;12(3):233-7.

[18] Donnelly LA, Doney AS, Tavendale R, Lang CC, Pearson ER, Colhoun HM, McCarthy MI, Hattersley AT, Morris AD, Palmer CN. Common nonsynonymous substitutions in SLCO1B1 predispose to statin intolerance in routinely treated individuals with type 2 diabetes: a go-DARTS study. *Clin Pharmacol Ther.* 2011 Feb;89(2):210-6.

[19] Carr DF, O'Meara H, Jorgensen AL, Campbell J, Hobbs M, McCann G, van Staa T, Pirmohamed M. SLCO1B1 Genetic Variant Associated With Statin-Induced Myopathy: A Proof-of-Concept Study Using the Clinical Practice Research Datalink. *Clin Pharmacol Ther.* 2013 Aug 13.

[20] Wilke RA, Ramsey LB, Johnson SG, Maxwell WD, McLeod HL, Voora D, Krauss RM, Roden DM, Feng Q, Cooper- Dehoff RM, Gong L, Klein TE, Wadelius M, Niemi M. The clinical pharmacogenomics implementation consortium: CPIC guideline for SLCO1B1 and simvastatin-induced myopathy. *Clin Pharmacol Ther.* 2012 Jul;92(1):112-7.

[21] Santos PC, Soares RA, Nascimento RM, Machado-Coelho GL, Mill JG, Krieger JE, Pereira AC. SLCO1B1 rs4149056 polymorphism associated with statin-induced myopathy is differently distributed according to ethnicity in the Brazilian general population: Amerindians as a high risk ethnic group. *BMC Med Genet.* 2011 Oct 12;12:136.

[22] Pasanen MK, Neuvonen M, Neuvonen PJ, Niemi M. SLCO1B1 polymorphism markedly affects the pharmacokinetics of simvastatin acid. *Pharmacogenet Genomics.* 2006 Dec;16(12):873-9.

[23] Akao H, Polisecki E, Kajinami K, Trompet S, Robertson M, Ford I, Jukema JW, de Craen AJ, Westendorp RG, Shepherd J, Packard C, Buckley BM, Schaefer EJ. Genetic variation at the SLCO1B1 gene locus and low density lipoprotein cholesterol lowering response to pravastatin in the elderly. *Atherosclerosis.* 2012 Feb;220(2):413-7.

[24] Bailey KM, Romaine SP, Jackson BM, Farrin AJ, Efthymiou M, Barth JH, Copeland J, McCormack T, Whitehead A, Flather MD, Samani NJ, Nixon J, Hall AS, Balmforth AJ. Hepatic metabolism and transporter gene variants enhance response to rosuvastatin in patients with acute myocardial infarction: the GEOSTAT-1 Study. *Circ Cardiovasc Genet.* 2010 Jun;3(3):276-85.

[25] Fu Q, Li YP, Gao Y, Yang SH, Lu PQ, Jia M, Zhang LR. Lack of association between SLCO1B1 polymorphism and the lipid-lowering effects of atorvastatin and simvastatin in Chinese individuals. *Eur J Clin Pharmacol.* 2013 Jun;69(6):1269-74.

[26] Generaux GT, Bonomo FM, Johnson M, Doan KM. Impact of SLCO1B1 (OATP1B1) and ABCG2 (BCRP) genetic polymorphisms and inhibition on LDL-C lowering and myopathy of statins. *Xenobiotica.* 2011 Aug;41(8):639-51.

[27] Chasman DI, Giulianini F, MacFadyen J, Barratt BJ, Nyberg F, Ridker PM. Genetic determinants of statin-induced low-density lipoprotein cholesterol reduction: the

Justification for the Use of Statins in Prevention: an Intervention Trial Evaluating Rosuvastatin (JUPITER) trial. *Circ Cardiovasc Genet.* 2012 Apr 1;5(2):257-64.

[28] Hopewell JC, Parish S, Offer A, Link E, Clarke R, Lathrop M, Armitage J, Collins R. Impact of common genetic variation on response to simvastatin therapy among 18,705 participants in the Heart Protection Study. *Eur Heart J.* 2013 Apr;34(13):982-92. PubMed PMID:23100282.

[29] Stewart A, SLCO1B1 Polymorphisms and Statin-Induced Myopathy. *PLoS Curr.* 2013 Dec 4;5.

[30] Wilke RA, Ramsey LB, Johnson SG, Maxwell WD, McLeod HL, Voora D, Krauss RM, Roden DM, Feng Q, Cooper- Dehoff RM, Gong L, Klein TE, Wadelius M, Niemi M. The clinical pharmacogenomics implementation consortium: CPIC guideline for SLCO1B1 and simvastatin-induced myopathy. *Clin Pharmacol Ther.* 2012 Jul;92(1):112-7.

[31] Niemi M. Transporter pharmacogenetics and statin toxicity. *Clin Pharmacol Ther.* 2010 Jan;87(1):130-3.

[32] Stewart A, SLCO1B1 Polymorphisms and Statin-Induced Myopathy. *PLoS Curr.* 2013 Dec 4;5

[33] Chasman DI, Posada D, Subrahmanyan L, Cook NR, Stanton Jr VP, Ridker PM. Pharmacogenetic study of statin therapy and cholesterol reduction. *JAMA* 2004;291(23):2821–7.

[34] Donnelly LA, Doney AS, Dannfald J, Whitley AL, Lang CC, Morris AD, et al. A paucimorphic variant in the HMG-CoA reductase gene is associated with lipid-lowering response to statin treatment in diabetes: a GoDARTS study. *Pharmacogenet Genomics* 2008;18(12):1021–6.

[35] Krauss RM, Mangravite LM, Smith JD, Medina MW, Wang D, Guo X, et al. Variation in the 3-hydroxyl-3-methylglutaryl coenzyme a reductase gene is associated with racial differences in low-density lipoprotein cholesterol response to simvastatin treatment. *Circulation* 2008;117(12):1537–44.

[36] Medina MW, Gao F, Ruan W, Rotter JI, Krauss RM. Alternative splicing of 3-hydroxy-3-methylglutaryl coenzyme A reductase is associated with plasma low-density lipoprotein cholesterol response to simvastatin. *Circulation* 2008;118(4):355–62.

[37] Chung JY, Cho SK, Oh ES, Lee DH, Lim LA, Jang SB, et al. Effect of HMGCR variant alleles on low-density lipoprotein cholesterol-lowering response to atorvastatin in healthy Korean subjects. *J Clin Pharmacol* 2012;52(3):339–46.

[38] Burkhardt R, Kenny EE, Lowe JK, Birkeland A, Josowitz R, Noel M, et al. Common SNPs in HMGCR in micronesians and whites associated with LDL-cholesterol levels affect alternative splicing of exon13. *Arterioscler Thromb Vasc Biol* 2008;28(11):2078–84.

[39] Mega JL, Morrow DA, Brown A, Cannon CP, Sabatine MS. Identification of genetic variants associated with response to statin therapy. *Arterioscler Thromb Vasc Biol* 2009;29(9):1310–5.

[40] Shiffman D, O'Meara ES, Bare LA, Rowland CM, Louie JZ, Arellano AR, et al. Association of gene variants with incident myocardial infarction in the Cardiovascular Health Study. *Arterioscler Thromb Vasc Biol* 2008;28(1):173–9.

[41] Iakoubova OA, Tong CH, Rowland CM, Kirchgessner TG, Young BA, Arellano AR, et al. Association of the Trp719Arg polymorphism in kinesin-like protein 6 with

myocardial infarction and coronary heart disease in 2 prospective trials: the CARE and WOSCOPS trials. *J Am Coll Cardiol* 2008;51(4):435–43.

[42] Iakoubova, O.A.; Sabatine, M.S.; Rowland, C.M.; Tong, C.H.; Catanese, J.J.; Ranade, K.; Simonsen, K.L.; Kirchgessner, T.G.; Cannon, C.P.; Devlin, J.J.; et al. Polymorphism in kif6 gene and benefit from statins after acute coronary syndromes: Results from the prove it-timi 22 study. *J. Am. Coll. Cardiol.* 2008, 51, 449–455.

[43] Iakoubova, O.A.; Robertson, M.; Tong, C.H.; Rowland, C.M.; Catanese, J.J.; Blauw, G.J.; Jukema, J.W.; Murphy, M.B.; Devlin, J.J.; Ford, I.; et al. Kif6 trp719arg polymorphism and the effect of statin therapy in elderly patients: Results from the prosper study. *Eur. J. Cardiovasc. Prev. Rehabil.* 2010, 17, 455–461.

[44] Ference, B.A.; Yoo, W.; Flack, J.M.; Clarke, M. A common kif6 polymorphism increases vulnerability to low-density lipoprotein cholesterol: Two meta-analyses and a meta-regression analysis. *PLoS One* 2011, 6, e28834.

[45] Hopewell, J.C.; Parish, S.; Clarke, R.; Armitage, J.; Bowman, L.; Hager, J.; Lathrop, M.; Collins, R. No impact of kif6 genotype on vascular risk and statin response among 18,348 randomized patients in the heart protection study. *J. Am. Coll. Cardiol.* 2011, 57, 2000–2007.

[46] Arsenault, B.J.; Boekholdt, S.M.; Hovingh, G.K.; Hyde, C.L.; DeMicco, D.A.; Chatterjee, A.; Barter, P.; Deedwania, P.; Waters, D.D.; LaRosa, J.C.; et al. The 719arg variant of kif6 and cardiovascular outcomes in statin-treated, stable coronary patients of the treating to new targets and incremental decrease in end points through aggressive lipid-lowering prospective studies. *Circ. Cardiovasc. Genet.* 2012, 5, 51–57.

[47] Ridker, P.M.; MacFadyen, J.G.; Glynn, R.J.; Chasman, D.I. Kinesin-like protein 6 (kif6) polymorphism and the efficacy of rosuvastatin in primary prevention. *Circ. Cardiovasc. Genet.* 2011, 4, 312–317.

[48] Charland SL, Agatep BC, Herrera V, Schrader B, Frueh FW, Ryvkin M, et al. Providing patients with pharmacogenetic test results affects adherence to statin therapy: results of the Additional KIF6 Risk Offers Better Adherence to Statins (AKROBATS) trial. *Pharmacogenomics J* 2013.

[49] Takemoto M, Liao JK. Pleiotropic effects of 3-hydroxy-3methylglutaryl coenzyme a reductase inhibitors. *Arterioscler Throm Vasc Biol* 2001; 21: 1712-19.

[50] Istvan ES, Deisenhofer J. Structural mechanism for statin inhibition of HMG-CoA reductase. *Science* 2001; 292:1160.

[51] Arad Y, Ramakrishnan R, Ginsberg HN. Lovastatin therapy reduces low density lipoprotein apoB levels in subjects with combined hyperlipidemia by reducing the production of apoB-containing lipoproteins: implications for the pathophysiology of apoB production. *J Lipid Res* 1990; 31:567.

[52] Terblanche M, Almog Y, Rosenson R, et al. Statins and sepsis : multiple modification at multiple levels. *Lancet Infect Dis* 2007 ;7 :358-68.

[53] Jacobson JR, Barnard JW, Grigoryev DN, et al. Simvastatin atenuates vascular leak and inflammation in murine inflammatory lung injury. *AM J Physiol Lung Cell Mol Physiol* 2005; 288: 1026- 32.

[54] Kallen J, Welzenbach K, Ramage P, et al. Structural basis for LFA-1 inhibition upon lovastatin binding to the CD11a I-domain. *J Mol Biol* 1999; 292: 1- 9.

[55] Weitz-Schmidt G, Welzenbach K, Brinkmann V, et al. Statins selectively inhibit leukocyte function antigen-1 by binding to a novel regulatory integrin site. *Nature Med* 2001; 7: 687- 92.

[56] Methe H, Kim J-O, Kofler S., et al. Statins decrease Toll-like receptor 4 expression and downstream signaling in human CD14+ moncytes. *Arteriosclerosis, Thrombosis, and Vascular Biology* 2005; 25: 1439- 45.

[57] Niessner A., Steiner S., Speidl W.S, et al. Simvastatin suppresses endotoxin-induced upregulation of Toll-like receptors 4 and 2 in vivo. *Atherosclerosis* 2006; 189: 408-413.

[58] Hodgkinson C.P. and Ye S. Statins inhibit Toll-like receptor 4-mediated lipopolysaccharide signalling and cytokine expression. *Pharmacogenetics and Genomics* 2008; 18: 803- 13.

[59] Kirsch C., Eckert G.P., and Meller W.E. Statin effects on cholesterol microdomains in brain plasma membranes. *Biochemical Pharmacology* 2003; 65: 843- 56.

[60] Shi J, Wang J, Zheng H, et al. Statins increase thrombomodulin expression and function in human endothelial cells by a nitric oxide-dependent mechanism and counteract tumor necrosis factor alpha-induced thrombomodulin downregulation. *Blood Coagul Fibrinolysis* 2003; 14: 575-85.

[61] Bernard GR, Vincent JL, Laterre PF, et al. Efficacity and safety of recombinant human activated protein C for severe sepsis. *N Engl J Med* 2001: 344; 699- 709.

[62] Huang KC, Chen CW, Chen JC, at al. MHG-CoA reductase inhibitors inhibits inducible nitric oxide synthase gene expression in macrophages. *J Biomed Sci* 2003; 10: 396-405.

[63] Guiti_Paiva A, Martinez MR, Felix JV, et al. Simvastatine decreases noictric oxide overproduction and reverts the impaired vascular responsivness induced by endotoxic shock in rats. *Shock* 2004; 21: 271-75.

[64] Pruefer D, Makowski J, Schell M., et al. Simvastatin inhibits inflammatory properties of Staphylococcus aureus alpha-toxin. *Circulation* 2002 ; 106 : 2104-10.

[65] Grover R, Zaccardelli D, Colice G, et al. An open-label dose escalation of the nitric oxide synthase inhibitor, N(G)-methyl-L-arginine hydrochloride (546C88), in patients with septic shock. *Crit Care Med* 1999; 27:913- 22.

[66] Cowley HC, Bacon PJ, Goode HF, et al. Plasma antioxidant potential in severe sepsis : a comparison of survivors and non-survivors. *Crit Care Med* 1996 ; 24 : 1179- 83.

[67] Goode HF, Cowley HC, Walker BE, et al. Decreased anti-oxidant status and increased lipid peroxidation in patients with septic shock and secondary organ dysfunction. *Crit Care Med* 1995; 23: 646- 51

[68] Motoyama T, Okamoto K, Kukita I, et al. Possible role of increased oxidant stress in multiple organ failure after systemic inflammatory response syndrome. *Crit Care Med* 2003; 31: 1048- 52

[69] Wassmann S, Laufs U, Muller K, et al. Cellular antioxidant effects of atorvastatin in vitro and in vivo. *Arteriosci Thromb Vasc Biol* 2002; 22: 300- 05

[70] Lee TS, Chang CC, Zhu Y, et al. Simvastatin induces heme oxygenase-1 : a novel mechanism of vessel protection. *Circulation* 2004; 110:1296- 302

[71] Grosser N, Erdamnn K, Hemmerle A, et al. Rosuvastatin upregulates the antioxidant defense protein heme oxygenase-1. *Biochem Biophys Res Commun* 2004; 325: 871- 76

[72] Grosser N, Hemmerle A, Berndt G., et al. The antioxidant defense protein heme oxygenase 1 is a novel target for statins in endothelial cells. *Free Radic Biol Med* 2004; 37:2064- 71

[73] Hashiba T, Suzuki M, Nagashima Y, et al. Adenovirus-mediated transfer of heme oxygenase-1 cDNA attenuates severe lung injury induced by the influenza virus in mice. *Gene Ther* 2001; 8: 1499- 507.
[74] Mascitelli L., Grant W. B., Goldstein MR. Letter to the editor: Statins, vitamin D, and severe sepsis. *Eur J Intern Med* 2011; 22 :25- 26.
[75] Liu PT, Stenger S, Li H., et al. Toll-like receptor triggering of a vitamin D-mediated human antimicrobial response. *Science* 2006: 311; 1770-3.
[76] Grimes DS. Statins and vitamin D. *Cardiovasc Drugs Ther* 2009; 23: 261-62.
[77] Goldstein MR, Mascitelli L, Pezzetta F. Rosuvastatin and vitamin D : might there be hypovitaminosis D on JUPITER ? *Int J Cardiol* 2001; 145:556- 57.
[78] Rosen CJ. Clinical Practice : Vitamin D insufficiency. *N Engl J Med* 2011 ; 364 : 248-54.
[79] Jeng L, Yamshchikov AV, Judd SE, et al. Alterations in vitamin D status and anti-microbial peptide levels in patients in the intensive care unit with sepsis. *J Transl Med* 2009; 7: 28.
[80] [80] Joy TR, Hegele RA. Narrative review: statin-related myopathy. *Ann Intern Med.* 2009 Jun 16;150(12):858-68.
[81] Abd TT, Jacobson TA. Statin-induced myopathy: a review and update. *Expert Opin Drug Saf.* 2011 May;10(3):373-87.
[82] Bleske BE, Willis RA, Anthony M, et al. The effect of pravastatin and atorvastatin on coenzyme Q10. *Am Heart J* 2001; 142:E2.
[83] Päivä H, Thelen KM, Van Coster R, et al. High-dose statins and skeletal muscle metabolism in humans: a randomized, controlled trial. *Clin Pharmacol Ther* 2005; 78:60.
[84] Laaksonen R, Jokelainen K, Laakso J, et al. The effect of simvastatin treatment on natural antioxidants in low-density lipoproteins and high-energy phosphates and ubiquinone in skeletal muscle. *Am J Cardiol* 1996; 77:851.
[85] Lamperti C, Naini AB, Lucchini V, et al. Muscle coenzyme Q10 level in statin related myopathy. *Arch Neurol* 2005; 62:1709.
[86] Larsen S, Stride N, Hey-Mogensen M, et al. Simvastatin effects on skeletal muscle: relation to decreased mitochondrial function and glucose intolerance. *J Am Coll Cardiol* 2013; 61:44.
[87] Phillips PS, Ciaraldi TP, Kim DL, et al. Myotoxic reactions to lipid-lowering therapy are associated with altered oxidation of fatty acids. *Endocrine* 2009; 35:38.
[88] Iacobazzi V, Convertini P, Infantino V, et al. Statins, fibrates and retinoic acid upregulation mitochondrial acylcarnitine carrier gene expression. *Biochem Biophys Res Commun* 2009; 388:643.
[89] Hanai J, Cao P, Tanksale P, et al. The muscle-specific ubiquitin ligase atrogin 1/MAFbx mediates statin-induced muscle toxicity. *J Clin Invest* 2007; 117:3940.
[90] Thompson PD, Clarkson PM, Rosenson RS, National Lipid Association Statin Safety Task Force Muscle Safety Expert Panel. An assessment of statin safety by muscle experts. *Am J Cardiol* 2006; 97:69C.
[91] Mohaupt MG, Karas RH, Babiychuk EB, Sanchez-Freire V, Monastyrskaya K, Iyer L, Hoppeler H, Breil F, Draeger A. Association between statin-associated myopathy and skeletal muscle damage. *CMAJ.* 2009 Jul 7;181(1-2):E11-8.

[92] Hansen KE, Hildebrand JP, Ferguson EE, Stein JH. Outcomes in 45 patients with statin-associated myopathy. *Arch Intern Med* 2005; 165:2671.

[93] Sathasivam S, Lecky B. Statin induced myopathy. BMJ 2008; 337:a2286.

[94] Dujovne CA, Chremos AN, Pool JL, et al. Expanded clinical evaluation of lovastatin (EXCEL) study results: IV. Additional perspectives on the tolerability of lovastatin. *Am J Med* 1991; 91:25S.

[95] Boccuzzi SJ, Bocanegra TS, Walker JF, et al. Long-term safety and efficacy profile of simvastatin. *Am J Cardiol* 1991; 68:1127.

[96] Pedersen TR, Berg K, Cook TJ, et al. Safety and tolerability of cholesterol lowering with simvastatin during 5 years in the Scandinavian Simvastatin Survival Study. *Arch Intern Med* 1996; 156:2085.

[97] "The Pink Sheet" *FDC Reports.* 2002; 64(vol 23):5.

[98] Graham DJ, Staffa JA, Shatin D, et al. Incidence of hospitalized rhabdomyolysis in patients treated with lipid-lowering drugs. *JAMA* 2004; 292:2585

[99] Physicians' Desk Reference, Medical Economics, Montvale, NJ 2002

[100] Zinman L, Sadeghi R, Gawel M, et al. Are statin medications safe in patients with ALS? *Amyotroph Lateral Scler* 2008; 9:223.

[101] Cartwright MS, Jeffery DR, Nuss GR, Donofrio PD. Statin-associated exacerbation of myasthenia gravis. *Neurology* 2004; 63:2188.

[102] Patel AM, Shariff S, Bailey DG, et al. Statin toxicity from macrolide antibiotic coprescription: a population-based cohort study. *Ann Intern Med* 2013; 158:869.

[103] Kashani A, Phillips CO, Foody JM, et al. Risks associated with statin therapy: a systematic overview of randomized clinical trials. *Circulation* 2006; 114:2788.

[104] Melli G, Chaudhry V, Cornblath DR. Rhabdomyolysis: an evaluation of 475 hospitalized patients. *Medicine (Baltimore)* 2005; 84:377.

[105] Craig Williams. Myopathy. In: Drug-Induced Diseases Prevention, Detection and Management, 2nd edition, James E. Tisdale, Douglas A. Miller. (Eds), American Society of Health-System Pharmacists, Inc., *Bethesda* 2010. p.1017.

[106] Joy TR, Hegele RA. Narrative review: statin-related myopathy. *Ann Intern Med* 2009;150:858.

[107] Caso G, Kelly P, McNurlan MA, Lawson WE. Effect of coenzyme q10 on myopathic symptoms in patients treated with statins. *Am J Cardiol* 2007; 99:1409.

[108] Ridker PM, Genest J, Boekholdt SM, Libby P, Gotto AM, Nordestgaard BG, et al. HDL cholesterol and residual risk of first cardiovascular events after treatment with potent statin therapy: an analysis from the JUPITER trial. *Lancet* 2012;376:333–9.

[109] Ruscica M, Macchi C, Morlotti B, Sirtori C., Magni P. Statin therapy and related risk of new-onset type 2 diabetes mellitus. *Eur J Intern Med* 2014; 25: 401- 406.

[110] Navarese EP, Buffon A, Andreotti F, Kozinski M, Welton N, Fabiszak T, et al. Meta-analysis of impact of different types and doses of statins on new-onset diabetes mellitus. *Am J Cardiol* 2013;111:1123–30.

[111] Sattar N, Taskinen MR. Statins are diabetogenic—myth or reality? *Atheroscler Suppl* 2012;13:1–10.

[112] J.C. LaRosa, S.M. Grundy, D.D. Waters, Treating to New Targets (TNT) Investigators, et al. Intensive lipid lowering with atorvastatin in patients with stable coronary disease *N Engl J Med,* 352 (2005), pp. 1425–1435

[113] T.R. Pedersen, O. Faergeman, J.J.K. Kastelein, Incremental Decrease in End Points Through Aggressive Lipid Lowering (IDEAL) Study Group, et al. High-dose atorvastatin vs usual-dose simvastatin for secondary prevention after myocardial infarction, *JAMA,* 294 (2005), pp. 2437–2445
[114] The Stroke Prevention by Aggressive Reduction in Cholesterol Levels (SPARCL) Investigators High-dose atorvastatin after stroke or transient ischemic attack *N Engl J Med,* 355 (2006), pp. 549–559
[115] Waters DD, Ho JE, Boekholdt SM, DeMicco DA, Kastelein JJ, Messig M, et al. Cardio-vascular event reduction versus new-onset diabetes during atorvastatin therapy: effect of baseline risk factors for diabetes. *J Am Coll Cardiol 2013*;61:148–52.
[116] Waters DD, Ho JE, DeMicco DA, Breazna A, Arsenault BJ, Wun CC, et al. Predictors of new-onset diabetes in patients treated with atorvastatin: results from 3 large randomized clinical trials. *J Am Coll Cardiol* 2011;57:1535–45.
[117] Shen L, Shah BR, Reyes EM, Thomas L, Wojdyla D, Diem P, et al. Role of diuretics, beta blockers, and statins in increasing the risk of diabetes in patients with impaired glucose tolerance: reanalysis of data from the NAVIGATOR study. *BMJ* 2013;347:f6745.
[118] Ballard KD, Quann EE, Kupchak BR, Volk BM, Kawiecki DM, Fernandez ML, et al. Dietary carbohydrate restriction improves insulin sensitivity, blood pressure, micro-vascular function, and cellular adhesion markers in individuals taking statins. *Nutr Res* 2013;33:905–12.
[119] Florentin M, Liberopoulos EN, Rizos CV, Kei AA, Liamis G, Kostapanos MS, et al. Colesevelam plus rosuvastatin 5 mg/day versus rosuvastatin 10 mg/day alone on markers of insulin resistance in patients with hypercholesterolemia and impaired fasting glucose. *Metab Syndr Relat Disord* 2013;11:152–6.
[120] Wierzbicki AS, Viljoen A, Hardman TC, Mikhailidis DP. New therapies to reduce low-density lipoprotein cholesterol. *Curr Opin Cardiol* 2013;28:452–7.
[121] Association. AD. Diagnosis and classification of diabetes mellitus. *Diabetes Care* 2012;35:S64–71.
[122] Saito Y, Yoshida S, Nakaya N, et al. Comparison between morning and evening dose of simvastatin in hyperlipidemic subjects. A double-blind comparative study. *Arterioscler Thromb* 1991; 11:816.
[123] Wallace A, Chinn D, Rubin G. Taking simvastatin in the morning compared with in the evening: randomised controlled trial. *BMJ* 2003; 327:788.
[124] Matalka MS, Ravnan MC, Deedwania PC. Is alternate daily dose of atorvastatin effective in treating patients with hyperlipidemia? The Alternate Day Versus Daily Dosing of Atorvastatin Study (ADDAS). *Am Heart J* 2002; 144:674.
[125] Rindone JP, Hiller D, Arriola G. A comparison of fluvastatin 40 mg every other day versus 20 mg every day in patients with hypercholesterolemia. *Pharmacotherapy* 1998; 18:836.
[126] Ferrer-García JC, Pérez-Silvestre J, Martínez-Mir I, Herrera-Ballester A. Alternate-day dosing of atorvastatin: effects in treating type 2 diabetic patients with dyslipidaemia. *Acta Diabetol* 2006; 43:75.
[127] FDA Drug Safety Communication: New restrictions, contraindications, and dose limitations for Zocor (simvastatin) to reduce the risk of muscle injury. 2011

[128] Fruchart JC, Brewer HB Jr, Leitersdorf E. Consensus for the use of fibrates in the treatment of dyslipoproteinemia and coronary heart disease. Fibrate Consensus Group. *Am J Cardiol* 1998; 81:912.

[129] Birjmohun RS, Hutten BA, Kastelein JJ, Stroes ES. Efficacy and safety of high density lipoprotein cholesterol-increasing compounds: a meta-analysis of randomized controlled trials. *J Am Coll Cardiol* 2005; 45:185.

[130] Rubins HB, Robins SJ, Collins D, et al. Gemfibrozil for the secondary prevention of coronary heart disease in men with low levels of high-density lipoprotein cholesterol. Veterans Affairs High-Density Lipoprotein Cholesterol Intervention Trial Study Group. *N Engl J Med* 1999; 341:410.

[131] Saha SA, Kizhakepunnur LG, Bahekar A, Arora RR. The role of fibrates in the prevention of cardiovascular disease--a pooled meta-analysis of long-term randomized placebo-controlled clinical trials. *Am Heart J* 2007; 154:943.

[132] Jun M, Foote C, Lv J, et al. Effects of fibrates on cardiovascular outcomes: a systematic review and meta-analysis. *Lancet* 2010; 375:1875.

[133] Frick MH, Elo O, Haapa K, et al. Helsinki Heart Study: primary-prevention trial with gemfibrozil in middle-aged men with dyslipidemia. Safety of treatment, changes in risk factors, and incidence of coronary heart disease. *N Engl J Med* 1987; 317:1237.

[134] Bezafibrate Infarction Prevention (BIP) study. Secondary prevention by raising HDL cholesterol and reducing triglycerides in patients with coronary artery disease. *Circulation* 2000; 102:21.

[135] Miller DB, Spence JD. Clinical pharmacokinetics of fibric acid derivatives (fibrates). *Clin Pharmacokinet* 1998; 34:155.

[136] Pierce LR, Wysowski DK, Gross TP. Myopathy and rhabdomyolysis associated with lovastatin-gemfibrozil combination therapy. *JAMA* 1990; 264:71.

[137] Shepherd J, Packard CJ, Morgan HG, et al. The effects of cholestyramine on high density lipoprotein metabolism. *Atherosclerosis* 1979; 33:433.

[138] Brown G, Albers JJ, Fisher LD, et al. Regression of coronary artery disease as a result of intensive lipid-lowering therapy in men with high levels of apolipoprotein B. *N Engl J Med* 1990; 323:1289.

[139] Comparative efficacy and safety of pravastatin and cholestyramine alone and combined in patients with hypercholesterolemia. Pravastatin Multicenter Study Group II. *Arch Intern Med* 1993; 153:1321.

[140] Knapp HH, Schrott H, Ma P, et al. Efficacy and safety of combination simvastatin and colesevelam in patients with primary hypercholesterolemia. *Am J Med* 2001; 110:352.

[141] Illingworth DR, Stein EA, Mitchel YB, et al. Comparative effects of lovastatin and niacin in primary hypercholesterolemia. A prospective trial. *Arch Intern Med* 1994; 154:1586.

[142] Canner PL, Berge KG, Wenger NK, et al. Fifteen year mortality in Coronary Drug Project patients: long-term benefit with niacin. *J Am Coll Cardiol* 1986; 8:1245.

[143] AIM-HIGH Investigators, Boden WE, Probstfield JL, et al. Niacin in patients with low HDL cholesterol levels receiving intensive statin therapy. *N Engl J Med* 2011; 365:2255.

[144] HPS2-THRIVE Collaborative Group, Landray MJ, Haynes R, et al. Effects of extended-release niacin with laropiprant in high-risk patients. *N Engl J Med* 2014; 371:203.

[145] Illingworth DR, Stein EA, Mitchel YB, et al. Comparative effects of lovastatin and niacin in primary hypercholesterolemia. A prospective trial. *Arch Intern Med* 1994; 154:1586.

[146] Sudhop T, Lütjohann D, Kodal A, et al. Inhibition of intestinal cholesterol absorption by ezetimibe in humans. *Circulation* 2002; 106:1943.

[147] Davidson MH, McGarry T, Bettis R, et al. Ezetimibe coadministered with simvastatin in patients with primary hypercholesterolemia. *J Am Coll Cardiol* 2002; 40:2125.

[148] Ginsberg HN, Elam MB, Lovato LC et al. Effects of combination lipid therapy in type 2 diabetes mellitus. *N Engl J Med* 2010; 362(17):1563-74.

[149] Boden WE, Probstfield JL, Anderson T et al. Niacin in patients with low HDL cholesterol levels receiving intensive statin therapy. *N Engl J Med* 2011; 365(24):2255-67.

[150] Cannon CP, Giugliano RP, Blazing MA, Harrington RA, et. al. IMPROVE-IT Investigators. Rationale and design of IMPROVE-IT (IMProved Reduction of Outcomes: Vytorin Efficacy International Trial): comparison of ezetimbe/simvastatin versus simvastatin monotherapy on cardiovascular outcomes in patients with acute coronary syndromes. *Am Heart J.* 2008; 156(5):826-32.

[151] Stone NJ, Robinson J, Lichtenstein AH, Merz CN, Blum CB, Eckel RH, Goldberg AC, Gordon D, Levy D, Lloyd-Jones DM, McBride P, Schwartz JS, Shero ST, Smith SC Jr, Watson K, Wilson PW. 2013ACC/AHA Guideline on the Treatment of Blood Cholesterol to Reduce Atherosclerotic Cardiovascular Risk in Adults: A Report of the American College of Cardiology/American Heart Association Task Force on Practice Guidelines. *J Am Coll Cardiol.* 2014 Jul 1;63(25 Pt B):2889-93.

[152] Ray KK, Kastelein JJ, Boekholdt SM, Nicholls SJ, Khaw KT, Ballantyne CM, Catapano AL, Reiner Ž, Lüscher TF. The ACC/AHA 2013 guideline on the treatment of blood cholesterol to reduce atherosclerotic cardiovascular disease risk in adults: the good the bad and the uncertain: a comparison with ESC/EAS guidelines for the management of dyslipidaemias 2011. *Eur Heart J.* 2014 Apr;35(15):960-8.

[153] Reiner Z, Catapano AL,DeBacker G, Graham I, Taskinen MR,Wiklund O, Agewall S, Alegria E, Chapman MJ, Durrington P, Erdine S, Halcox J, Hobbs R, Kjekshus J, Filardi PP, Riccardi G, Storey RF, Wood D. ESC/EAS Guidelines for the management of dyslipidaemias: the Task Force for the management of dyslipidaemias of the European Society of Cardiology (ESC) and the European Atherosclerosis Society (EAS). *Eur Heart J* 2011;32:1769–1818.

[154] Abud-Mendoza C, de la Fuente H, Cuevas-Orta E, Baranda L, Cruz-Rizo J, González-Amaro R. Therapy with statins in patients with refractory rheumatic diseases: a preliminary study. *Lupus.* 2003;12(8):607-11.

[155] McCarey DW, McInnes IB, Madhok R, Hampson R, Scherbakov O, Ford I,et al. Trial of atorvastatin in rheumatoid arthritis (TARA): double-blind, randomised placebo-controlled trial. *Lancet* 2004;363:2015–21.

[156] Cojocaru L, Rusali AC, Suta C, Radulescu AM, Suta M, Craiu E. The role of simvastatin in the therapeutic approach of rheumatoid arthritis. *Autoimmune Dis* 2013;2013:326258.

[157] Okamoto H, Koizumi K, Kamitsuji S, Inoue E, Hara M, Tomatsu T, et al. Beneficial action of statins in patients with rheumatoid arthritis in a large observational cohort. *J Rheumatol* 2007;34:964–8.

[158] Lodi S, Evans SJ, Egger P, Carpenter J. Is there an anti-inflammatory effect of statins in rheumatoid arthritis? Analysis of a large routinely collected claims database. *Br J Clin Pharmacol* 2010;69:85–94.

[159] Ferri N, Corsini A. Clinical evidence of statin therapy in non-dyslipidemic disorders. *Pharmacol Res.* 2014 Feb 15

[160] V Arts EE, Jansen TL, Den Broeder A, Vonkeman HE, Dutmer E, Van de Laar MA, et al. Statins inhibit the antirheumatic effects of rituximab in rheumatoid arthritis: results from the Dutch Rheumatoid Arthritis Monitoring (DREAM)registry. *Ann Rheum Dis* 2011;70:877–8.

[161] Prandoni P, Ghirarduzzi A, Prins MH, Pengo V, Davidson BL, Sorensen H, et al. Venous thromboembolism and the risk of subsequent symptomatica therosclerosis. J Thromb Haemost 2006;4:1891–6.

[162] Undas A, Celinska-Lowenhoff M, Domagala TB, Iwaniec T, Dropinski J, Lowen-hoff T, et al. Early anti-thrombotic and anti-inflammatory effects of simvastatin versus fenofibrate in patients with hypercholesterolemia. *Thromb Haemost* 2005;94:193–9.

[163] Szczeklik A, Musial J, Undas A, Gajewski P, Gora P, Swadzba J, et al. Inhibition of thrombin generation by simvastatin and lack of additive effects of aspirin in patients with marked hypercholesterolemia. *J Am Coll Cardiol* 1999;33:1286–93.

[164] Pai M, Evans NS, Shah SJ, Green D, Cook D, Crowther MA. Statins in the prevention of venous thromboembolism: a meta-analysis of observational studies. *Thromb Res* 2011;128:422–30.

[165] Squizzato A, Galli M, Romualdi E, Dentali F, Kamphuisen PW, Guasti L, et al. Statins, fibrates, and venous thromboembolism: a meta-analysis. *Eur Heart J* 2010;31:1248–56.

[166] Glynn RJ, Danielson E, Fonseca FA, Genest J, Gotto Jr AM, Kastelein JJ, et al. A randomized trial of rosuvastatin in the prevention of venous thromboembolism. *N Engl J Med* 2009;360:1851–61.

[167] Li L, Sun T, Zhang P, Tian J, Yang K. Statins for primary prevention of venous thromboembolism. *Cochrane Database Syst Rev* 2011:CD008203.

[168] Freeman DJ, Robertson M, Brown EA, Rumley A, Tobias ES, Frolich M, et al. Incident venous thromboembolic events in the prospective study of pravastatin the elderly at risk (PROSPER). *BMC Geriatr* 2011;11:8.

[169] Rahimi K, Bhala N, Kamphuisen P, Emberson J, Biere-Rafi S, Krane V, et al. Effect of statins on venous thromboembolic events: a meta-analysis of published and unpublished evidence from randomised controlled trials. *PLoS Med* 2012;9:e1001310.

[170] Ehrmann DA. Polycystic ovary syndrome. *N Engl J Med* 2005;352:1223–36.

[171] Azziz R, Woods KS, Reyna R, Key TJ, Knochenhauer ES, Yildiz BO. The prevalence and features of the polycystic ovary syndrome in an unselected population. *J Clin Endocrinol Metab* 2004;89:2745–9.

[172] Dobs AS, Schrott H, Davidson MH, Bays H, Stein EA, Kush D, et al. Effects of high-dose simvastatin on adrenal and gonadal steroidogenesis in men with hypercholesterolemia. *Metabolism* 2000;49:1234–8.

[173] Gao L, Zhao FL, Li SC. Statin is a reasonable treatment option for patients with polycystic ovary syndrome: a meta-analysis of randomized controlled trials. *Exp Clin Endocrinol Diabetes* 2012;120:367–75.

[174] Sathyapalan T, Kilpatrick ES, Coady AM, Atkin SL. The effect of atorvastatin in patients with polycystic ovary syndrome: a randomized double-blind placebo-controlled study. *J Clin Endocrinol Metab* 2009;94:103–8.

[175] Sathyapalan T, Smith KA, Coady AM, Kilpatrick ES, Atkin SL. Atorvastatin therapy decreases androstenedione and dehydroepiandrosterone sulphate concentrations in patients with polycystic ovary syndrome: randomized controlled study. *Ann Clin Biochem* 2012;49:80–5.

[176] Banaszewska B, Pawelczyk L, Spaczynski RZ, Dziura J, Duleba AJ. Effects of simvastatin and oral contraceptive agent on polycystic ovary syndrome: prospective, randomized, crossover trial. *J Clin Endocrinol Metab* 2007;92:456–61.

[177] Banaszewska B, Pawelczyk L, Spaczynski RZ, Duleba AJ. Comparison of simvastatin and metformin in treatment of polycystic ovary syndrome: prospective randomized trial. *J Clin Endocrinol Metab* 2009;94:4938–45.

[178] Banaszewska B, Pawelczyk L, Spaczynski RZ, Duleba AJ. Effects of simvastatin and metformin on polycystic ovary syndrome after six months of treatment. *J Clin Endocrinol Metab* 2011;96:3493–501.

[179] Kaya C, Cengiz SD, Berker B, Demirtas S, Cesur M, Erdogan G. Comparative effects of atorvastatin and simvastatin on the plasma total homocysteine levels in women with polycystic ovary syndrome: a prospective randomized study. *Fertil Steril* 2009;92:635–42.

[180] Hotchkiss RS, Karl IE. The pathophysiology and treatment of sepsis. *N Engl J Med* 2003; 348 : 138- 50

[181] Padkin A, Goldfrad C, Brady A, et al. Epidemiology of severe sepsis occurring in the first 24 hrs in intensive care units in England, Wales, and Nothern Ireland. *Crit Care Med* 2003; 31 : 2332- 38

[182] Weycker D, Akhras KS, Edelsberg J, et al. Long-term mortality and medical care charges in patients with severe sepsis. *Crit Care Med* 2003 ; 31 : 2316- 23

[183] Finfer S, Bellomo R, Lipman J, et al. Adult-population incidence of severe sepsis in AUstralian and New-Zealand intensive care units. *Intensive Care Med* 2004 ; 30 : 589- 96.

[184] Ando H, Takamura T, Ota T., et al. Cerivastatine improves survival of mice with lipopolysaccharide-induced sepsis. *J Pharmacol Exp Ther* 2000; 294:1043- 6.

[185] Merx MW, Liehn EA, Janssens U, et al. HMG-CoA reductase inhibitor simvastatin profoundly improves survival in a murine model of sepsis. *Circualtion* 2004; 109: 2560- 5.

[186] Giusti-Paiva A, Martinez MR, Felix JV, et al. Simvastatin decreases nitric oxide overproduction and reverts the impaired vascular responsiveness induced by endotoxic shock in rats. *Shock* 2004; 21: 271- 5.

[187] Merx MW, Liehn EA, Graf J, et al. Statin treatment after onset of sepsis in a murine model improves survival. *Circulation* 2005; 112: 117- 24.

[188] Janda S., Young A., Fitzgerald JM., et al. The effect of statins on mortality from severe infections and sepsis: A systematic review and meta-analysis. *J Crit Care* 2010; 25: 656 e7-22.

[189] Almog Y, Novack V, Eisinger M, et al. The effect of statins therapy on infection-related mortality in patients with atherosclerotic diseases. *Crit Care Med* 2007; 35 : 372–78.

[190] Chalmers JD, Singanayagam A, Murray MP, et al. Prior statin use is associated with improved outcomes in community-acquired pneumonia. *Am J Med* 2008; 121:1002-1007 e1001.

[191] P.P. Dobesh, D.G. Klepser and T.R. McGuire, et al. Reduction in mortality associated with statin therapy in patients with severe sepsis. *Pharmacotherapy* 2009 ; 29 : 621–630.

[192] M.W. Donnino, M.N. Cocchi and M. Howell, et al. Statin therapy is associated with decreased mortality in patients with infection. *Acad Emerg Med* 2009 ; 16 : 230–234.

[193] F.J. Frost, H. Petersen and K. Tollestrup, et al. Influenza and COPD mortality protection as pleiotropic, dose-dependent effects of statins. *Chest* 2007 ; 131 :1006–1012.

[194] D.G. Hackam, M. Mamdani and P. Li, et al. Statins and sepsis in patients with cardiovascular disease: a population-based cohort analysis. *Lancet* 2006 ; 367 : 413–418.

[195] J. Hsu, D.R. Andes and V. Knasinski, et al. Statins are associated with improved outcomes of bloodstream infection in solid-organ transplant recipients. *Eur J Clin Microbiol Infect Dis* 2009 ; 28 : 1343–1351.

[196] P. Kruger, K. Fitzsimmons and D. Cook, et al. Statin therapy is associated with fewer deaths in patients with bacteraemia. *Intensive Care Med*, 32 (2006), pp. 75–79.

[197] A.P. Liappis, V.L. Kan and C.G. Rochester, et al. The effect of statins on mortality in patients with bacteremia. *Clin Infect Dis,* 33 (2001), pp. 1352–1357.

[198] E.M. Mortensen, M.I. Restrepo and A. Anzueto, et al. The effect of prior statin use on 30-day mortality for patients hospitalized with community-acquired pneumonia. *Respir Res* 2005; 6 : 82.

[199] E.M. Mortensen, M.I. Restrepo and L.A. Copeland, et al. Impact of previous statin and angiotensin II receptor blocker use on mortality in patients hospitalized with sepsis. *Pharmacotherapy* 2007 ; 27 : 1619–1626.

[200] E.M. Mortensen, M.J. Pugh and L.A. Copeland, et al. Impact of statins and angiotensin-converting enzyme inhibitors on mortality of subjects hospitalised with pneumonia. *Eur Respir J* 2008 ; 31 : 611–617.

[201] R.G. Schlienger, D.S. Fedson and S.S. Jick, et al. Statins and the risk of pneumonia: a population-based, nested case-control study. *Pharmacotherapy* 2007 ; 27 : 325–332.

[202] R.W. Thomsen, A. Riis and J.B. Kornum, et al. Preadmission use of statins and outcomes after hospitalization with pneumonia: population-based cohort study of 29,900 patients. *Arch Intern Med* 2008 ; 168 : 2081–2087.

[203] M.Y. Tseng, P.J. Hutchinson and M. Czosnyka, et al. Effects of acute pravastatin treatment on intensity of rescue therapy, length of inpatient stay, and 6-month outcome in patients after aneurysmal subarachnoid hemorrhage. *Stroke* 2007 ; 38 : 1545–1550.

[204] S.R. Majumdar, F.A. McAlister and D.T. Eurich, et al. Statins and outcomes in patients admitted to hospital with community acquired pneumonia: population based prospective cohort study. *BMJ* 2006 ; 333 : 999.

[205] C.P. Martin, R.L. Talbert and D.S. Burgess, et al. Effectiveness of statins in reducing the rate of severe sepsis: a retrospective evaluation. *Pharmacotherapy* 2007 ; 27 : 20–26.

[206] R.W. Thomsen, H.H. Hundborg and S.P. Johnsen, et al. Statin use and mortality within 180 days after bacteremia: a population-based cohort study. *Crit Care Med* 2006 ; 34 : 1080–1086.

[207] K.C. Yang, J.Y. Chien and W.K. Tseng, et al. Statins do not improve short-term survival in an oriental population with sepsis. *Am J Emerg Med* 2007 ; 25 : 494–501.

[208] R. Fernandez, V.J. De Pedro and A. Artigas, Statin therapy prior to ICU admission: protection against infection or a severity marker? *Intensive Care Med* 2006 ; 32 : 160–164.

[209] Novack V., Eisinger M., Frenkel A., et al. The effects of statin therapy on inflammatory cytokines in patients with bacterial infections: a randomized double-blind placebo controlled clinical trial. *Intensive Care Med* 2009; 35: 1255- 60.

[210] Simvastatin and severe sepsis trial (SIMSEPT), ISRCTN 92093279, Eudra CT number 2005-003438-17.

[211] Statins in sepsis study ACTRN 12607000028404.

[212] Statins for the Early Treatment of Sepsis (SETS). NCT 00528580.

[213] Study of Statin Therapy in the Treatment of Sepsis. NCT 00676897.

[214] Ware LB, Matthay MA. The acute respiratory distress syndrome. *N Engl J Med* 2000; 342: 1334- 49.

[215] The Acute Respiratory Distress Syndrome Network. Ventilation with lower tidal volumes as compared with traditional tidal volumes for acute lung injury and the acute respiratory distress syndrome. *N Engl J Med* 2000; 342: 1301- 08.

[216] Hager DN, Krishnan JA, Hayden JL, et al. Tidal volume reduction in patients with acute lung injury when plateau pressures are not high. *Am J Respir Crit Care Med* 2005; 354: 2464-75.

[217] Craig T., O'Kane C. and McAuley D. Potential Mechanism by which Statins Modulate the Development of Acute Lung Injury. In Yearbook of Intensive Care and Emergency Medicine Edited by JL Vincent. *Springer;* 2007: 276-88.

[218] Naidu BV, Woolley SM, Farivar AS, et al. Simvastatine ameliorates injury in an experimental model of lung ischemia-reperfusion. *J Thorac Cardiovasc Surg* 2003; 126: 482- 9.

[219] Fischetti F., Carretta R., Borotto G., et al. Fluvastatin treatment inhibits leucocyte adhesion and extravasation in models of complement-mediated acute inflammation. *Clin Exp Immunol* 2004; 135:186- 93.

[220] Jacobson JR, Barnard JW, Grigoryev DN, et al. Simvastatin attenuates vascular leak and inflammation in murine inflammatory lung injury. *Am J Physiol Lung Cell Mol Biol* 2004; 30: 662- 70.

[221] Fessler MB, Young SK, Jeyaseelan S, et al. A role for hydroxymethylglutaryl coenzyme A reductase in pulmonary inflammation and host defense. *Am J Respir Crit Care Med* 2005; 171: 606- 15.

[222] Thomsen RW., Riis A, Kornum JB., et al. Preadmission use of statins and outcomes after hospitalization with pneumonia : population-based cohort study of 29,900 patients. *Arch Intern Med* 2008; 168: 2081- 87.

[223] Chalmers JD, Singanayagam A, Murray MP, et al. Prior statin use is associated with improved outcomes in community-acquired pneumonia. *Am J Med* 2008; 168: 2081-87.

[224] Mortensen EM, Restrepo MI, Anzueto A, et al. The effect of prior statin use on 30-day mortality for patients hospitalized with community-acquired pneumonia. *Respi Res* 2005; 6: 82.

[225] Shyamsundar M., McKweon S., O'Kane C., et al. Simvastatin decreases lipopolysaccharide-induced pulmonary inflammation in healthy volunteers. *Am J Respir Crit Care Med* 2009; 179: 1107- 14.

[226] Li Q, Park PW, Wilson CL, et al. Matrilysin shedding of syndecan-1 regulates chemokine mobilization and transepithelial efflux of neutrophils in acute lung injury. *Cell* 2002; 111: 635- 46.

[227] Thomsen RW., Riis A, Kornum JB., et al. Preadmission use of statins and outcomes after hospitalization with pneumonia : population-based cohort study of 29,900 patients. *Arch Intern Med* 2008; 168: 2081- 87.

[228] Chalmers JD, Singanayagam A, Murray MP, et al. Prior statin use is associated with improved outcomes in community-acquired pneumonia. *Am J Med* 2008; 168: 2081-87.

[229] Mortensen EM, Restrepo MI, Anzueto A, et al. The effect of prior statin use on 30-day mortality for patients hospitalized with community-acquired pneumonia. *Respi Res* 2005; 6: 82.

[230] The Irish Critical Care Trials Group. Acute lung injury and the acute respiratory distress syndrome in Ireland: a prospective audit of epidemiology and management. *Crit Care* 2008; 12: R30

[231] Kor D., Iscimen R., Yilmaz M., et al. Statin administration did not influence the progression of lung injury or associated organ failures in a cohort of patients with acute lung injury. *Intensive Care Med* 2009; 35: 1494- 95.

[232] Craig T., Duffy M., Shyamsundar M., et al. A randomized clinical trial of hydroxymethylglutaryl-coenzyme A reductase inhibition for acute lung injury (The HARP study). *Am J Respir Crit Care Med* 2001; 183: 620-6.

[233] The National Heart, Lung, and Blood Institute ARDS Clinical Trials Network, Rosuvastatin for Sepsis-Associated Acute Respiratory Distress Syndrome, *N Engl J Med* 2014; 370:2191-2200

[234] Origitano TC, Wascher TM, Reichman OH, et al. Sustained increased cerebral blood flow with prophylactic hypertensive hypervolemic hemodilution (triple-H therapy) after subarachnoid hemorrhage. *Neurosurgery* 1990; 27: 729- 39

[235] Dorhout Mees SM, Rinkel GJ, Feigin VL, et al. Calcium antagonists for aneurysmal subarachnoid haemorrhage. *Cochrane Database Syst. Rev.* 2007; 3: CD000277.

[236] Sugawara T, Ayer R, Zhang JH. Role of statins in cerebral vasospasm. *Acta Neurochir Suppl.* 2008; 104:287-90.

[237] Sillberg VA, Wells GA and Perry JJ. Do statins improve outcomes and reduce the incidence of vasospasm after aneurismal subarachnoid hemorrhage: a meta-analysis. *Stroke* 2008; 39: 2622- 26.

[238] Cook AM, Hessel EA II. Meta-analysis of statins for aneurismal subarachnoid hemorrhage falls short. *Stroke* 2009; 40:e79.

[239] Kramer AH. Statins in the management of aneurismal subarachnoid hemorrhage – not (yet) a standard of care. *Stroke* 2009; 40: e80-81.

[240] Lynch JR, Wang H, McGirt MJ, et al. Simvastatin reduces vasospasm after aneurysmal subarachnoid hemorrhage: results of a pilot randomized clinical trial. *Stroke* 2005; 36: 2024-26

[241] Tseng MY, Czosnyka M, Richards H, et al. Effects of acute pravastatin treatment on cerebral vasospasm, autoregulation, and delayed ischemic deficits after aneurismal subarachnoid hemorrhage: a phase II randomized placebo-controlled trial. *Stroke* 2005; 36: 1627-32.

[242] Tseng MY, Hutchinson PJ, Czosnyka M, et al. Effects of acute pravastatin treatment on intensity of rescue therapy, length of inpatient stay, and 6-month outcome in patients after aneurismal subarachnoid hemorrhage. *Stroke* 2007; 38:1545-50.

[243] Chou SHY, Smith EE, Badjatia N, et al. A randomised, double-blind, placebo-controlled pilot study of simvastatin in aneurismal subarachnoid hemorrhage. *Stroke* 2008; 39: 2891- 93.

[244] Vergouwen MD, Meijers JC, Geskus RB, et al. Biological effects of simvastatin in patients with aneurismal subarachnoid hemorrhage - a double-blind, placebo-controlled randomized trial. *J Cereb Blood Flow Metab.* 2009; 29: 1444- 53.

[245] Vergouwen MD, de Haan RJ, Vermeulen M, et al. Effect of statin treatment on vasospasm, delayed cerebral ischemia, and functional outcome in patients with aneurismal subarachnoid hemorrhage: a systematic review and meta-analysis update. *Stroke* 2010; 41:e47-52.

[246] Kramer AH, Fletcher JJ. Statins in the management of patients with aneurysmal subarachnoid hemorrhage: a systematic review and meta-analysis. *Neurocritical care* 2010 Apr; 12(2): 285-296.

[247] Jachinski U, Scherer K, Lichtwark M, et al. Impact of treatment with pravastatin on delayed ischemic disease and mortality after aneurysmal subarachnoid hemorrhage. *Crit Care* 2008; 12 (Suppl 2): 112.

[248] Macedo S., Bello Y., Silva A, et al. Effects of simvastatin in prevention of vasospasm in nontraumatic subarachnoid hemorrhage: preliminary data. *Crit Care* 2009; 13 (Suppl 1): 103.

[249] Kramer AH, Gurka MJ, Nathan B, et al. Statin use was not associated with less vasospasm or improved outcome after subarachnoid hemorrhage. *Neurosurgery* 2008; 62: 422- 7.

[250] Kerz T., Victor A., Beyer C., et al. A case control study of statin and magnesium administration in patients after aneurismal subarachnoid hemorrhage: incidence of delayed cerebral ischemia and mortality. *Neurol Res.* 2008; 30: 893- 7.

[251] Kern M, Lam MM, Knuckey MW, et al. Statins may not protect against vasospasm in subarachnoid hemorrhage. *J Clin Neurosci.* 2009; 16: 527- 30.

[252] McGirt MJ, Garces Ambrossi GL, Huang J, et al. Simvastatin for the prevention of symptomatic cerebral vasospasm following aneurysmal subarachnoid hemorrhage: a single institution prospective cohort study. *J Neurosurg.* 2009; 110: 968- 74.

[253] Mokowitz SI, Ahrens C, Provencio JJ, et al. Prehemorrhage statin use and the risk of vasospasm after aneurysmal subarachnoid hemorrhage. *Surg Neurol.* 2009; 71: 311-8.

[254] Singhal AB, Topcuoglu MA, Dorer DJ, et al. SSRI and statin increases the risk of vasospasm after subarachnoid hemorrhage. *Neurology* 2005; 64: 1008- 13.

[255] Simvastatin in Aneurysmal Subarachnoid Haemorrhage (STASH) a Multicentre Randomised Controlled Clinical Trial; ClinicalTrials.gov: NCT00731627.

[256] Statins and Cerebral Blood Flow in Subarachnoid Hemorrhage (SAH); ClinicalTrials.gov: NCT00795288.

[257] High-dose Simvastatin for Aneurysmal Subarachnoid Haemorrhage (HDS-SAH); ClinicalTrials.gov identifier: NCT01077206.
[258] The Role of Statins in Preventing Cerebral Vasospasm Secondary to Subarachnoid Hemorrhage; ClinicalTrials.gov: NCT01346748.

In: Statins
Editor: Eric R. Travers

ISBN: 978-1-63463-057-3

Chapter 4

STATINS AND THE BRAIN: GOOD, BAD OR BOTH?

Simran D. S. Maggo and John C. Ashton*
Department of Pharmacology and Toxicology, School of Medical Sciences,
University of Otago, Dunedin, New Zealand

ABSTRACT

Statins are widely used drugs that reduce mortality associated with cardiovascular disease. Despite an extensive evidence base for both their efficacy and adverse effects, the effect of statins on the brain and behaviour remains controversial, with some types of data suggesting harmful effects from statins but with other types of data suggesting beneficial effects. This article reviews these diverse sources of evidence, combining information from randomised clinical trials, case studies and adverse reaction monitoring programs, preclinical research, and epidemiological studies. Statins are discussed for potential psychiatric effects, effects on learning and memory, neuroprotective effects, effects on Alzheimer's disease, and on cerebral blood flow. We conclude that although there is some evidence that high doses of statins may have adverse psychiatric effects in some people, these are rare and can be managed through dose alteration or change in statin, and should not impact on current practice for the use of statins management of cardiovascular disease.

Keywords: Adverse effects, Central nervous system (CNS), Cholesterol lowering medication, Hippocampus, Memory, Psychiatric adverse effects, Statins

---

* Corresponding author: Dr John C. Ashton; Address: Department of Pharmacology and Toxicology, School of Medical Sciences, University of Otago, P.O. Box 913, Dunedin, New Zealand. Email: john.ashton@otago.ac.nz; Phone: + 64 3 479 7266; Fax: +64 3 479 9140.

INTRODUCTION – THE STATIN/BRAIN CONTROVERSY

It is now clear that 3-hydroxy-3-methylglutaryl-coenzyme A (HMG CoA) inhibitors (statins) significantly reduce mortality associated with cardiovascular disease (CVD). Both the efficacy of statins [1-4], and their adverse reactions (adverse drug reactions, ADRs) [5-8] are well documented.

All statins have a HMG CoA like moiety present in their structure, (Figure 1.) As a result of this property statins competitively inhibit the HMG CoA reductase enzyme. The primary clinical effect of this is to reduce total cholesterol and low-density lipoprotein cholesterol (LDL-C) levels in the plasma, which in turn inhibits plaque formation in the pathogenesis of atherosclerosis, thus reducing CVD. However, HMG CoA reductase and its metabolic products are involved in a variety of cellular processes, such that tolerated doses are limited by adverse drug reactions (ADRs) that include myopathies and myalgia, liver dysfunction and, very rarely, rhabdomyolysis.

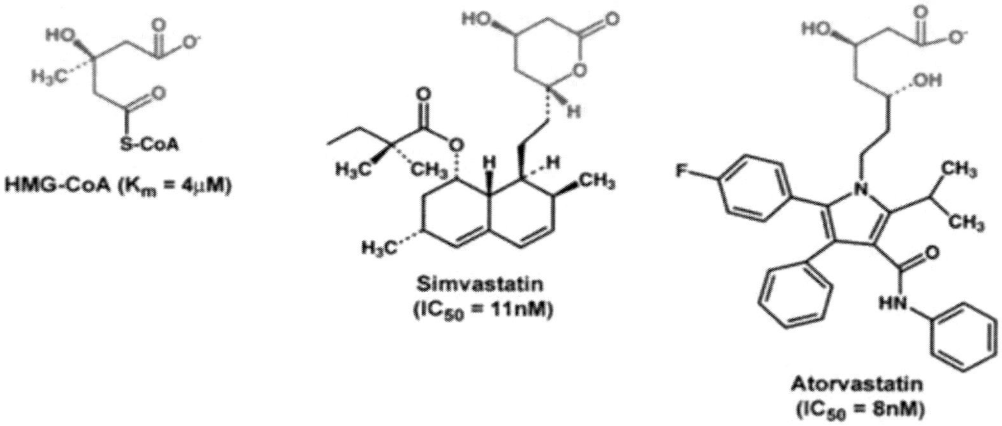

Figure 1. Chemical structures of statins. The chemical structures of the HMG CoA moiety and two commonly marketed statins, simvastatin and atorvastatin. The solo structure in red illustrates the HMG CoA moiety. A structurally similar red moiety present on statins competes for the binding site of the HMG CoA reductase enzyme with high potency indicated by the low IC50 values. Adapted from Istavan & Deisenhofer, 2001.

Along with these established clinical benefits and ADRs there has been much debate over the effect of statins on the brain. Statins have been suggested by various researchers and investigations to cause anything from memory loss to cognitive impairment to hallucinations. Much of the evidence for this has been anecdotal, or based on uncontrolled case-studies. Stronger evidence has come from ADR monitoring programs, but reviews of clinical trials have often failed to find convincing evidence of neurological or psychiatric effects, whether they are beneficial or harmful. In particular, the relationship between statin use and Alzheimer's disease (AD) has been particularly ambiguous, with some studies suggesting that statins are protective against AD whereas others have suggested that AD may be exacerbated by statins. Because of on-going concerns over the possible effects of statins on the brain and behaviour such as memory loss, forgetfulness and confusion, the US Food and Drug Administration (FDA) expanded its advisory statement on statin risks in 2012 [9].

It is the aim of this chapter to review the evidence for effects by statins on the brain. A wide body of evidence will be reviewed, including preclinical experiments, clinical trials and systematic reviews, pharmacovigilance data, and case studies. A variety of possible effects will be considered, including effects on memory, learning and synaptic plasticity, effects on mood and behaviour, as well as the evidence pertaining to effects on the onset and symptoms of AD. In order to place such evidence in its proper context, however, first the evidence for the benefits of statins will be reviewed and discussed.

THE UNDISPUTED CARDIOVASCULAR BENEFITS OF STATINS

CVDs are the most common cause of death globally. In 2008, the World Health Organisation (WHO) reported 17.3 million deaths attributed to CVDs, representing 30 % of all deaths worldwide. Further, WHO estimates 23.6 million deaths in 2030 will be attributed to CVD, particularly, from heart disease and stroke [10]. The Framingham heart study group, started in 1948, established the most common factors and/or characteristics in the development of CVD. Castelli et al., (1986) performed a follow-up study lasting 12 years on a cohort of 2489 men and 2856 women. At the end of the 12 year follow up, a total of 383 men and 277 women developed coronary heart disease (CHD) which was attributable to factors such as hypertension, and hypercholesterolemia [11]. In the study population, 27 % and 34 % of CHD in men and women, respectively, were attributed to elevated total cholesterol (TC) of ≥ 5.2 mmol/L [11]. Since then, meta-analysis of prospective studies has shown a linear relationship between increasing CVD risk and TC levels between 4.5-7.5 mmol/L [12].

The Framingham study group demonstrated that a low level of high-density lipoprotein cholesterol (HDL-C) could be a predictor of CVD risk [13, 14], but later studies suggested that the Total Cholesterol : High-density lipoprotein cholesterol (TC : HDL-C) ratio was a better and more accurate predictor of CVD risk compared to TC, LDL-C, or HDL-C individually [15]. Meta-analysis of prospective studies has provided evidence that a 1.0 mmol/L reduction in LDL-C results in a 30-35% risk reduction of CVD, specifically CHD and stroke [16].

Since the approval of the first statin in 1987, there have been numerous clinical trials that have established the benefits of reducing TC and LDL-C and how this translates to reduce CVD risk. That is, not only is lipid modification by statins associated with significant reductions in CVD, but a number of these high quality randomized clinical trials (RCTs) have shown directly that statins significantly reduce mortality associated with CVD in both primary and secondary prevention [17-19]. This has been demonstrated in particular by the Scandinavian Simvastatin Survival Study (4S) [20] and the Heart Protection Study [21], among other RCTs [22-25].

The Scandinavian Simvastatin Survival Study (4S) was the first of a series of landmark clinical trials and was conducted using 4444 patients with established CHD [26]. Patients were randomised to 20-40 mg of simvastatin or placebo and followed up for a median of 5.4 years. Simvastatin reduced TC and LDL-C up to 25 % and 35 % respectively which was attributed a 30 % and 34 % reduction in risk of death and major cardiovascular events respectively in the simvastatin group. The West of Scotland Coronary Prevention Study (WOSCOPS) was the first landmark *primary* prevention study [25]. Men with a fasting LDL-

C level of ≥ 4.0 mmol/L and ≤ 6.0 mmol/L but without any symptomatic CVD were randomised to receive 40 mg of pravastatin or placebo for 5 years. Pravastatin but not placebo lowered TC, LDL-C (26 %) and triglycerides as well as increasing HDL-C and resulted in a 24 % decrease in major coronary events in the pravastatin arm.

The 4S study and WOSCOPS study were followed by two *secondary* prevention trials, Cholesterol and Recurrent Events trial (CARE) [23], Long-term Intervention with Pravastatin Ischaemic Disease (LIPID) trial [27] and one primary prevention trial, the Air Force/Texas Coronary Atherosclerosis prevention Study (AFCAPS/TexCAPS) [22]. All showed that statin treatment was efficacious in improving lipid profiles and reducing the risk of CVD. A further landmark clinical trial, the Heart Protection Study was designed to investigate the long-term benefits of cholesterol-lowering therapy in patients at risk of death from CVD [21]. In the main study, inclusion criteria were that patients were aged 40-80 years with coronary disease or any other occlusive arterial disease or diabetes. In this largest reported study to date, 20,536 patients were randomised to receive 40 mg of simvastatin or placebo and followed up for 5 years. All-cause mortality was significantly reduced in the simvastatin group (12.9 %) compared with the placebo group (14.7 %) [21].

More recently, the Justification for the use of statins in prevention, an intervention trial evaluating rosuvastatin (JUPITER) (primary prevention trial) was terminated early based on unequivocal evidence for reduction of CVD and related mortality. In addition, 20 mg rosuvastatin treatment reduced LDL-C levels by 50 % and C-reactive protein (CRP by 37 %). C-reactive protein is an inflammatory biomarker that has been shown to predict vascular events independently of LDL-C [28]. However, a genetic study later in 2009 suggested that there was no association between CHD, *CRP* genotype and CRP plasma levels. This result suggests that CRP may just be an indicator and not a direct causal factor for developing CHD. Furthermore, the protective effects in the JUPITER trial can be attributed to LDL-C lowering [29, 30]. Since the JUPITER trial, several clinical trials of statins have demonstrated significant reductions in CVD events compared to placebo. Overall, the risk of CVD compared appears to be reduced by statins by about 25-33 %. This has prompted the design of studies to aggressively lower LDL-C levels, which usually requires higher doses (intensive therapy).

The TNT (Treating to New Targets trial and PROVE-IT (Pravastatin or Atorvastatin Evaluation and Infection Therapy) compared standard versus intensive statin therapy [31, 32]. In the TNT trial, patients were randomised to receive either 10mg or 80mg atorvastatin and followed up for a median of 5 years. Higher doses resulted in enhanced LDL-C reduction that was associated with a 22 % and 25 % relative risk reduction in myocardial infarction and stroke respectively. However, intensive therapy was significantly ($p<0.001$) associated with persistent elevations in plasma alanine amino transferase (ALT) but not creatine kinase (CK), markers of statin toxicity (see below) [31]. The PROVE-IT trial investigated the effect of 40 mg pravastatin therapy compared with 80 mg atorvastatin therapy in patients with acute coronary syndrome. Atorvastatin treatment resulted in significantly reduced LDL-C (1.6 mmol/L) compared with pravastatin treatment (2.46 mmol/L). Similar to the TNT trial, a greater number of patients (3.3 %) on intensive atorvastatin therapy had persistent elevation in ALT compared with pravastatin therapy (1.1 %). However, intensive atorvastatin therapy also resulted in 3.3 % of patients with myalgia, muscle aches or elevations in CK in comparison to 2.7 % in the pravastatin arm [33]. These studies made it clear that increasing statin dose increases the likelihood of adverse drug reactions. Increasing the statin dose is suggested for high-risk patients with a 5-year cardiovascular risk profile greater than 15 % (i.e., a 0.15 probability of having a cardiovascular event within 5 years) [34]. In this population it is suggested that the advantages of lipid lowering therapy outweigh the moderately increased risk of ADRs. Lipid targets are based on calculated 5-year CVD risk tables. For example, the New Zealand Primary Care Handbook [34] suggests a target lipid profile of TC of < 4.0 mmol/L and LDL-C < 2.0 mmol/L in a patient with established CVD or at CVD risk of >15 %. Achieving such goals may require intensive treatment, which, as discussed above, is likely to increase the risk of statin-associated adverse events. These are discussed further in the section below.

Established Adverse Drug Reactions of Statins

The most commonly reported statin-associated ADRs are indicated by elevations in ALT and CK levels, which are associated with liver toxicity and muscle myalgia, respectively. Even though they are the most commonly reported ADRs of statin therapy, myopathies and hepatotoxicity are classed as rare events and are reported to occur in 1-5 % of all patients initiated on statin therapy [35, 36]. Both types of ADRs are reported to become more frequent in a dose dependent manner [37-39]. A meta-analysis of 18 randomised controlled trials revealed a total of 1017 ADRs in statin-treated patients compared with 811 in the placebo group, such that statin therapy increased the risk of any adverse event by 39 % compared with placebo [38]. More specifically, 316 incidents of myopathy were reported in the statin group compared with 253 in the placebo group. Abnormal liver function tests (609 reports) (i.e., transaminase levels >3X the upper limit of normal [ULN] were reported in the statin group compared with 487 cases in the placebo group [38]. However, another meta-analysis of 35 randomized clinical trials, including >70 000 patients, revealed that the risk of myalgia (15.4 % and 18.6 % in the statin-treated and placebo groups, respectively) and rhabdomyolysis (0.2 % and 0.1 % in the statin-treated and placebo groups, respectively) with statin (simvastatin, atorvastatin, fluvastatin, rosuvastatin and lovastatin) therapy was not significantly increased in the statin-treatment groups [40]. The meta-analysis did, however, reveal a significantly increased risk of elevated ALT levels in the statin-treated group (1.4 % and 1.1 % in the statin-treated and placebo groups, respectively) [40]. Despite these ADRs, statins continue to be the drug of first choice in the treatment of hypercholesterolemia, and as long ago as 2004 were prescribed to over 20 million people worldwide [35]. In other words, the benefits of statin use with respect to CVD risk are considered to clearly outweigh the risks and severity of adverse events.

Mechanism of Action of Statins

Statins competitively inhibit HMG CoA reductase, which is the rate-limiting step during the process of cholesterol biosynthesis (Figure 2) [41]. By this means statins cause a reduction in the amount of endogenously synthesised cholesterol. This results in the up-regulation of LDL-receptors on most mammalian cells and therefore an increase in the uptake of cholesterol and LDL-C from systemic circulation [42].

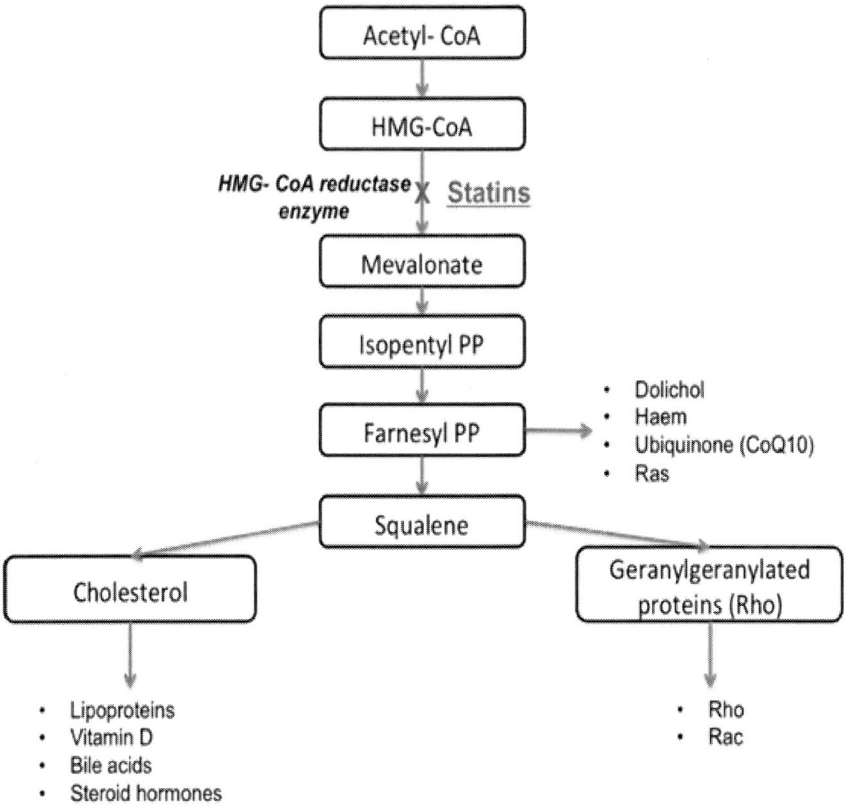

Figure 2. Mevalonate pathway. The mevalonate pathway showing the endogenous synthesis of cholesterol. Statins competitively inhibit the rate limiting enzyme, HMG- CoA reductase, hence inhibiting the endogenous synthesis of cholesterol.

Lipid homeostasis is regulated by a group of transcription factors; sterol regulatory element binding proteins (SREBPs). SREBP2 and SREBP1c regulate genes involved in cholesterol metabolism and in fatty acid and triglyceride metabolism respectively [42]. Hence, the reduction in cholesterol synthesis that results from statin therapy causes the induction of SREBPs. These act as transcription factors within the nuclei of cells, activating genes that regulate the expression of LDL-receptors [42, 43]. These processes have been demonstrated experimentally in mice fed with a diet containing 0.1 % simvastatin for two weeks. This induced a 2-fold increase in the number of LDL receptors expressed on skeletal muscles and a 1.5-fold increase in HMG CoA reductase activity compared to mice on a normal diet [43]. When the SREB2 gene is transgenically overexpressed in mice, there is an 11-fold increase in the amount of cholesterol in the livers of the transgenic mice [44].

The linear relationship between increasing plasma LDL-C and CVD risk established by the Framingham study group makes it plausible that the lipid-lowering effect of statins is solely responsible for reducing the risk of CVD [45]. However, data from the Heart Protection Study (HPS) has suggested that patients in the simvastatin arm who did not achieve a substantial decrease in LDL-C still benefited from reduced mortality and morbidity [46]. Further analysis of both large scale randomised clinical trials (RCTs) and smaller statin studies has identified non-lipid lowering effects such as improvement in endothelial function, reduction in inflammation, antithrombotic activity and improvements in hypertension [46-48].

This suggests that statins may act in a variety of ways to reduce the risk of CVD, and not solely through lipid reduction.

Mechanisms of Statin-Induced Adverse Drug Reactions

Several different mechanisms have been hypothesised to explain the hepatotoxicity and myopathy caused by statins. The most probable mechanism of muscle myopathy is depletion of cholesterol within the myocyte cell wall and/or the depletion of key intermediates from the mevalonate pathway (Figure 2) [49]. Statin-induced psychiatric ADRs have been hypothesised to result from reductions in cholesterol within cell membranes, particularly within the brain [50-52]. *In vitro* studies have also demonstrated deleterious effects such as inhibiting the formation of neuronal synapses [53] and impairing synaptic plasticity [54] (see below).

Brain tissue only accounts for 2-3 % of the body's total mass but has such a high metabolic demand that it uses 20 % of the body's oxygen and 50 % of total body glucose [55]. As has been suggested for muscle and liver ADRs, depletion of one intermediary of the mevalonate pathway, ubiquinone (often referred to as Co-enzyme Q10, (CoQ10)) [49] and mitochondrial dysfunction has been suggested to have a role in statin-induced psychiatric ADRs [56, 57]. Co-enzyme Q10 is an essential anti-oxidant, and is part of the oxidative phosphorylation system that generates ATP in mitochondria [58]. Some animal studies have demonstrated that statins can reduce CoQ10 levels in cardiac muscle [59], but other studies have produced inconsistent results [60]. For example, one study using rabbits reported significant reductions in skeletal muscle CoQ10 (72 %) with simvastatin or pravastatin treatment [61] whereas another in study high dose statin treatment (50 mg/kg) was associated with severe skeletal muscle lesions on biopsy but not with reduced levels of CoQ10 [62].

Tavintharan (2007) investigated the role of simvastatin on hepatic cells. Hepatic cells (HepG2) were incubated with simvastatin ranging from 0-10 μM for 18 hours. As was expected, simvastatin dose dependently inhibited the activity of HMG CoA reductase enzyme. However, simvastatin also significantly increased cell death (by 13 % compared to control) at the highest dose (10 μM). Cell-death was inhibited if cells were co-incubated with CoQ10 (10 μg/ml), which reduced cell death by 6-fold. Simvastatin also dose-dependently reduced mitochondrial CoQ10 and significantly increased oxidative damage to nuclear DNA. Again, co-incubation with 10 μg/ml CoQ10 provided significant protection [63].

No clinical study has yet established that reduction in CoQ10 enzyme levels by statin therapy correlate with severity of myopathy, although one study has shown that CoQ10 enzyme levels were significantly lower in statin-treated patients (0.75±0.04 mg, n=40) compared to untreated hypercholesteraemic patients (0.95± 0.09 mg, n=20) [64]. Two further RCTs were designed to specifically to assess the protective effect of CoQ10 supplementation. The first study was conducted in 41 patients and investigated the effect of 400 IU of Vitamin E or 100 mg of CoQ10 for 30 days. These patients had improved subjectively assessed pain scores and fewer muscle-related symptoms [65]. The second study used 44 dyslipidaemic patients that had been previously assessed for statin-induced myalgia. These patients were allocated into groups administered simvastatin (10-40 mg/d) together with 200 mg/d CoQ10. This study found no difference in myalgia scores or statin tolerance with the addition of CoQ10.

STATINS AND ALZHEIMER'S DISEASE – EVIDENCE IN FAVOUR

Alzheimer's disease (AD) is a neurodegenerative disease with progressive memory loss and abnormal psychological behaviour. Various researchers have attempted to determine whether statin treatment can prevent or delay the onset of AD [66-70]. There are theoretical reasons for expecting a protective effect by statins with respect to AD, which is characterised by aggregations of amyloid beta (Aβ) plaques in the brain. These result from altered proteolytic processing of the amyloid precursor protein (APP). The resulting Aβ aggregations are neurotoxic [71, 72].

Cholesterol homeostasis is known to correlate with various stages of AD. Observations that have been made with 24(*s*)-hydroxy-cholesterol (the major breakdown product of brain cholesterol) have revealed that patients in the early stages of AD have increased plasma levels of 24s-hydroxycholesterol, whereas patients in the late stages of AD have low levels of 24s-hydroxycholesterol [73, 74]. This may be partially explained through the demyelination of neurons in the early stages of AD and hence higher plasma concentrations of 24(*s*)-hydroxy-cholesterol. In later stages of AD the lower 24(*s*)-hydroxy-cholesterol plasma levels may be explained by atrophy of the structures responsible for producing the enzyme 24(*s*)-hydroxylase [73, 74].

The aetiology of AD is thought to be multifactorial and to involve a (highly debated) genetic component. Genetic mutations in genes coding for *APP, presenilin 1* and *2* are associated with the rare, early onset form of AD. In addition, a genetic risk factor, the *APOE* gene, specifically the E4 allele is associated with an increased risk of both familial late-onset and sporadic late onset AD [75]. Apolipoprotein E (APOE) binds to lipids and lipoprotein receptors and modulates cellular lipoprotein levels by altering the mobilisation and redistribution of cholesterol. In the CNS, cholesterol is required for repair, growth and remodelling of axons and synapses, processes that are crucial for memory and learning. In particular, cholesterol is thought to have a role in the activity of β-Secretase which is involved in processing of APP and, hence, accumulation of Aβ aggregates [73]. Therefore, it has been suggested that elevated levels of cholesterol may promote Alzheimer's disease pathology by inducing an aggregation of amyloid beta plaques [76, 77].

Because of these considerations, and because some statins are able to cross the blood-brain barrier [78-82], it has been suggested that statins may help prevent the progression of AD. It is important to stress that statins do not directly reduce central nervous system (CNS) cholesterol, but rather alter CNS cholesterol *homeostasis*. A further consideration is that elevated levels of plasma cholesterol have been well established as a significant risk factor for cerebrovascular disease [11, 83] and patients suffering from cerebral infarcts with existing Alzheimer's disease pathology are at 20-fold increased risk of developing dementia [84].

It has therefore seemed plausible that lowering cholesterol through statin therapy may be a therapeutic option in the treatment and prevention of Alzheimer's disease [85] and indeed experiments using rodent models have shown that statins improve pathophysiological features of AD in these models - such as reductions in extracellular depositions of amyloid beta and intracellular accumulation of hyper-phosphorylated Tau protein - as well as causing behavioural improvements such as reversal of memory deficits [86-88]. In other studies, statins have also shown to improve cognitive measures in rodent models. For example, simvastatin (40 mg/kg for 3 months) fully restored short- and long-term memory in six-month-old transgenic mice. While this finding was not replicated in 12-month-old mice, simvastatin treatment was reported to rescue markers of cerebrovascular activity and endothelial nitric oxide synthesis [89]. Other studies have demonstrated improvement in learning and memory in rats orally administered atorvastatin (10 or 20 mg/kg/d) or rosuvastatin (20 mg/kg/d) for 90 days using the "shuttle box", a tool used to assess memory retention and active avoidance in rodents [90]. Similarly, the same authors have demonstrated that atorvastatin (10 mg/kg/d) or rosuvastatin (10mg/kg/d) reversed the effects of diazepam-induced amnesia, and preserved long-term memory [90].

There is also now a considerable body of epidemiological evidence that support a protective role for statins in AD [68, 91-93]. A meta-analysis incorporating seven studies was used to quantify the risk of AD with statin use and revealed that the risk of cognitive impairment was significantly reduced in patients on statin therapy compared to non-statin users (Relative Risk=0.43). Similarly, in a further meta-analysis of 20 studies, statin use was associated with a reduced risk of AD and all-type dementia (Relative Risk = 0.70) [94], and in a meta-analysis comparing short-term vs long-term treatment, short-term patients were associated with no cognitive adverse reactions, while long-term patients were associated with a beneficial effect with respect to dementia. Pooled results showed an average 29 % reduction in the incidence of dementia [95].

STATINS AND ALZHEIMER'S DISEASE – EVIDENCE AGAINST

Despite the theoretical, arguments and the pre-clinical, and epidemiological evidence favouring the use of statins for AD prevention, two large RCTs involving statins, the Heart Protection Study (HPS) [21] involving over 20,000 patients prescribed simvastatin and the Prospective Study of Pravastatin in the Elderly at Risk (PROSPER) study involving over 5000 patients showed there was no effect of statin therapy on the prevalence of dementia or development of AD [21, 25]. A Cochrane review of these two trials (HPS and PROSPER) concluded that there was no benefit of statin treatment with respect to the prevention of dementia [96]. The preclinical experiments in support of statins for AD have also been criticised, particularly the aggressive nature of animal models used in Alzheimer's disease research [97-99].

Padala et al., (2012) have published the results of a 12-week prospective pilot study investigating the effect of statin therapy in patients with AD. Patients were recruited if they were 60 years of age with a history or new diagnosis of AD with an MMSE (mini-mental state examination) score of > 10 and currently on statin therapy for at least six weeks. At the start of the study patients underwent an MMSE and a CERAD (Consortium to Establish a Registry for Alzheimer's Disease) neuropsychological battery of testing. Thereafter, patients were advised to stop taking statin therapy for six weeks. After six weeks, patients underwent neuropsychological testing again, and then were re-started on statin therapy at their previous dose for a period of six weeks. At the end of the 12-week study patients underwent the battery of neuropsychological testing. The results of this pilot study showed that patients with pre-existing dementia whom were *withdrawn from statin treatment* showed a significant improvement in MMSE scores but no improvement in the CERAD neuropsychological battery score. Furthermore, when patients were re-challenged with statin therapy, MMSE scores deteriorated to levels at the beginning of the study [100]. Even though only 18 patients completed this study, the results appear to suggest that statins can negatively affect cognition in patients with *existing* dementia.

To sum up the last two sections, with respect to epidemiological studies there are no studies that suggest statins *increase* the risk of AD. Overall, there is equivocal evidence with respect to AD and statins, and therefore as previously concluded by the Cochrane review, there is insufficient evidence to recommend statins for the treatment and/or prevention of AD [101].

STATINS AND NEUROPROTECTION

Preclinical experiments into the effects of statins on AD have been part of a wider research program aimed at investigating the neuroprotective properties of statins. A number of studies have now been carried out to assess the effect of statins after CNS trauma, such as traumatic brain injury and stroke [102-106]. A review published by van der Most (2009) identified studies that showed a neuroprotective effect of statins. Twelve studies were identified which investigated the effects of statins on memory function before or after brain insult, either chemically or mechanically. All twelve studies demonstrated an improvement or beneficial effect of statin treatment in models of behaviour and learning. As an example, a recent study showed that simvastatin protects against kainite-induced excitotoxicity and memory impairments in mice [107]. Although this study has important implications for stroke and TBI, what can one conclude in a non-pathologic state? The authors suggested that statins attenuate kainate-induced overstimulation of glutamate receptors (kainate and α–amino-3-hydroxy-5-methyl-4-isoxazolepropionic acid receptors (AMPARs)) by direct interaction with the receptors.

Stroke is a major area of research intensively looking for neuroprotective agents, and statins have been an agent used in several pre-clinical trials. For example, Endres et al., (1998) assessed the effect of 14 days of pre-treatment with statins in a murine stroke model. This study was the first to show that, compared with controls, pre-treatment with statins reduced infarct size, improved cerebral blood flow and improved neurologic function [108]. The concept of pre-treatment of statins offering a degree of protection against the neurotoxic insult of stroke has since been replicated [109, 110]. Statins have also been trialled after the induction of stroke. A study by Sironi et al., (2003) showed that compared with controls, administration of simvastatin (20 mg/kg) after the onset of stroke significantly reduced infarct size and increased the expression of endothelial nitric oxide (eNOS) on blood vessels in the brain. Similarly, this has been reproduced in various animal models of stroke with varying doses of statins [111-113]. Statins have also shown to enhance the time-window of tissue plasminogen activator (tPA – Alteplase) in a rat model of embolic stroke [114]. One possible mechanism through which statins may be neuroprotective is by suppressing inflammation. For example, Pahan and colleagues reported that lovastatin (10 μM) and mevastatin (10 μM) inhibited lipopolysaccharide (LPS) induced inflammation in the CNS [115]. Mediators of inflammation were not, however, reduced when compared with control animals.

The potential of statins as possible neuroprotective agents continues to be a field of active research interest [86-88]. However, the significant improvements seen in animal models have not been replicated in clinical trials [97-99, 116].

STATINS AND PSYCHIATRIC ADVERSE EFFECTS

Patient case histories and post-marketing surveillance by pharmacovigilance authorities have documented mood disorders, cognitive disorders (amnesia), sleep disorders (insomnia and nightmares) and perception disorders (including hallucinations) in patients receiving statins [51, 117-119, 120, 121]. However, the association of statin therapy with psychiatric events has not at the time of writing been specifically assessed through clinical trials. Specifically, clinical trials have provided no evidence of statin-induced depression or suicidal behaviour associated with cholesterol reduction [122, 123].

Pharmacovigilance monitoring and patient case histories have indicated that statins may induce amnesia [117, 118, 120]. Statins have also been reported to induce psychiatric or CNS-related ADRs. The New Zealand Pharmacovigilance Centre (NZPhvC) reported an increase in the number of statin-induced psychiatric adverse events over the period of 2000-2005 [120]. Up to 2005, 21 % [145] of all reported simvastatin-induced ADRs were psychiatric in nature. Specifically, 26 psychiatric adverse event reports with atorvastatin, 24 with fluvastatin and 8 with pravastatin had been reported in New Zealand [120]. Additionally, of the 203 psychiatric reports received, 40 reports describe how the psychiatric condition regressed upon withdrawal of the statin and recurred upon re-challenge [120].

These data are controversial however. One recent review of the literature concluded that the evidence for psychiatric associations with statin treatment is ambiguous, and often conflicting, with negative, positive or no effect associated with statin treatment in different studies [124]. In fact it has been concluded by some authors that long-term statin use is associated with beneficial psychological outcomes [125].

Preclinical evidence of psychiatric ADRs is ambiguous. Some studies have suggested instead that that simvastatin has anxiolytic properties [126, 127]. Both of these cited studies utilised Sprague–Dawley rats using the anxiety-elevated plus maze or open field tests. The rats received a dose of 10 mg/kg/d, which equates to more than 100 mg/d in a 80 kg adult human, calculated using a literature standard dose translation tool of body surface area [128]. This is in excess of the maximal clinical dose and is associated with an increased risk of adverse effects [37]. By contrast, we [129] found that a comparatively low dose (0.5 mg/kg/d atorvastatin or 1 mg/kg/d simvastatin) treatment with statins had subtle effects on thigmotaxis in the Morris water maze (MWM), which may be interpreted as anxiogenic. The doses used in the contrast with Madsen et al., (2008) used 0.1-1.2 mg/kg cerivastatin, 50-200 mg/kg pravastatin, and 10-100 mg/kg rosuvastatin, and 25-250 mg/kg atorvastatin in guinea pig. In that study, total cholesterol and LDL-C reduction as well as an increase in CK levels were dose-dependent [130]. However, Madsen et al., (2008) only dosed over 10 days, and some animals that received 150 mg/kg atorvastatin died during the study. Baytan et al., (2008) administered 4 weeks of 10 mg/kg/day simvastatin to Sprague Dawley rats, which resulted in impaired performance in the Barnes maze test of spatial memory – though this did not appear to be a dose dependent effect, as behavioural deficits were not reported in rats dosed with 30 mg/kg/day simvastatin [130, 131].

Statins, Neuroplasticity and Memory

One of the main psychiatric ADRs attributed to statins in pharmacovigilance studies (see above) is memory loss. To take one case report as an illustration, a 65-year-old male had been prescribed atorvastatin (10 mg/day) for 1 year. A range of neurocognitive testing demonstrated significantly reduced performance in cognitive (Hopkins Verbal Learning Test, Visuospatial memory test and Wechsler Adult Intelligence Scale) and working memory (Sternberg Task) tests. Furthermore, functional magnetic resonance imaging (fMRI) showed impaired neuronal activation in the dorso-lateral prefrontal cortex and over activation in the pre-frontal cortex (key areas of memory, attention and executive cognitive functions) during the working memory test. Two months after stopping atorvastatin, all parameters assessed through cognitive and fMRI testing had returned to baseline levels. The patient reported further subjective improvements at a 5-month follow up [132]. This was the first clinical study to provide fMRI evidence of statin-induced memory and cognitive impairment, other case series and reports have documented similar objective and subjective symptoms of memory loss following initiation of statin therapy [118, 133-135].

There is also a growing body of evidence from rodent studies that statins, particularly simvastatin and atorvastatin, can cross the blood brain barrier (BBB) [136] and can affect memory as well as synaptic plasticity, irrespective of the presence of injury or AD. However, the impact of statins on processes of memory and learning has not been clearly established. Very few laboratory studies have directly aimed to investigate psychiatric effects of statins. In similar fashion to the human evidence, animal studies across differing rodent species and behavioural models have produced conflicting results [119, 131, 137, 138].

One type of evidence comes from examining the effects of statins on control animals in neuroprotection studies. In the review published by van der Most (2009) discussed above on the neuroprotective effect of statins, no changes were identified in statin-treated controls compared with untreated controls. On the other hand in *vitro* studies have demonstrated deleterious effects such as inhibiting the formation of neuronal synapses [53] and impairing synaptic plasticity [54]. Long-term potentiation (LTP), an extensively studied form of synaptic plasticity, and a candidate mechanism for memory formation within the CNS, specifically within the hippocampus [139, 140], has been shown to be both enhanced or inhibited by statins, depending on animal model used [141-143].

The majority of electrophysiological and behavioural assessment of statins has been conducted in rat or mouse models [141, 144]. However, the authors of this review have carried out a series of experiments using guinea pigs, which more closely model lipid metabolism in humans [129, 145]. In these studies we found that administration of statins (to a maximal dose of 1 mg/kg/d atorvastatin and 2 mg/kg/d simvastatin) adversely affected performance in working memory (short-term memory) but not reference (long-term) memory tests – as assessed through the Morris Water Maze (MWM). In dissected hippocampal slices, both atorvastatin and simvastatin impaired LTP in a dose dependent manner (1-10 μM bath application). In these experiments we found evidence that pre-synaptic activity is modified by statins. Specifically, LTP can cause an increase or a decrease in the paired pulse ratio (PPR) depending on the initial PPR [146, 147]. Higher PPR prior to the induction of LTP is likely to result in a larger PPR after LTP and vice versa [147]. In our experiments simvastatin and atorvastatin (3 μM) both resulted in a decrease in the PPR after the induction of LTP; this is characteristic of paired pulse depression. Postulated mechanisms of paired pulse depression include a decrease in amount of pre-synaptic neurotransmitter release through activation of metabotropic receptors or retrograde release of neuromodulators such as dopamine or retrograde messengers such as endogenous cannabinoids from the post-synaptic site [148].

In comparison to results obtained using guinea pigs, Mans et al., (2010) demonstrated that a 20-minute incubation of hippocampal slices from C57Bl/6 mice in 10 μM simvastatin had no effect on the induction of LTP in area CA1. However, that study reported that a 2-4 hour incubation in simvastatin (10 μM) *enhanced* LTP by 21 % [141]. By contrast, in our experiments there was a 41 % attenuation of LTP by 10 μM simvastatin and 53 % attenuation by atorvastatin after only a 10-minute bath application [145]. Mans et al., (2010) utilised C57Bl/6 mice that express robust LTP compared with other mouse strains [149]. In addition, Mans et al., used a different LTP induction paradigm from our experiments [145]. This is important because it has been suggested that different LTP induction protocols induce LTP of varying strength and persistence [150, 151].

Pro-cognitive effects have been demonstrated in statin-treated rats, using both MWM and T-maze tasks. It has been demonstrated that atorvastatin and simvastatin attenuate alprazolam- and scopolamine-induced spatial memory deficits [119]. Also, Allami et al., (2011) demonstrated a reversal of scopolamine-induced memory impairment by atorvastatin treatment (1 and 5 mg/kg) in mice. Atorvastatin administered 30 minutes prior to scopolamine administration reversed scopolamine (1 mg/kg) induced spatial memory deficits as measure using a Y-Maze test [137]. These results have been reproduced by the same laboratory [137, 138].

Similarly a study conducted in male Wistar rats showed that pre-treatment with atorvastatin and rosuvastatin (10 and 20 mg/kg respectively) significantly attenuated diazepam-induced cognitive deficits as assessed through various neurocognitive tasks (shuttle box test and the step through & step down task) [90]. A further study compared the effects of commercially available statins (simvastatin, lovastatin, fluvastatin, pravastatin, and atorvastatin) on neuron damage and memory impairment in a mouse model of systemic administration of kainate. Simvastatin was the most effective statin in reducing the deleterious effects caused by kainate, including the severity of seizures, excitotoxicity, oxidative damage, neuritic dystrophy and apoptosis in the hippocampus and other limbic structures of the brain cortex.

Lovastatin was beneficial with respect to preventing seizures and histopathological signs of excitotoxicity. Other statins studied (fluvastatin, pravastatin, and atorvastatin) did not show any antiepileptic nor neuroprotective effects. Furthermore, it was reported that simvastatin enhanced episodic-like memory [107]. Another recent study demonstrated that statin (simvastatin – 20 mg/kg/d bw or pravastatin – 25 mg/kg/d bw) treatment for four months but not 15 days showed a significant increase in memory function using the elevated plus maze and step down passive avoidance tasks [152].

Statins, Cerebrovascular Blood Flow and Post-operative Delirium

Statins can alter the tone of smooth muscle through modulation of the expression of endothelial nitric oxide (eNOS). An increase in eNOS activity can result in vasodilation of the arterioles and redistribution of blood flow to the microvasculature [153, 154]. While this mechanism has reported benefits in stroke and neurologic trauma, altered cerebral blood-flow has been reported to predispose patients to delirium after anaesthesia [155]. Redelmeier et al., (2008) investigated this effect of statins in patients undergoing elective surgery. Using a retrospective cohort design, the investigators isolated 284,158 patients 65 years or older who had undergone elective surgery in the Canadian Institutes for Health Information database. Out of these, 7 % (19 501) of patients were reported to be taking statins prior to surgery. The investigators used a multivariate model to account for preceding predictors such as surgery type and duration, and concluded that patients on statin therapy prior to surgery had a 28 % increased risk of post-operative delirium. This study was conducted in the elderly population who often take neuropsychiatric medicine for anxiety or sleep. Therefore, the investigators attempted to control for this confound, and did not find an increased risk in patients taking concomitant neuropsychiatric medication [156].

Conclusion

Reports of statin-associated cognitive impairment have been found primarily in observational studies (i.e., case reports/series). One randomised controlled trial has demonstrated that simvastatin impaired some measures of cognition compared to placebo. However, the majority of randomised controlled trials and observational studies, statins were found to have either a neutral or beneficial effect on cognition. Some data suggest that statins that are less lipophilic (pravastatin and rosuvastatin) may be less likely to contribute to cognitive impairment due to limited penetration across the blood-brain barrier. These drugs would be a logical alternative in cases where cognitive impairment secondary to another statin is suspected. Therefore, if statin-associated cognitive impairment is suspected, a trial discontinuation may be attempted to evaluate if the statin is at fault and, switching from lipophilic to hydrophilic statins may resolve suspected cognitive adverse effects. The cardiovascular benefits have been repeatedly been assessed as outweighing the risk of cognitive impairment associated with statin use. Therefore, while the current evidence from human observational studies does not support changing practice with respect to statin use, emerging animal data which suggest that statins may induce cognitive deficits needs further evaluation.

Conflict of Interest

None.

REFERENCES

[1] Balk EM, Karas, Richard H., Jordan, Harmon S., Kupelnick, Bruce., Chew, Priscilla., Lau, Joseph. Effects of statins on vascular structure and function: A systematic review. *The American Journal of Medicine.* 2004;117(10):775-90.

[2] Bays H. Statin Safety: An Overview and Assessment of the Data--2005. *The American Journal of Cardiology.* 2006;97(8, Supplement 1):S6-S26.

[3] Ross SD, Allen IE, Connelly JE, Korenblat BM, Smith ME, Bishop D, et al. Clinical Outcomes in Statin Treatment Trials: A Meta-analysis. *Arch Intern Med.* 1999;159(15):1793-802.

[4] Wierzbicki AS, Mikhailidis DP. Dose-response effects of atorvastatin and simvastatin on high-density lipoprotein cholesterol in hypercholesterolaemic patients: a review of five comparative studies. *Int J Cardiol.* 2002;84(1):53-7.

[5] Pasternak RC, Smith SC, Jr., Bairey-Merz CN, Grundy SM, Cleeman JI, Lenfant C. ACC/AHA/NHLBI clinical advisory on the use and safety of statins. *J Am Coll Cardiol.* 2002;40(3):567-72.

[6] Davidson MH, Clark JA, Glass LM, Kanumalla A. Statin Safety: An Appraisal from the Adverse Event Reporting System. *The American Journal of Cardiology.* 2006;97(8, Supplement 1):S32-S43.

[7] Wilke RA, Lin DW, Roden DM, Watkins PB, Flockhart D, Zineh I, et al. Identifying genetic risk factors for serious adverse drug reactions: current progress and challenges. *Nat Rev Drug Discov.* 2007;6(11):904-16.

[8] Bolego C, Baetta R, Bellosta S, Corsini A, Paoletti R. Safety considerations for statins. *Curr Opin Lipidol.* 2002;13(6):637-44.

[9] FDA. FDA Drug Safety Communication: Important safety label changes to cholesterol-lowering statin drugs 2012 [cited 2012 09.02.14]. Available from: http://www.fda.gov/forconsumers/consumerupdates/ucm293330.htm.

[10] WHO. Global Atlas on Cardiovascular Disease Prevention and Control. Mendis S PP, Norrving, Backx PH, editors. Geneva: WHO; 2011 2011.

[11] Castelli WP, Garrison RJ, Wilson PW, Abbott RD, Kalousdian S, Kannel WB. Incidence of coronary heart disease and lipoprotein cholesterol levels. The Framingham Study. *JAMA: The Journal of the American Medical Association.* 1986;256(20):2835-8.

[12] Law MR, Wald NJ, Thompson SG. By how much and how quickly does reduction in serum cholesterol concentration lower risk of ischaemic heart disease? *BMJ.* 1994;308(6925):367-72.

[13] Kannel W, Castelli W, Gordon T, McNamara P. Serum cholesterol, lipoproteins, and the risk of coronary heart disease. The Framingham study. *Ann Intern Med.* 1971;74 (1):1-12.

[14] Wilson PWF, D'Agostino RB, Levy D, Belanger AM, Silbershatz H, Kannel WB. Prediction of Coronary Heart Disease Using Risk Factor Categories. *Circulation.* 1998;97(18):1837-47.

[15] Haq IU, Ramsay LE, Jackson PR, Wallis EJ. Prediction of coronary risk for primary prevention of coronary heart disease: a comparison of methods. *QJM.* 1999;92(7):379-85.

[16] Qizilbash N, Lewington S, Duffy S, Peto R. Cholesterol, diastolic blood pressure, and stroke: 13 000 strokes in 450 000 people in 45 prospective cohorts. *The Lancet.* 1995;346(8991-8892):1647-53.

[17] Vrecer M, Turk S, Drinovec J, Mrhar A. Use of statins in primary and secondary prevention of coronary heart disease and ischemic stroke. Meta-analysis of randomized trials. *International Journal of Clinical Pharmacolgy and Therapeutics.* 2003;41(12):567-77.

[18] Cheung BMY, Lauder IJ, Lau C-P, Kumana CR. Meta-analysis of large randomized controlled trials to evaluate the impact of statins on cardiovascular outcomes. *Br J Clin Pharmacol.* 2004;57(5):640-51.

[19] Brugts JJ, Yetgin T, Hoeks SE, Gotto AM, Shepherd J, Westendorp RGJ, et al. The benefits of statins in people without established cardiovascular disease but with cardiovascular risk factors: meta-analysis of randomised controlled trials. *BMJ.* 2009;338(jun30_1):b2376.

[20] Pedersen TR. Randomised trial of cholesterol lowering in 4444 patients with coronary heart disease: the Scandinavian Simvastatin Survival Study (4S). *Atherosclerosis Supplements.* 2004;5(3):81-7.

[21] Collins R, Armitage J, Parish S, Sleight P, Peto R. MRC/BHF Heart Protection Study of cholesterol lowering with simvastatin in 20 536 high-risk individuals: a randomised placebo controlled trial. *The Lancet.* 2002;360(9326):7-22.

[22] Downs JR, Clearfield M, Weis S, Whitney E, Shapiro DR, Beere PA, et al. Primary prevention of acute coronary events with lovastatin in men and women with average cholesterol levels: results of AFCAPS/TexCAPS. Air Force/Texas Coronary Atherosclerosis Prevention Study. *JAMA.* 1998;279(20):1615-22.

[23] Sacks FM, Pfeffer MA, Moye LA, Rouleau JL, Rutherford JD, Cole TG, et al. The effect of pravastatin on coronary events after myocardial infarction in patients with average cholesterol levels. Cholesterol and Recurrent Events Trial investigators. *N Engl J Med.* 1996;335(14):1001-9.

[24] Shepherd J, Blauw GJ, Murphy MB, Bollen ELEM, Buckley BM, Cobbe SM, et al. Pravastatin in elderly individuals at risk of vascular disease (PROSPER): a randomised controlled trial. *The Lancet.* 2002;360(9346):1623-30.

[25] Shepherd J, Cobbe SM, Ford I, Isles CG, Lorimer AR, MacFarlane PW, et al. Prevention of coronary heart disease with pravastatin in men with hypercholesterolemia. West of Scotland Coronary Prevention Study Group. *N Engl J Med.* 1995;333(20):1301-7.

[26] Wright RA, Flapan AD. Scandinavian simvastatin study (4S). *Lancet.* 1994;344(8939-8940):1765; author reply 7-8.

[27] Sharpe N, Hunt, D., West, M., Thomson, P & White, H. Prevention of cardiovascular events and death with pravastatin in patients with coronary heart disease and a broad range of initial cholesterol levels. The Long-Term Intervention with Pravastatin in Ischaemic Disease (LIPID) Study Group. *N Engl J Med.* 1998;339(19):1349-57.

[28] Ridker PM, Danielson E, Fonseca FAH, Genest J, Gotto Jr AM, Kastelein JJP, et al. Reduction in C-reactive protein and LDL cholesterol and cardiovascular event rates after initiation of rosuvastatin: a prospective study of the JUPITER trial. *The Lancet.* 2009;373(9670):1175-82.

[29] De Lorgeril M, Salen P, Abramson J, Dodin S, Hamazaki T, Kostucki W, et al. Cholesterol lowering, cardiovascular diseases, and the rosuvastatin-JUPITER controversy: a critical reappraisal. *Arch Intern Med.* 2010;170(12):1032-6.
[30] Elliott P, Chambers JC, Zhang W, Clarke R, Hopewell JC, Peden JF, et al. Genetic Loci associated with C-reactive protein levels and risk of coronary heart disease. *JAMA.* 2009;302(1):37-48.
[31] LaRosa JC, Grundy SM, Kastelein JJP, Kostis JB, Greten H. Safety and Efficacy of Atorvastatin-Induced Very Low-Density Lipoprotein Cholesterol Levels in Patients With Coronary Heart Disease (a Post Hoc Analysis of the Treating to New Targets [TNT] Study). *The American Journal of Cardiology.* 2007;100(5):747-52.
[32] Ray KK, Cannon CP, Cairns R, Morrow DA, Rifai N, Kirtane AJ, et al. Relationship between uncontrolled risk factors and C-reactive protein levels in patients receiving standard or intensive statin therapy for acute coronary syndromes in the PROVE IT-TIMI 22 trial. *J Am Coll Cardiol.* 2005;46(8):1417-24.
[33] Ray KK, Cannon CP, McCabe CH, Cairns R, Tonkin AM, Sacks FM, et al. Early and late benefits of high-dose atorvastatin in patients with acute coronary syndromes: results from the PROVE IT-TIMI 22 trial. *J Am Coll Cardiol.* 2005;46(8):1405-10.
[34] NZGG. New Zealand primary care handbook 2012. 3 ed. Wellington, New Zealand: Ministry of Health; 2012 February 2012.
[35] Davidson MH, Toth PP. Comparative effects of lipid-lowering therapies. *Prog Cardiovasc Dis.* 2004;47(2):73-104.
[36] Knopp RH. Drug Treatment of Lipid Disorders. *The New England Journal of Medicine.* 1999;341(7):498-511.
[37] Silva M, Matthews ML, Jarvis C, Nolan NM, Belliveau P, Malloy M, et al. Meta-analysis of drug-induced adverse events associated with intensive-dose statin therapy. *Clin Ther.* 2007;29(2):253-60.
[38] Silva MA, Swanson AC, Gandhi PJ, Tataronis GR. Statin-related adverse events: A meta-analysis. *Clin Ther.* 2006;28(1):26-35.
[39] Afilalo J, Majdan AA, Eisenberg MJ. Intensive statin therapy in acute coronary syndromes and stable coronary heart disease: a comparative meta-analysis of randomised controlled trials. *Heart.* 2007;93(8):914-21.
[40] Jones P, Kafonek S, Laurora I, Hunninghake D. Comparative Dose Efficacy Study of Atorvastatin Versus Simvastatin, Pravastatin, Lovastatin, and Fluvastatin in Patients With Hypercholesterolemia (The CURVES Study). *The American Journal of Cardiology.* 1998;81:582-7.
[41] Pahan K. Lipid-lowering drugs. *Cell Mol Life Sci.* 2006;63(10):1165-78.
[42] Horton JD, Goldstein JL, Brown MS. SREBPs: activators of the complete program of cholesterol and fatty acid synthesis in the liver. *J Clin Invest.* 2002;109(9):1125-31.
[43] Yokoyama M, Seo T, Park T, Yagyu H, Hu Y, Son NH, et al. Effects of lipoprotein lipase and statins on cholesterol uptake into heart and skeletal muscle. *J Lipid Res.* 2007;48(3):646-55.
[44] Horton JD, Shimomura I, Brown MS, Hammer RE, Goldstein JL, Shimano H. Activation of Cholesterol Synthesis in Preference to Fatty Acid Synthesis in Liver and Adipose Tissue of Transgenic Mice Overproducing Sterol Regulatory Element-binding Protein-2. *J Clin Invest.* 1998;101(11):2331-9.

[45] Cromwell WC, Otvos JD, Keyes MJ, Pencina MJ, Sullivan L, Vasan RS, et al. LDL Particle Number and Risk of Future Cardiovascular Disease in the Framingham Offspring Study - Implications for LDL Management. *Journal of clinical lipidology.* 2007;1(6):583-92.

[46] Pedersen TR. Pleiotropic effects of statins: evidence against benefits beyond LDL-cholesterol lowering. *American journal of cardiovascular drugs: drugs, devices, and other interventions.* 2010;10 Suppl 1:10-7.

[47] Zhou Q, Liao JK. Pleiotropic effects of statins. - Basic research and clinical perspectives. *Circulation journal: official journal of the Japanese Circulation Society.* 2010;74(5):818-26.

[48] Liao JK, Laufs U. Pleiotropic effects of statins. *Annu Rev Pharmacol Toxicol.* 2005;45:89-118.

[49] Vaughan CJ, Gotto AM. Update on Statins: 2003. *Circulation.* 2004;110(7):886-92.

[50] Evans MA, Golomb BA. Statin-Associated Adverse Cognitive Effects: Survey Results from 171 Patients. *Pharmacotherapy.* 2009;29(7):800-11.

[51] Golomb BA, Criqui MH, White HL, Dimsdale JE. The UCSD Statin Study: a randomized controlled trial assessing the impact of statins on selected noncardiac outcomes. *Control Clin Trials.* 2004;25(2):178-202.

[52] Golomb BA, Dimsdale JE, White HL, Criqui MH. Abstract 1501: Do Low Dose Statins Affect Cognition? Results of the UCSD Statin Study. *Circulation.* 2006;114(18_MeetingAbstracts):II_289-d.

[53] Mauch DH, Nagler K, Schumacher S, Goritz C, Muller E-C, Otto A, et al. CNS Synaptogenesis Promoted by Glia-Derived Cholesterol. *Science.* 2001;294(5545):1354-7.

[54] Koudinov AR, Koudinova NV. Essential role for cholesterol in synaptic plasticity and neuronal degeneration. *The FASEB Journal.* 2001;15(10):1858-60.

[55] Fehm HL, Kern W, Peters A. The selfish brain: competition for energy resources. *Prog Brain Res.* 2006;153:129-40.

[56] Fattal O, Budur K, Vaughan AJ, Franco K. Review of the literature on major mental disorders in adult patients with mitochondrial diseases. *Psychosomatics.* 2006;47(1):1-7.

[57] Golomb BA, Evans MA. Statin adverse effects : a review of the literature and evidence for a mitochondrial mechanism. *American journal of cardiovascular drugs: drugs, devices, and other interventions.* 2008;8(6):373-418.

[58] Crane FL. Biochemical Functions of Coenzyme Q10. *J Am Coll Nutr.* 2001;20(6):591-8.

[59] Willis RA, Folkers K, Tucker JL, Ye CQ, Xia LJ, Tamagawa H. Lovastatin decreases coenzyme Q levels in rats. *Proc Natl Acad Sci U S A.* 1990;87(22):8928-30.

[60] Marcoff L, Thompson PD. The Role of Coenzyme Q10 in Statin-Associated Myopathy: A Systematic Review. *J Am Coll Cardiol.* 2007;49(23):2231-7.

[61] Nakahara K, Kuriyama M, Sonoda Y, Yoshidome H, Nakagawa H, Fujiyama J, et al. Myopathy induced by HMG-CoA reductase inhibitors in rabbits: a pathological, electrophysiological, and biochemical study. *Toxicol Appl Pharmacol.* 1998;152(1):99-106.

[62] Fukami M, Maeda N, Fukushige J, Kogure Y, Shimada Y, Ogawa T, et al. Effects of HMG-CoA reductase inhibitors on skeletal muscles of rabbits. *Res Exp Med* (Berl). 1993;193(5):263-73.

[63] Tavintharan S, Ong CN, Jeyaseelan K, Sivakumar M, Lim SC, Sum CF. Reduced mitochondrial coenzyme Q10 levels in HepG2 cells treated with high-dose simvastatin: A possible role in statin-induced hepatotoxicity? *Toxicol Appl Pharmacol.* 2007;223(2):173-9.

[64] De Pinieux G, Chariot P, Ammi-Said M, Louarn F, Lejonc JL, Astier A, et al. Lipid-lowering drugs and mitochondrial function: effects of HMG-CoA reductase inhibitors on serum ubiquinone and blood lactate/pyruvate ratio. *Br J Clin Pharmacol.* 1996;42(3):333-7.

[65] Kelly P, Vasu S., Getato M, McNurlan M, Lawson WE. Coenzyme Q10 improves myopathic pain in statin treated patients. *J Am Coll Cardiol.* 2005;45:3A.

[66] Arvanitakis Z, Schneider JA, Wilson RS, Bienias JL, Kelly JF, Evans DA, et al. Statins, incident Alzheimer disease, change in cognitive function, and neuropathology. *Neurology.* 2008;70(19_Part_2):1795-802.

[67] Cucchiara B, Kasner SE. Use of statins in CNS disorders. *J Neurol Sci.* 2001;187(1-2):81-9.

[68] Hajjar I, Schumpert J, Hirth V, Wicland D, Eleazer GP. The Impact of the Use of Statins on the Prevalence of Dementia and the Progression of Cognitive Impairment. *Journals of Gerontology Series A: Biological Sciences and Medical Sciences.* 2002;57(7):M414-8.

[69] Kandiah N, Feldman HH. Therapeutic potential of statins in Alzheimer's disease. J Neurol Sci. 2009;283(1-2):230-4.

[70] Rockwood K. Epidemiological and clinical trials evidence about a preventive role for statins in *Alzheimer's disease.* 2006. p. 71-7.

[71] Buckner RL, Snyder AZ, Shannon BJ, LaRossa G, Sachs R, Fotenos AF, et al. Molecular, Structural, and Functional Characterization of Alzheimer's Disease: Evidence for a Relationship between Default Activity, Amyloid, and Memory. *J Neurosci.* 2005;25(34):7709-17.

[72] Mattson MP. Pathways towards and away from Alzheimer's disease. *Nature.* 2004;430(7000):631-9.

[73] Bjorkhem I, Meaney S. Brain Cholesterol: Long Secret Life Behind a Barrier. *Arterioscler Thromb Vasc Biol.* 2004;24(5):806-15.

[74] Bretillon L, Siden A, Wahlund L-O, Lutjohann D, Minthon L, Crisby M, et al. Plasma levels of 24S-hydroxycholesterol in patients with neurological diseases. *Neurosci Lett.* 2000;293(2):87-90.

[75] Dufouil C, Richard F, Fievet N, Dartigues JF, Ritchie K, Tzourio C, et al. APOE genotype, cholesterol level, lipid-lowering treatment, and dementia: The Three-City Study. *Neurology.* 2005;64(9):1531-8.

[76] Ian JM, Tamar B, Matthew JS, Giuseppe V, Stephanie JF, Ralph NM. Cholesterol metabolism and transport in the pathogenesis of Alzheimer's disease. 2009. p. 1275-308.

[77] Wolozin B, Iii JB, Theisler C, Silberman S. The Cellular Biochemistry of Cholesterol and Statins: Insights into the Pathophysiology and Therapy of Alzheimer's Disease. *CNS Drug Reviews.* 2004;10(2):127-46.

[78] Sierra S, Ramos MC, Molina P, Esteo C, Vazquez JA, Burgos JS. Statins as neuroprotectants: a comparative in vitro study of lipophilicity, blood-brain-barrier penetration, lowering of brain cholesterol, and decrease of neuron cell death. *Journal of Alzheimer's disease: JAD.* 2011;23(2):307-18.
[79] Ghribi O. Preservation of the blood brain barrier integrity may underlie neuroprotective effects of statins in Alzheimer's disease. *Journal of Alzheimer's disease: JAD.* 2006;10(4):407-8.
[80] Stuve O. Statins and the blood-brain barrier: plugging the holes. *Ann Neurol.* 2006;60(1):1-2.
[81] Vuletic S, Riekse RG, Marcovina SM, Peskind ER, Hazzard WR, Albers JJ. Statins of different brain penetrability differentially affect CSF PLTP activity. *Dement Geriatr Cogn Disord.* 2006;22(5-6):392-8.
[82] Kirsch C, Eckert GP, Koudinov AR, Muller WE. Brain cholesterol, statins and Alzheimer's Disease. *Pharmacopsychiatry.* 2003;36 Suppl 2:S113-9.
[83] Lindenstrom E, Boysen G, Nyboe J. Influence of total cholesterol, high density lipoprotein cholesterol, and triglycerides on risk of cerebrovascular disease: the Copenhagen City Heart Study. *BMJ.* 1994;309(6946):11-5.
[84] Schneider JA, Wilson RS, Bienias JL, Evans DA, Bennett DA. Cerebral infarctions and the likelihood of dementia from Alzheimer disease pathology. *Neurology.* 2004;62(7):1148-55.
[85] Sparks DL, Connor DJ, Browne PJ, Lopez JE, Sabbagh MN. HMG-CoA reductase inhibitors (statins) in the treatment of Alzheimer's disease and why it would be ill-advise to use one that crosses the blood-brain barrier. *The journal of nutrition, health & aging.* 2002;6(5):324-31.
[86] Boimel M, Grigoriadis N, Lourbopoulos A, Touloumi O, Rosenmann D, Abramsky O, et al. Statins reduce the neurofibrillary tangle burden in a mouse model of tauopathy. *J Neuropathol Exp Neurol.* 2009;68(3):314-25.
[87] Kurata T, Miyazaki K, Kozuki M, Panin VL, Morimoto N, Ohta Y, et al. Atorvastatin and pitavastatin improve cognitive function and reduce senile plaque and phosphorylated tau in aged APP mice. *Brain Res.* 2011;1371:161-70.
[88] Refolo LM, Pappolla MA, LaFrancois J, Malester B, Schmidt SD, Thomas-Bryant T, et al. A cholesterol-lowering drug reduces beta-amyloid pathology in a transgenic mouse model of Alzheimer's disease. *Neurobiol Dis.* 2001;8(5):890-9.
[89] Tong XK, Lecrux C, Rosa-Neto P, Hamel E. Age-dependent rescue by simvastatin of Alzheimer's disease cerebrovascular and memory deficits. *J Neurosci.* 2012;32(14):4705-15.
[90] Georgieva-Kotetarova MT, Kostadinova, II. Effect of atorvastatin and rosuvastatin on learning and memory in rats with diazepam-induced amnesia. *Folia Med* (Plovdiv). 2013;55(2):58-65.
[91] Abbas T, Faivre E, Holscher C. Impairment of synaptic plasticity and memory formation in GLP-1 receptor KO mice: Interaction between type 2 diabetes and Alzheimer's disease. *Behav Brain Res.* 2009;205(1):265-71.
[92] Haag MDM, Hofman A, Koudstaal PJ, Stricker BHC, Breteler MMB. Statins are associated with a reduced risk of Alzheimer disease regardless of lipophilicity. The Rotterdam Study. *J Neurol Neurosurg Psychiatry.* 2009;80(1):13-7.

[93] Hussain HM, Zakria M, Arshad AR, Arvanitakis Z, Bennett DA, Pappolla MA, et al. Statins, Incident Alzheimer Disease, Change In Cognitive Function, And Neuropathology. *Neurology.* 2008;71(24):2019-20.

[94] Wong WB, Lin VW, Boudreau D, Devine EB. Statins in the prevention of dementia and Alzheimer's disease: a meta-analysis of observational studies and an assessment of confounding. *Pharmacoepidemiology and drug safety.* 2013;22(4):345-58.

[95] Swiger KJ, Manalac RJ, Blumenthal RS, Blaha MJ, Martin SS. Statins and cognition: a systematic review and meta-analysis of short- and long-term cognitive effects. *Mayo Clin Proc.* 2013;88(11):1213-21.

[96] McGuinness B, O'Hare John, Craig David, Bullock Roger, Malouf Reem, Peter. P. Statins for the treatment of dementia. *Cochrane Database of Systematic Reviews.* 2010;4(8).

[97] Woodruff-Pak DS. Animal models of Alzheimer's disease: therapeutic implications. *Journal of Alzheimer's disease: JAD.* 2008;15(4):507-21.

[98] Macleod M, van der Worp HB. Animal models of neurological disease: are there any babies in the bathwater? *Practical neurology.* 2010;10(6):312-4.

[99] van der Worp HB, Howells DW, Sena ES, Porritt MJ, Rewell S, O'Collins V, et al. Can animal models of disease reliably inform human studies? *PLoS medicine.* 2010;7(3):e1000245.

[100] Padala KP, Padala PR, McNeilly DP, Geske JA, Sullivan DH, Potter JF. The Effect of HMG-CoA Reductase Inhibitors on Cognition in Patients With Alzheimer's Dementia: A Prospective Withdrawal and Rechallenge Pilot Study. *The American journal of geriatric pharmacotherapy.* 2012;10(5):296-302.

[101] McGuinness B, O'Hare J, Craig D, Bullock R, Malouf R, Passmore P. Cochrane review on 'Statins for the treatment of dementia'. *Int J Geriatr Psychiatry.* 2013;28(2):119-26.

[102] Balduini W, De Angelis V, Mazzoni E, Cimino M. Simvastatin Protects Against Long-Lasting Behavioral and Morphological Consequences of Neonatal Hypoxic/Ischemic Brain Injury. *Stroke.* 2001;32(9):2185-91.

[103] van der Most PJ, Dolga AM, Nijholt IM, Luiten PGM, Eisel ULM. Statins: Mechanisms of neuroprotection. *Prog Neurobiol.* 2009;88(1):64-75.

[104] Vaughan CJ, Delanty N. Neuroprotective Properties of Statins in Cerebral Ischemia and Stroke. *Stroke.* 1999;30(9):1969-73.

[105] Qu C, Lu D, Goussev A, Schallert T, Mahmood A, Chopp M. Effect of atorvastatin on spatial memory, neuronal survival, and vascular density in female rats after traumatic brain injury. *J Neurosurg.* 2005;103(4):695-701.

[106] Wang H, Lynch JR, Song P, Yang H-J, Yates RB, Mace B, et al. Simvastatin and atorvastatin improve behavioral outcome, reduce hippocampal degeneration, and improve cerebral blood flow after experimental traumatic brain injury. *Exp Neurol.* 2007;206(1):59-69.

[107] Ramirez C, Tercero I, Pineda A, Burgos JS. Simvastatin is the statin that most efficiently protects against kainate-induced excitotoxicity and memory impairment. *Journal of Alzheimer's disease: JAD.* 2011;24(1):161-74.

[108] Endres M, Laufs U, Huang Z, Nakamura T, Huang P, Moskowitz MA, et al. Stroke protection by 3-hydroxy-3-methylglutaryl (HMG)-CoA reductase inhibitors mediated by endothelial nitric oxide synthase. *Proc Natl Acad Sci U S A.* 1998;95(15):8880-5.

[109] Cakmak A, Yemisci M, Koksoy C, Yazgan U, Dincer D, Dalkara T. Statin pre-treatment protects brain against focal cerebral ischemia in diabetic mice. *J Surg Res.* 2007;138(2):254-8.

[110] Kawashima S, Yamashita T, Miwa Y, Ozaki M, Namiki M, Hirase T, et al. HMG-CoA reductase inhibitor has protective effects against stroke events in stroke-prone spontaneously hypertensive rats. *Stroke.* 2003;34(1):157-63.

[111] Kilic U, Bassetti CL, Kilic E, Xing H, Wang Z, Hermann DM. Post-ischemic delivery of the 3-hydroxy-3-methylglutaryl coenzyme A reductase inhibitor rosuvastatin protects against focal cerebral ischemia in mice via inhibition of extracellular-regulated kinase-1/-2. *Neuroscience.* 2005;134(3):901-6.

[112] Prinz V, Laufs U, Gertz K, Kronenberg G, Balkaya M, Leithner C, et al. Intravenous rosuvastatin for acute stroke treatment: an animal study. *Stroke.* 2008;39(2):433-8.

[113] Sironi L, Cimino M, Guerrini U, Calvio AM, Lodetti B, Asdente M, et al. Treatment with statins after induction of focal ischemia in rats reduces the extent of brain damage. *Arterioscler Thromb Vasc Biol.* 2003;23(2):322-7.

[114] Zhang L, Chopp M, Jia L, Cui Y, Lu M, Zhang ZG. Atorvastatin extends the therapeutic window for tPA to 6 h after the onset of embolic stroke in rats. *J Cereb Blood Flow Metab.* 2009;29(11):1816-24.

[115] Pahan K, Sheikh FG, Namboodiri AM, Singh I. Lovastatin and phenylacetate inhibit the induction of nitric oxide synthase and cytokines in rat primary astrocytes, microglia, and macrophages. *J Clin Invest.* 1997;100(11):2671-9.

[116] McKinney JS, Kostis WJ. Statin therapy and the risk of intracerebral hemorrhage: a meta-analysis of 31 randomized controlled trials. *Stroke.* 2012;43(8):2149-56.

[117] Galatti L, Polimeni G, Salvo F, Romani M, Sessa A, Spina E. Short-term memory loss associated with rosuvastatin. *Pharmacotherapy.* 2006;26(8):1190-2.

[118] King DS, Wilburn AJ, Wofford MR, Harrell TK, Lindley BJ, Jones DW. Cognitive impairment associated with atorvastatin and simvastatin. *Pharmacotherapy.* 2003;23(12):1663-7.

[119] Parle M, Singh N. Reversal of Memory Deficits by Atorvastatin and Simvastatin in Rats. Yakugaku Zasshi. 2007;127(7):1125-37.

[120] Tatley M, Savage R. Psychiatric adverse reactions with statins, fibrates and ezetimibe: implications for the use of lipid-lowering agents. *Drug Saf.* 2007;30(3):195-201.

[121] Tuccori M, Lapi F, Testi A, Coli D, Moretti U, Vannacci A, et al. Statin-Associated Psychiatric Adverse Events: A Case/Non-Case Evaluation of an Italian Database of Spontaneous Adverse Drug Reaction Reporting. *Drug Saf.* 2008;31:1115-23.

[122] Yang CC, Jick SS, Jick H. Lipid-lowering drugs and the risk of depression and suicidal behavior. *Arch Intern Med.* 2003;163(16):1926-32.

[123] Stewart RA, Sharples KJ, North FM, Menkes DB, Baker J, Simes J. Long-term assessment of psychological well-being in a randomized placebo-controlled trial of cholesterol reduction with pravastatin. The LIPID Study Investigators. *Arch Intern Med.* 2000;160(20):3144-52.

[124] While A, Keen L. The effects of statins on mood: A review of the literature. *European Journal of Cardiovascular Nursing.* 2010; In Press, Corrected Proof.

[125] Young-Xu Y, Chan KA, Liao JK, Ravid S, Blatt CM. Long-term statin use and psychological well-being. *J Am Coll Cardiol.* 2003;42(4):690-7.

[126] Wang Q, Zengin A, Deng C, Li Y, Newell KA, Yang GY, et al. High dose of simvastatin induces hyperlocomotive and anxiolytic-like activities: The association with the up-regulation of NMDA receptor binding in the rat brain. *Exp Neurol.* 2009;216(1):132-8.

[127] Yan J, Xu Y, Zhu C, Zhang L, Wu A, Yang Y, et al. Simvastatin Prevents Dopaminergic Neurodegeneration in Experimental Parkinsonian Models: The Association with Anti-Inflammatory Responses. *PloS one*. 2011;6(6):e20945.

[128] Reagan-Shaw S, Nihal M, Ahmad N. Dose translation from animal to human studies revisited. *The FASEB Journal.* 2008;22(3):659-61.

[129] Maggo S, Clark D, Ashton JC. The effect of statins on performance in the Morris water maze in guinea pig. *Eur J Pharmacol.* 2012;674(2-3):287-93.

[130] Madsen CS, Janovitz E, Zhang R, Van N-T, Ryan CS, Yin X, et al. The Guinea Pig as a Preclinical Model for Demonstrating the Efficacy and Safety of Statins. *J Pharmacol Exp Ther.* 2008;324(2):576-86.

[131] Baytan SH, Alkanat M, Okuyan M, Ekinci M, Gedikli E, Ozeren M, et al. Simvastatin Impairs Spatial Memory in Rats at a Specific Dose Level. *The Tohoku Journal of Experimental Medicine.* 2008;214(4):341-9.

[132] Parker AB, Polk MD, Rabdiya V, Meda SA, Anderson K, Hawkins KA, et al. Changes in Memory Function and Neuronal Activation Associated with Atorvastatin Therapy. *Pharmacotherapy.* 2010;30(6):236e-40e.

[133] Orsi A, Sherman O, Woldeselassie Z. Simvastatin-associated memory loss. *Pharmacotherapy.* 2001;21(6):767-9.

[134] Padala KP, Padala PR, Potter JF. Simvastatin-Induced Decline in Cognition. *The Annals of Pharmacotherapy.* 2006;40(10):1880-3.

[135] Wagstaff LR, Mitton MW, Arvik BM, Doraiswamy PM. Statin-associated memory loss: analysis of 60 case reports and review of the literature. *Pharmacotherapy.* 2003;23(7):871-80.

[136] Saheki A, Terasaki T, Tamai I, Tsuji A. In Vivo and in Vitro Blood–Brain Barrier Transport of 3-Hydroxy-3-Methylglutaryl Coenzyme A (HMG-CoA) Reductase Inhibitors. *Pharm Res.* 1994;11(2):305-11.

[137] Allami N, Javadi-Paydar M, Rayatnia F, Sehhat K, Rahimian R, Norouzi A, et al. Suppression of nitric oxide synthesis by L-NAME reverses the beneficial effects of pioglitazone on scopolamine-induced memory impairment in mice. *Eur J Pharmacol.* 2011;650(1):240-8.

[138] Rayatnia F, Javadi-Paydar M, Allami N, Zakeri M, Rastegar H, Norouzi A, et al. Nitric oxide involvement in consolidation, but not retrieval phase of cognitive performance enhanced by atorvastatin in mice. *Eur J Pharmacol.* 2011;666(1-3):122-30.

[139] Bliss TVP, Collingridge GL. A synaptic model of memory: long-term potentiation in the hippocampus. *Nature.* 1993;361(6407):31-9.

[140] Neves G, Cooke SF, Bliss TV. Synaptic plasticity, memory and the hippocampus: a neural network approach to causality. *Nature reviews Neuroscience*. 2008;9(1):65-75.

[141] Mans RA, Chowdhury N, Cao D, McMahon LL, Li L. Simvastatin enhances hippocampal long-term potentiation in C57BL/6 mice. *Neuroscience.* 2010; 166(2):435-44.

[142] Frank C, Giammarioli AM, Pepponi R, Fiorentini C, Rufini S. Cholesterol perturbing agents inhibit NMDA-dependent calcium influx in rat hippocampal primary culture. *FEBS Lett.* 2004;566(1-3):25-9.

[143] Frank C, Rufini S, Tancredi V, Forcina R, Grossi D, D'Arcangelo G. Cholesterol depletion inhibits synaptic transmission and synaptic plasticity in rat hippocampus. *Exp Neurol.* 2008;212(2):407-14.

[144] Kotti TJ, Ramirez DMO, Pfeiffer BE, Huber KM, Russell DW. Brain cholesterol turnover required for geranylgeraniol production and learning in mice. *Proc Natl Acad Sci U S A.* 2006;103(10):3869-74.

[145] Maggo S, Ashton JC. Effects of HMG-CoA reductase inhibitors on learning and memory in the guinea pig. *Eur J Pharmacol.* 2014;723:294-304.

[146] Kleschevnikov AM, Sokolov MV, Kuhnt U, Dawe GS, Stephenson JD, Voronin LL. Changes in paired-pulse facilitation correlate with induction of long-term potentiation in area CA1 of rat hippocampal slices. *Neuroscience.* 1997;76(3):829-43.

[147] Schulz PE, Cook EP, Johnston D. Changes in paired-pulse facilitation suggest presynaptic involvement in long-term potentiation. *J Neurosci.* 1994;14(9):5325-37.

[148] Zucker RS, Regehr WG. Short-term synaptic plasticity. *Annu Rev Physiol.* 2002;64:355-405.

[149] Nguyen PV, Abel T, Kandel ER, Bourtchouladze R. Strain-dependent differences in LTP and hippocampus-dependent memory in inbred mice. *Learn Mem.* 2000;7(3):170-9.

[150] Lisman J. Long-term potentiation: outstanding questions and attempted synthesis. *Philos Trans R Soc Lond B Biol Sci.* 2003;358(1432):829-42.

[151] Larson J, Lynch G. Theta pattern stimulation and the induction of LTP: the sequence in which synapses are stimulated determines the degree to which they potentiate. *Brain Res.* 1989;489(1):49-58.

[152] Ghodke RM, Tour N, Devi K. Effects of statins and cholesterol on memory functions in mice. *Metab Brain Dis.* 2012;27(4):443-51.

[153] McGown CC, Brookes ZL. Beneficial effects of statins on the microcirculation during sepsis: the role of nitric oxide. *Br J Anaesth.* 2007;98(2):163-75.

[154] Chen J, Zacharek A, Zhang C, Jiang H, Li Y, Roberts C, et al. Endothelial nitric oxide synthase regulates brain-derived neurotrophic factor expression and neurogenesis after stroke in mice. *J Neurosci.* 2005;25(9):2366-75.

[155] Redelmeier D. New thinking about postoperative delirium. *CMAJ.* 2007;177(4):424.

[156] Redelmeier DA, Thiruchelvam D, Daneman N. Delirium after elective surgery among elderly patients taking statins. *CMAJ.* 2008;179(7):645-52.

In: Statins
Editor: Eric R. Travers

ISBN: 978-1-63463-057-3

Chapter 5

STATINS IN CARDIAC SURGERY: THE CURRENT EVIDENCE

Elmar W. Kuhn*[*,1], M.D., Yeong H. Choi[1], M.D., Thorsten Wahlers[1], M.D., and Oliver J. Liakopoulos[2], M.D.

[1]Department of Cardiothoracic Surgery, Heart Center,
University of Cologne, Germany
[2]Department of Thoracic and Cardiovascular Surgery,
West-German Heart Center Essen, Germany

ABSTRACT

Cardiac surgery is associated with excellent results for patients treated for acquired cardiac disease such as coronary artery or valve disease. However, the constantly ageing patient population presents with a rising prevalence of relevant co-morbidities leading to a significant risk for postoperative major adverse cardiovascular events. This trend implies the importance of an optimal perioperative medical treatment. In this context, statins have shown to be linked with beneficial effects after on-pump coronary artery bypass graft procedures while less evidence is available for patients referred to valve surgery. This chapter aims to summarize the current evidence for perioperative statin therapy for various kinds of surgery.

INTRODUCTION

Heart surgery is the optimal therapy for patients with advanced coronary artery disease or severe aortic valve stenosis and offers excellent therapeutical options for acquired cardiac disease. However, heart surgery is far more invasive compared to other alternatives and is therefore associated with the development of postoperative major adverse cardiovascular

[*] Corresponding author: Elmar W. Kuhn, MD, Department of Cardiothoracic Surgery, Heart Center, University of Cologne, Germany, Kerpener Strasse 62, 50924 Cologne, Germany, Phone: +49 (221) 478 32406; Fax: +49 (221) 478 32648, Email: elmar.kuhn@uk-koeln.de.

events. The Adult Cardiac Surgical Database Report of the year 2010 of the European Association for Cardio-Thoracic Surgery (EACTS) ranged the in-hospital mortality for patients undergoing coronary artery bypass grafting (CABG) at 2.2% and 3.4% for patients undergoing isolated valve procedures [1]. On the one hand, mortality rates remained stable over the past years enabled by important improvements in surgical techniques and perioperative management of patients. On- or off-pump procedures, minimal-invasive approaches and myocardial protection strategies allow to personalize planning and execution of the procedures. On the other hand, these advantageous developments are challenged by the increasing incidence of relevant co-morbidities in the constantly ageing patient population. Therefore, implementation of better strategies that limit the risk for major adverse events after cardiac procedures is imperative if outcomes among cardiac surgery patients are aimed to be improved.

Concerning the optimization of care especially in patients presenting with cardiovascular risk factors, both basic researchers and clinicians focused on the effects of statins in the last decades. Statins competitively inhibit the 3-hydroxy 3-methylglutaryl (HMG-) CoA reductase that catalyzes the rate-limiting step in cholesterol synthesis and, consequently, reduce the concentration of mevalonate and further down-stream products (*figure*) [2]. As a result, expression of low-density lipoprotein (LDL) receptors on hepatocytes is increased and uptake of LDL-cholesterol from the blood into the liver is augmented thereby leading to a decrease of LDL in the blood.

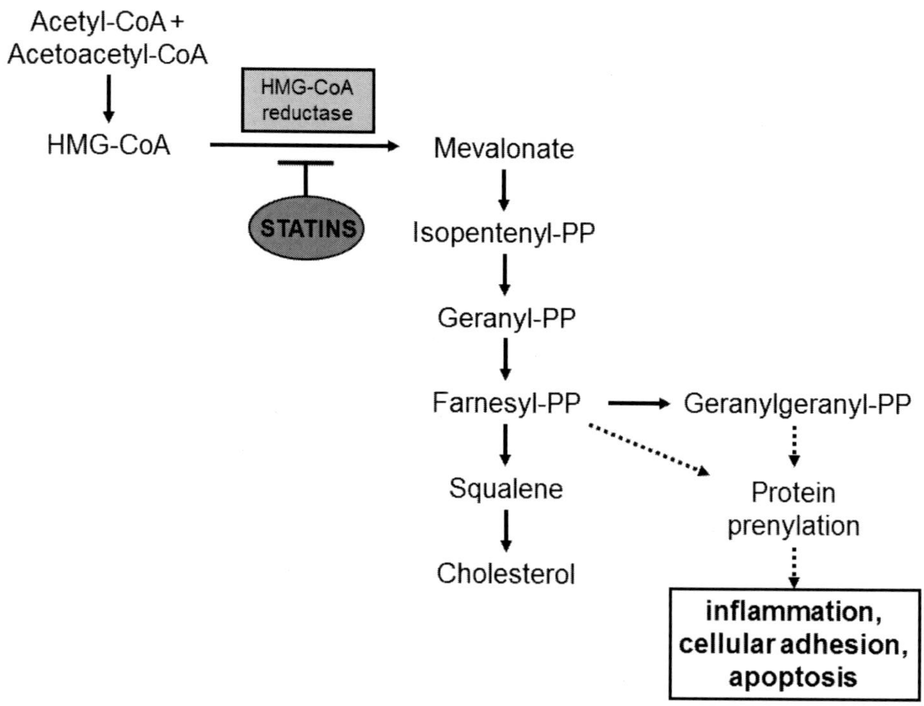

Figure. Statins inhibit cholesterol biosynthesis and exert pleiotropic effects such as reducing inflammation, cellular adhesion and apoptosis by blocking the key enzyme HMG-CoA-reductase. CoA – coenzyme A; HMG – hydroxy-methylglutaryl; PP-pyrophosphate.

Since elevated LDL blood concentration is one of the major risk factors for the development and progression of coronary artery disease, statin therapy has become an inherent part of the primary and secondary prevention of cardiovascular disease [3]. With regard to primary prevention, there is a number of debates about the usefullness of statins in "healthy" people with no signs for coronary heart disease and normal cholesterol levels [4]. A review conducted by Taylor et al. rises doubts in this matter since expecially people with a low cardiovascular risk profile do not clearly profit by statin therapy in terms of preventing cardiovascular events [5]. Since primary prevention implies prescribing statins to people that have not developed coronary artery disease (yet), benefits and risks need to be balanced out.

But even irrespective of the patients´ initial lipid profile or other presenting characteristics, a meta-analysis of more than 90,000 participants demonstrated that statins reduce the incidence of major coronary events, myocardial revascularization and stroke in a wide range of individuals [6]. Further more, high-risk patients with established coronary artery disease benefit from a statin therapy with regard to a significant reduction in all-cause mortality and stroke rates [7]. Therefore, current guidelines of the ACC/AHA and NCEP recommend the use of statins patients with established coronary artery disease when serum LDL-levels exceed 100 mg/dl [8].

Beyond their lipid-lowering actions, statins exert lipid-independent (´pleiotropic´) effects that offer additional cardiovascular protection [9, 10]. These effects may be beneficial for the prevention of plaque rupture and thrombotic occlusion in coronary artery disease by inhibition of inflammatory cascades, endothelial dysfunction and platelet activation [11-15]. Evidence for potentially relevant effects of non-lipid statin actions is mainly driven by results from animal and cell culture studies and various clinical trials. Accumulating evidence from randomized controlled trials have demonstrated the efficacy of a preoperative statin therapy in reducing periprocedural cardiovascular events after PCI and non-cardiac surgery when compared to statin-naïve patients, thereby making a preoperative treatment with statins a promising approach to reduce postoperative morbidity and mortality in patients scheduled for cardiac surgery [16-18]. However, in patients undergoing cardiac procedures results are conflicting, with several studies reporting a decrease in short-term mortality and major cardiovascular events including myocardial infarction, atrial fibrillation, stroke and renal failure in patients receiving preoperative statins [19, 20] while others have failed to show a beneficial effect of statins on these endpoints [21-24].

Statins in Patients Undergoing Myocardial Revascularization Procedures or Combined Cardiac Surgery

The evaluation of potential statin effects in cardiac surgerical patients is mainly focused on coronary artery bypass graft surgery since statin therapy is a corner stone in the treatment of coronary artery disease. However, large and relevant studies include patients undergoing various kinds of surgical procedures. These investigations add valuable evidence about the effectiveness of statins in cardiac surgery in general, but impede at the same time precise conclusions for specific patient populations. Therefore, the value of statin treatment in cardiac surgery is elucidated in the following with focus on myocardial revascularization procedures.

The first link of statin therapy and superior survival rates among patients with coronary heart disease was established in the Scandinavian Simvastatin Survival Study (4S). A total of 4,444 patients with myocardial ischemia and elevated serum cholesterol levels were randomized to simvastatin or placebo. During the median follow-up of 5.4 years simvastatin intake was not only associated with a drop in total and low-density cholesterol but even in a significant survival benefit compared to placebo treatment. Statin treated patients suffered less frequently from coronary and noncardiovascular causes of deaths, including a significant reduction in the risk of myocardial revascularization [25]. A consecutive study investigating the effect of statins prior to coronary artery bypass graft surgery was published in 1999 by Christenson and colleagues. The authors randomized 77 patients with symptomatic coronary artery disease and elevated cholesterol levels to either lipid-control with simvastatin (40 patients) or control (37 patients) for a preoperative duration of 4 weeks. Not surprisingly, statin intake resulted in a reduction of total cholesterol levels before CABG surgery. But moreover, the incidence of postoperative thrombocytosis as the primary endpoint was significantly reduced in statin-treated patients which was associated to a reduction of postoperative myocardial infarction and transient renal failure when compared to statin-naïve patients [22]. One-year follow-up after myocardial revascularization revealed that the incidence of bypass graft lesions of patients in the simvastatin group was significantly lower compared to control [26]. These results initiated a broad investigation of statin effects on patients presenting with elevated cholesterol levels with coronary artery disease who were scheduled for myocardial revascularization.

All patients included into the first studies investigating statin effects on outcomes in patients undergoing myocardial revascularization suffered from hypercholesterolemia, however, even normolipemic patients appear to benefit from a statin therapy. Mannacio et al. randomized 200 patients with normal LDL-cholesterol levels (mean LDL range: 121 to 127 mg/dL) to treatment with rosuvastatin or placebo 1 week prior to CABG. Incidence of myocardial damage defined as an elevation of cardiac troponin I, myoglobin and creatine kinase-MB was significantly lower in statin-treated patients when compared to the placebo group. The authors concluded that perioperative statin therapy may improve short- and long-term results after CABG procedures in patients with normal cholesterol levels [19]. Similarly, Thielmann and colleagues assessed the impact of statin intake in patients with different preoperative cholesterol levels in a retrospective analysis. Patients referred to first-time elective coronary bypass grafting (3,346 patients) were classified into three groups; those with statin-*un*treated hyperlipemia (group 1, control), patients with statin-treated hyperlipemia (group 2) and a group of normolipemic patients without statin therapy (group 3). The authors found that statin thyerpy of hyperlipemia reduced the risk of major cardiovascular events in CABG patients to similar levels of untreated normolipemic patients when compared to controls [27]. Thus, beneficial statin effects are not necessarily bound to high cholesterol levels emphasizing that lipid lowering is at least not the only mechanism of providing superior outcomes. The CASCADE (Clopidogrel after Surgery for Coronary Artery Disease) trial initially investigated the additional effect of clopidogrel added to a standard medical therapy including aspirin and statin treatment after myocardial revascularization. After the 1-year follow-up of all patients, results of the study-related coronary andiogram was evaluated based on the serum LDL level achieved with statin therapy. The authors found higher graft patency rates for patients with LDL levels of less than 100 mg/dL compared with those presenting with higher LDL levels, but no further improvement was detected in patients with LDL levels of less than 70 mg/dL [28]. This conclusion follows current guidelines of the European Society of Cardiology (ESC), American College of Cardiology (ACC) and the American Heart Association (AHA) recommending that patients with established coronary artery disease undergoing CABG surgery should receive an intensified statin treatment (target LDL-levels <100 mg/dL) unless otherwise contraindicated [29]. Otherwise, Quin et al., found a survival benefit of patients receiving lipid lowering medication after CABG, but did not find an association of LDL-levels <100 mg/dL and superior outcomes compared to patients with higher levels. The authors retrospectively analyzed records of 2,203 patients regarding LDL-levels, incidences of acute myocardial infarction, repeat revascularization and graft patency and principilly concluded that discharge on lipid-lowering medication was associated with superior survival but independently of LDL-levels [30].

Statins for Reduction of Mortality

Although these studies show benefits of a preoperative statin therapy for patients referred to CABG procedures, a surprisingly sparse evidence is available from large-scale RCTs that analyse the impact of a preoperative statin therapy on hard clinical outcomes including postoperative mortality. The ARMYDA-3 trial could not find an influence of preoperative atorvastatin administration on mortality in patients undergoing myocardial revascularization. Two-hundred patients were randomized to receive either atorvastatin (101 patients) or placebo (99 patients) 7 days before the procedure. Of note, the study was clearly underpowered to reveal a significant difference among groups with regard to postoperative mortality, but showed a clear reduction in the incidence of postoperative atrial fibrillation in statin-treated patients [20]. Comparable results to the ARYMDA-3 trial were presented by Mannacio et al. in 200 CABG patients with a preoperative random allocation to rosuvastatin or placebo for 7 days [19]. The first report of a significant reduction of postoperative mortality associated with statin therapy was presented by Pan et al. in a retrospective cohort study of patients undergoing CABG surgery. The investigators compared 943 patients with antihyperlipemic therapy to 720 statin-naïve patients and multivariate logistic regression analysis revealed that statin treatment was independently linked with a reduced incidence of 30-day all-cause mortality. Even after propensity-matching statin therapy turned out to be an independent predictor for a lower incidence of the composite endpoint consisting of 30-day all-cause mortality and stroke (7.1% vs. 4.6%; $p<0.05$) [31]. This finding was supported by another large retrospective analysis comprising 2,377 patients undergoing isolated CABG. While only 42% of patients admitted to receive coronary surgery received statin therapy preopratively, statin users showed a lower operative mortality of 1.7% compared to 2.8% for statin-naïve patients. Among high-risk patients, statin intake was found to be an independent predictor of superior survival rates [32].

Statins for Reduction of Stroke, Atrial Fibrillation and Renal Failure

Postoperative occurrence of stroke, atrial fibrillation or renal failure relevantly influence patients´ outcome. Therefore, many studies have investigated the respective incidences in dependence of statin intake. Aboyans et al. analysed factors predicting the incidence of stroke in patients referred to CABG surgery and demonstrated a protective effect of statins with a reduction in postoperative cerebrovascular events (odds ratio (OR): 0.26; 95% conficence interval (CI): 0.06-0.86) [33].

New-onset atrial fibrillation is a common phenomenon after heart surgery and is associated with raised morbidity and mortality. The impact of statins on the postoperative incidence of atrial fibrillation was elucidated in a meta-analysis of our group. This systematic review gathered data from 3 RCTs and 10 observational studies comprising about 17,000 cardiac surgery patients. Preoperative statin use finally lead to an unadjusted odds reduction of 22% for atrial fibrillation (OR: 0.78; 95%CI: 0.67-0.90) and 34% for new-onset atrial fibrilliation (OR: 0.66; 95%CI: 0.51-0.84). This finding persisted after pooled analysis of risk-adjusted treatment effects from RCTs and observational trials [34]. These results were supported by another meta-analysis conducted by Winchester et al. showing a significant reduction in the occurrence of atrial fibrillation after CABG (OR: 0.54; 95%CI: 0.43-0.68) in statin pretreated patients [35]. The influence of statin therapy on success rates after surgical ablation for atrial fibrillation was evaluated in a prospective cohort study on patients with (n=73) and without (n=76) preoperative statin therapy. The total cohort of patients received on-pump cardiac procedures with concomitant surgical ablation for atrial fibrillation. Improved conversion rates were associated with statin treatment at discharge from hospital ($p=0.07$) and after 3 and 6 months ($p<0.05$ for both) [36].

Renoprotective properties of statins have been presented by Tabata et al. in a study of 1,802 CABG patients. The investigators reviewed data from 641 matched patients in terms of statin and non-statin treatment and detected a link between preoperative statin therapy and a lower incidence of postoperative renal injury (OR: 0.54; 95%CI: 0.18-0.99) [37]. Since acute kidney injury holds an inherent part of postoperative morbidity and mortality, Singh and coworkers performed a meta-analysis of studies investigating the association of preoperative statin therapy and postoperative renal failure. They included a total of 17 studies comprising about 45,000 patients undergoing various types of cardiac surgery and found a significant lower need for renal replacement therapy in the subset of patients with CABG procedures (OR: 0.56; 95%CI: 0.41-0.76). Furthermore, the authors describe a lower mortality rate among all patients treated with statins irrespective of the type of surgery what might mainly be driven by the lower rate of dialysis in the large cohort of CABG patients [38]. In a complex analysis accomplished by Layton and colleagues focusing on acute kidney injury after surgical myocardial revascularization, the authors identified about 17,000 patients using healthcare databases referred to non-emergency CABG that either newly received statin therapy within 20 days before surgery or were not taking statins at least for 200 days prior to surgery. The overall incidence of acute kidney injury in the statin group was 3.4% and 6.2% in the non-statin group. After adjustment for baseline characteristics, a protective effect of statin therapy was detected with the final conclusion that statin prescription even immediately prior to CABG may prevent the incidence of acute kidney injury [39].

Meta-Analyses on Statins in Cardiac Surgery

Large randomized controlled trials assessing the evidence of statin therapy in cardiac surgery are lacking up to date, therefore, the most robust evidence for the effect of statin treatment prior to cardiac surgery is summarized in comprehensive meta-analyses. One of the first systematic reviews consisted of 31,725 patients undergoing predominately CABG procedures (92%). Statin pretreatment was associated with a substantial postoperative reduction in the odds of early mortality (OR: 0.57; 95%CI: 0.49-0.6), stroke (OR: 0.74, 95%CI: 0.60-0.91) and atrial fibrillation (OR: 0.67, 95%CI: 0.51-0.88) when compared to non-treated patients [40]. The updated version of this meta-analysis even included 54 trials (12 RCT, 42 observational trials) with over 90,000 patients undergoing various types of cardiac surgery and could confirm these results with an absolute risk reduction for early all-cause mortality in statin treated patients compared to those without statin therapy (2.6 versus 3.5%). Similarly, incidence rates of atrial fibrillation and stroke as well as lenghts of stay on the intensive care unit and in-hospital stay were reduced in the statin group [41]. The separate analysis of patients undergoing isolated CABG procedures (32 studies) revealed a comparable benefit in terms of favourable outcomes [42].

Results from meta-analyses containing observational trials usually imply a certain methodological imprecision, whereas reviews according to the high standards of the Cochrane Collaboration represent the highest level of evidence available. The review of our group consisted of eleven randomized controlled studies including a total of 984 patients undergoing on- or off-pump cardiac surgical procedures. Pooled analysis showed that statin pretreatment before surgery reduced the incidence of postoperative atrial fibrillation (OR 0.40; 95%-CI: 0.29 to 0.55; $p<0.01$), but failed to influence short-term mortality or postoperative stroke. In addition, statin therapy was associated with a shorter length of stay of patients on the ICU and in-hospital. There was no reduction in myocardial infarction or renal failure. These results were unaffected after subgroup analysis. Interestingly, no major or minor perioperative statin side-effects were reported from trials investigating this safety endpoint [43]. Since this meta-analysis included mainly patients undergoing myocardial revascularizations the results cannot be extrapolated to patients undergoing other cardiac procedures such as heart valve or aortic surgery.

In contrast to the above mentioned meta-analysis with more than 90,000 patients, the Cochrane review exclusively comprising RCTs included a surprisingly low number of 984 patients. This huge difference highlights the fact that large RCTs are not available and most evidence about statin effects in cardiac surgery is derived from observational trials or retrospective analyses with potential methodological flaws.

Conflicting Evidence for Reduction of Postoperative Outcomes

In contrast to the above mentioned investigations showing superior clinical outcomes for patients treated with statins in the perioperative period, data from other studies could not demonstrate any benefit from statin treatment with regard to mortality and morbidity in patients subjected to cardiac surgery. Ali et al. analysed postoperative endpoints of patients referred to different kinds of cardiac surgery and assessed the effect of preoperative statin intake in a total of 3,555 patients and compared the result to individuals without statin treatment (1,914 patients). The authors discribed lower rates of mortality, stroke and ventilation time, but this result was no more detectable after adjustment for relevant covariates [21]. Likewise, Powell et al. detected benefitial results of statins in patients undergoing myocardial revascularization in terms of lower mortality in 2,334 patients on statins compared with 2,405 patients not on statins. However, this effect did not persist after multivariate analysis [44]. Propensity score matching of 654 patients per group revealed similar incidences of perioperative mortality, cardiac, neurologic, renal and respiratory morbidity and atrial fibrillation in an observational cohort study [24].

Whereas the above mentioned studies showed lower incidence rates of renal failure among patients undergoing revascularization procedures, Mithani et al., failed to reproduce the finding in a population of 2,104 patients undergoing various kinds of cardiac surgery including coronary artery bypass graft or valve surgery. And even after propensity adjustment statin treatment was not associated with postoperative incidence of acute kidney injury [45].

Statins in Patients Undergoing Isolated Valve Surgery

The role of statins for patients with valvular heart disease is less well defined compared to the large amount of studies investigating their impact on perioperative outcomes in myocardial revascularization. Compared to coronary artery disease, the linkage between lipid metabolism and calcified aortic valve disease or bioprosthetic valve degeneration remains to be determined. In this field, new results from basic science and clinical investigations add important aspects for a further understanding. For example, genetic contribution to valvular calcification was elucidated by searching for genomewide associations with aortic and mitral valve calcification. A single nucleotide polymorphism in the lipoprotein(a) locus was found to be combined with aortic valve stenosis in European, African-American and Hispanic-American cohorts. The central role for lipoprotein(a) in the development of aortic valve calcification was furthermore underlined as lipoprotein(a) levels that were predicted from the genotype could be directly linked with the amount of calcification of the aortic valve [46]. Such new findings show that our understanding of the pathophysiology of valve calcification and the implications for subsequent therapeutic options regarding lipid metabolism remains limited.

Statins and Their Effect on Non-Clinical Outcome Variables

The linkage between LDL-cholesterol levels and the progression of valve calcification was investigated by Pohle et al., showing that lipid-lowering therapy beneficially influences aortic valve degeneration. A patient population including 104 individuals was subdivided into two groups in accordance to their LDL-levels. A more rapid increase of valve calcification was found during follow-up in patients with cholesterol levels of more than 130 mg/dL in contrast to patients with lower levels. However, since the applied statin therapy was inhomogeneous among both groups the impact of this analysis is limited [47]. Nevertheless, cholesterol levels of more than 200 mg/dL were associated to a higher degree of aortic or mitral valve calcification in patients referred to valve replacement surgery in an analysis published by Farivar et al. (OR: 3.9; 95%CI: 1.7-8.9) [48].

Clinical evidence for the impact of statins on the progression of degenerative aortic valve stenosis was first provided by Antonini-Canterin et al. who demonstrated a slower progression of aortic stenosis in patients treated with statins compared with untreated individuals assessed by the change in peak aortic velocity by echocardiography during follow-up examinations [49].

Such results are summarized in a systematic review including data of about 1,000 patients with aortic stenosis accumulated from seven studies analysing the effect of statin intake on progression of aortic stenosis. Pooled analysis of the treatment effect of statins versus control revealed a benefit of a statin therapy in terms of aortic jet velocity and regression of aortic valve area [50].

For patients after bioprosthetic aortic valve replacement the potential influence of statin therapy on popstoperative development of valve degeneration was evaluated in a study including more than 1,000 patients with a mean follow-up of 4.5 years by echocardiographic re-examinations. Patients were stratified into two groups according to the presence of lipid-lowering therapy including statin treatment. In this study, there was finally no benefit for patients receiving statins regarding the progression of trans-valvular preesure gradients (0.9±7.7 mmHg vs. 1.1±10.9 mmHg; p=0.87) or 10-year freeedom from re-operation (98.9% vs. 95.4%; p=0.72) [51].

Statins and Their Effect on Clinical Outcome Variables

The role of statins in the progression of non-rheumatic calcific aortic stenosis was investigated in a meta-analysis by Parolari et al. that reviewed 10 studies (7 non-RCTs, 3 RCTs) with a total of 3,822 patients. The authors did neither find any marked difference with regard to all-cause (OR: 0.98; 95%CI: 0.74-1.30) or cardiovascular (OR: 0.79; 95%CI: 0.54-1.15) mortality nor to the need for aortic valve surgery (OR: 0.92; 95%CI: 0.76-1.10) between both groups. Furthermore, statin therapy had no impact on the progression of peak aortic jet velocity and mean aortic pressure gradient [52]. Likewise, no relevant advantages were found in the subset of patients with aortic valve replacement that were included in the meta-analysis of our group. Of the 3,091 patients, 1,043 were treated with statins before surgery and in summary, no favourable outcomes were detectable in terms of mortality, myocardial infarction, stroke and renal failure [42]. As Singh et al. focused on the incidence of acute kidney injury, they neither reported about beneficial statin effects in their subgroup of patients referred to isolated valve replacement procedures [38].

The trials mentioned above not showing a detectable benefit mediated by statin therapy after valve surgery are opposed to further investigations with favourable results. In patients undergoing valvular procedures preoperative statin therapy was linked with a significant lower 30-day and longer-term mortality after a mean follow-up of 33 months. The investigated patient cohort consisted of 381 matched pairs addressing baseline risk imbalances [53].

The final question about the pro and contra of statin therapy in the prevention of bioprosthetic aortic valve degeneration after surgical valve replacement was the focus of a literature review of Gilmanov et al. leading to the result that the current evidence derived from clinical studies is insufficient to recommend statin therapy [54]. On the other hand, the presence of potentially beneficial pleiotropic effects might in turn argue for a routine statin use for patients undergoing aortic valve replacement as it was recommended by Paraskevas et al. [55]. This recommendation is supported by a retrospective study including 447 patients undergoing valvular procedures. The group of patients with perioperative statin treatment consisted of 203 individuals and presented with more comorbidities including preoperative stroke, diabetes and cerebrovascular disease. Despite of the increased risk profile of the statin group, the incidence of a composite endpoint including death, stroke and renal failure was lower in patients with statin treatment pointing to beneficial perioperative pleiotropic effects (OR: 1.9; 95%CI: 0.96-3.76) [56]. Data derived from 1,400 patients undergoing cardiac valve surgery yielded in the same direction showing that preoperative statin intake correlated significantly with lower mortality for statin-patients (OR: 0.25; 95%CI: 0.12-0.54), but the raw operative mortality rate and the incidences of stroke and perioperative myocardial infarction were not markedly lower for patients in the statin group compared to statin-naïve patients. But of note, risk profiles and preoperative medications were distributed inhomogeneously [57].

Since these investigations not clearly distinguish between various valvular procedures, statin therapy is especially linked with favourable long-term survival after biologic aortic valve replacement according to a database analysis published by Pullan et al. in a cohort of about 5,000 patients. Otherwise, statin treatment had no advantageous effect after mitral valve replacement or repair [58].

Finally, the routine use of statins in patients at risk for degenerative valve disease or after bioprosthetic valve replacement can not be recommended on the basis of the current evidence [59]. Since the theoretical mechanisms of potential benefits exerted through statins in patients with coronary artery disease and heart valve disease are fundamentally different, results derived from studies with patients undergoing myocardial revascularization should not be translated to valve surgery. Further elucidation of this issue is will be provided by a Cochrane review that is currently expected to be published [60]. In the meanwhile, current guidelines on the management of valvular heart disease do not recommend statin therapy in patients with aortic stenosis “where their only purpose is to slwo progression” [61].

Choice of Statin Medication and Dose

All different kinds of statins that are on the market have the same way of action in terms of a reduction of LDL-cholesterol by blocking the key enzyme HMG-CoA reductase. However, the degree of inhibition varies among all statins so that the maximal LDL-reduction that can be achieved with a specific statin determines its potency. The table depicts the average LDL-reduction of commonly prescribed statins and the dose-effect-relationship seems to be most favourable for rosuvastatin with a 40% reduction of LDL-cholesterol with 5 mg (*table*) [62]. Of note, a high potency to inhibit the enzyme HMG-CoA reductase with subsequent reduction of cholesterol biosynthesis is not necessarily associated with a high benefit for the individual patient exerted through pleiotropic effects. Since most clinical trials investigate the effects of a specific statin compared to placebo or control, the direct comparability of different types of statins remains limited.

Nevertheless, comparative surveys among cardiac surgical patients revealed that rosuvastatin and atorvastatin are likely to provide the greatest benefit with regard to cardiac procedures. This thesis is supported by studies from Tran and Ohsfeldt et al. investigating cost-effectiveness of various types of statins. The authors finally generated a sequence with decreasing cost-effectiveness starting with rosuvastatin following atorvastatin, simvastatin and pravastatin for patients with elevated lipid-levels. This results is mainly based on the finding that more patients with coronary heart disease reached the target LDL-levels in accordance to current guidelines if they were treated wicht rosuvastatin when compared to atorvastatin and simvastatin [63, 64]. Similarly, a literature review published by Conway et al. with special focus on CABG patients placed rosuvastatin over all other statins [65]. However, the attempt to order all available types of statins is unable to reflect differences in the exertion of beneficial pleiotropic actions that finally appear to be class-dependent since they are in fact attributed to suppressed production of downstream products of mevalonate [66].

Table. Reduction of low density lipoprotein (LDL) level in percent achieved by different statins in various available doses (modified after [62])

Statin	LDL reduction (%)			
	>40	30-40	20-30	<20
Atorvastatin	>20	10	-	-
Fluvastatin	-	80	40	20
Pravastatin	-	-	20/40	10
Rosuvastatin	>5	-	-	-
Simvastatin	>40	20	10	-

Beside variations in cost-effectiveness and potentially differences in pleiotropic effects, the central aspect of statin therapy remains to achieve the recommended LDL-levels. When statin treatment is started once in the perioperative period, the statin dose needs to be adopted appropriately.

The Post-CABG trial aimed to address the impact of different doses of statins in a cohort of 1,351 patients who had undergone CABG surgery. The population was subdivided in a group with “aggressive” statin treatment (40 mg lovastatin per day) and a group with “moderate” therapy (2.5 mg lovastatin per day) with a median follow-up of 4.3 years. The effect was a marked reduction in the progression of atherosclerosis in the bypass grafts of patients with aggressive lovastatin therapy going along with a significantly lower rate of repeat-revascularization (6.5%) in contrast to the group receiving moderate therapy (9.2%) [67].

Pravastatin and atorvastatin were compared in different doses in a study conducted by Cannon et al. in a cohort of more than 4,000 patients with acute coronary syndromes. The incidence of the composite endpoint including death, myocardial infarction, unstable angina, revascularization and stroke was recorded in dependence of a random allocation to “standard therapy” with 40 mg pravastatin or “high-dose” 80 mg atorvastatin. Finally, the high-dose atorvastatin treatment turned out to be associated with a 16%-reduction in the hazard ratio of death or major cardiovascular events in contrast to standard treatment after a total follow-up of three years [68]. The clearly evident drawback of this investigation is the comparison of two statins in two doses (two comparisons at once), since the dose-effect relationship of atorvastatin is different compared to pravastatin (see table). On the other side, there is no other way to find out the practical value of a given type of statin in a certain dose than to perform multiple comparisons. This is even more important since new statin medications have become available and need to be assessed. In conclusion, these findings underline the need for a continuous re-evaltuation of statin effects in various subsets of patients.

Results from studies were collected in a recent meta-analysis of randomized controlled trials comparing aggressive and moderate statin therapy. Although the pooled analysis combines various definitions of "aggressive" and "moderate" statin treatment, the higher dose therapy slowed the progression of graft disease after myocardial revascularization, reduced the incidence of postoperative myocardial infarction the the need for repeat revascularization with comparable statin-related side-effects [69].

The most important aspect around statins is the administration itself beyond considerations about optimal doses and pleiotropic effects since statins are underutilized in patients undergoing surgical myocardial revascularization although they might profit from this relative safe class of drugs [70, 71]. For every individual patient potential side-effects of statin therapy need to be estimated taking into account the preoperative risk profile. But if statin related adverse effects occur they can be handled easily provided that adequate diagnostic and therapeutic tools are implemented as summarized in the clinical advisory of the American College of Cardiology and the American Heart Association [72]. Statin side-effects include a reversible myopathy at a rate of 11 in 100,000 patient-years of follow-up and the incidence of rhabdomyolysis is reported at about 1 death per 1 million. An increase of liver enzymes can be measured in about 1% of patients treated with statins what is usually reversible after statin withdrawal [70, 73, 74]. But although statins are in gerenal a well tolerated class of medications, only half of the patients that are planned to undergo CABG surgery are receiving statin therapy and an even smaller part is treated effectively to reach the recommended lipid-levels prior to myocardial revascularization in accordance to existing guidelines [75].

The optimal timing for (re-)administration of statins in the postoperative period remains under debate due to the common elevation of creatin kinase or liver enzymes after the operation that may interfere with or mask statin side-effects. Moreover, there are many reasons for complaints diagnosed as myopathy in a patient after saphenectomy for CABG surgery that can be classified as statin-related adverse effects. Considering discontinuation of postoperative statin intake should therefore be well balanced according to the potential benefits. This aspect was investigated by Laufs et al. who reported about improved endothelial and vascular function mediated by atorvastatin therapy in men with normal cholesterol levels that was no more present after discontinuation of statin treatment. This effect was independent of the change of cholesterol levels [76]. Likewise, statin therapy reduced the incidences of death and nonfatal myocardial infarction in patients with acute coronary syndromes at 30-day follow-up in comparison to those who did not receive statins, but most importantly, the discontinuation of statin treatment after hospital admission lifted the risk to the level of statin-naïve patients [77]. A comparable result is provided from a study by Collard et al. that retrospectively analysed records of more than 2,600 patients referred to CABG surgery of which one half was treated with statins preoperatively and one half presented without statin therapy. While preoperative statin intake was linked with favourable survival, discontinuation of statin intake was independently associated with an increased all-cause (0.6% vs. 2.6%; $p<0.01$) and cardiac mortaliy (0.5% vs. 1.9%; $p<0.01$) at 30 days [78]. Especially the statin administration on the day before elective cardiac surgery seemed to be linked with a marked reduction of biomarkers for acute kidney injury [79].

In conclusion, continuous statin administration and early re-initiation is likely to provide beneficial outcomes in cardiac surgery and especially in CABG patients.

High-Dose Statin Administration and Reloading Statin Effects in Cardiovascular Medicine

The classical concept of long-term statin therapy aims to interfere with the metabolism of cholesterol. However, growing evidence from animal models is emerging about beneficial statin actions that become effective when given shortly before an ischemic event or at reperfusion. In a study conducted by Mensah et al. that provided new insights into statin actions, the authors recorded infarct sizes of isolated rat hearts subjected to regional ischemia with various timing patterns of statin exposure. Firstly, the authors observed reduced infarct sizes with atorvastatin treatment for only one and three days, and this favourable effect was not detectable after treatment for one and two weeks. The authors concluded that the protection mediated by pleiotropic statin effects fades away over time. Secondly, in two additional groups, atorvastatin was given for one and two weeks, respectively, with supplementary doses directly before post-ischemic heart reperfusion. These extra doses reactivated the protective effects of statins on infarct size when compared to chronic statin therapy alone [80].

The results mentioned above from laboratory and animal studies were transferred into the clinical life in patients undergoing percutaneous coronary interventions. The ARMYDA-Recapture trial included 383 patients that presented with stable angina or acute coronary syndromes. Key inclusion criterion was a preexisting chronic statin intake of more than 30 days. All patients were then ramdomized to either atorvastatin reloading therapy 12 hours and immediately before the procedure (192 patients) or placebo (191 patients). The authors found a striking difference in the incidence of a composite endpoint consisting of cardiac death, myocardial infarction or unplanned revascularization at 30 days with 9.4% in the placebo group compared to the statin reloading group with 3.7% ($p=0.037$). This intensive statin treatment was identified as an independent predictor for a reduced incidence of a composite endpoint including cardiac death, myocardial infarction and target vessel revascularization with a 82% relative risk reduction in patients with acute coronary syndromes [16].

The investigators of the ROMA II study compared the effect of statin recapturing to control in patients undergoing elective PCI. A total of 350 patients receiving long-term statin therapy was randomized to either rosuvastatin or atorvastatin reloading and these two groups were finally compared to 100 consecutive patients serving as a control group. Primary endpoint was the incidence of periprocedural myocardial infarction, and furthermore, the occurrence of MACCE was detected. Parallel to the findings of the ARMYDA-Recapture trial, the authors found a significant benefit for statin reloading therapy in terms of lower incidences of myocardial infarction in the statin treated groups with a remarkable reduction of MACCE occurrence at 12-month follow-up (41.0% for control, 11.4% for rosuvastatin, 12.0% for atorvastatin group). However, based on the results of this investigation, a direct comparison of rosuvastatin and atorvastatin is not possible due to the design of ths study [81].

Unfortunately, there is no comparable trial for patients referred to cardiac surgery or especially for those undergoing myocardial revascularization procedures available up to date.

However, the ongoing Statin Recapture Therapy before CABG (StaRT-CABG) trial seeks to provide evidence about the effectiveness of reloading statin effects prior to myocarial revascularization. The StaRT-CABG trial is a phase 4, multicenter (9 centers in Germany), randomized, double-blind and placebo-controlled, parallel-group study in a total of 2,630 patients scheduled for on- or off-pump CABG. The primary outcome measure is the incidence of a composite endpoint consisting of all-cause mortality, non-fatal myocardial infarction and cerebrovascular event at 30 days after CABG with a total follow-up of 12 months. Included patients will be ranodmized to receive either oral statin reloading therapy or matching placeo at two separate doses before CABG surgery. Reload and placebo therapy will be administered twice at 12 hours and 2 hours prior to surgery. The individual statin regimen will be maintained before the procedure in both groups ensuring the comparability to normal routine (clinicaltrials.gov identifier: NCT01715714).

While the ARMYDA-Recapture study, the ROMA II and the StaRT-CABG trial deal with the impact of reactivating statin effects, many studies examined the benefit of high-dose administration of statins prior to PCI in statin-naïve patients. The authors of the NAPLES II trial randomized 668 statin-naïve patients to atorvastatin or control and report about a 44% reduction in the odds for periprocedural myocardial infarction associated with atorvastatin administration [82]. Similarly, the ROMA trial assessed the impact of high-dose rosuvastatin prior to elective PCI compared to control. The main finding of this study was the significantly lower incidence of periprocedural myocardial infarction among statin treated patients [83]. The results of six trials with a cumulative population of 2,088 individuals about the effect of high-dose statin administration in statin-naïve PCI patients were collected in a meta-analysis by Zhang et al., showing a 49% reduction in the odds for periprocedural myocardial infarction of statin pretreated patients [84].

In summary, high-dose statin administration prior to cardiovascular procedures including cardiac surgery in patients with or without prior statin intake can provide additional benefit far beyond the lipid-lowering effects of statins.

Conclusion

All patients with established coronary artery disease scheduled for CABG surgery should be treated with statins before and after cardiac surgery unless in the presence of contraindications. Otherwise, untreated patients are deprived of a safe therapeutic option that reduces short and long-term cardiovascular mortality and morbidity.

For patients undergoing valve surgery without any other reason for statin therapy, there is currently no definite evidence for the administration of statins.

References

[1] Bridgewater B, Gummert J, Walton P, Kinsman R. *Fourth EACTS Adult Cardiac Surgical Database Report.* Henley-on-Thames, Oxfordshire, UK: Dendrite Clinical Systems Ltd., 2010.

[2] Andrews TC, Ballantyne CM, Hsia JA, Kramer JH. Achieving and maintaining National Cholesterol Education Program low-density lipoprotein cholesterol goals with five statins. *Am. J. Med.* 2001;111:185-91.

[3] Brugts JJ, Yetgin T, Hoeks SE et al., The benefits of statins in people without established cardiovascular disease but with cardiovascular risk factors: meta-analysis of randomised controlled trials. *Bmj* 2009;338:b2376.

[4] Joshi PH, Chaudhari S, Blaha MJ et al., A point-by-point response to recent arguments against the use of statins in primary prevention: this statement is endorsed by the American Society for Preventive Cardiology. *Clinical cardiology* 2012;35:404-9.

[5] Taylor F, Ward K, Moore TH et al., Statins for the primary prevention of cardiovascular disease. *Cochrane Database Syst. Rev.* 2011;1:CD004816.

[6] Baigent C, Keech A, Kearney PM et al., Efficacy and safety of cholesterol-lowering treatment: prospective meta-analysis of data from 90,056 participants in 14 randomised trials of statins. *Lancet* 2005;366:1267-78.

[7] MRC/BHF Heart Protection Study of cholesterol lowering with simvastatin in 20,536 high-risk individuals: a randomised placebo-controlled trial. *Lancet* 2002;360:7-22.

[8] Grundy SM, Cleeman JI, Merz CN et al., Implications of recent clinical trials for the National Cholesterol Education Program Adult Treatment Panel III guidelines. *Circulation* 2004;110:227-39.

[9] Davignon J. Beneficial cardiovascular pleiotropic effects of statins. *Circulation* 2004;109:III39-43.

[10] Ray KK, Cannon CP. The potential relevance of the multiple lipid-independent (pleiotropic) effects of statins in the management of acute coronary syndromes. *J. Am. Coll Cardiol.* 2005;46:1425-33.

[11] Liakopoulos OJ, Dorge H, Schmitto JD, Nagorsnik U, Grabedunkel J, Schoendube FA. Effects of preoperative statin therapy on cytokines after cardiac surgery. *Thorac. Cardiovasc. Surg.* 2006;54:250-4.

[12] Laufs U, La Fata V, Plutzky J, Liao JK. Upregulation of endothelial nitric oxide synthase by HMG CoA reductase inhibitors. *Circulation* 1998;97:1129-35.

[13] Chello M, Patti G, Candura D et al., Effects of atorvastatin on systemic inflammatory response after coronary bypass surgery. *Crit. Care Med.* 2006;34:660-7.

[14] Bonetti PO, Lerman LO, Napoli C, Lerman A. Statin effects beyond lipid lowering--are they clinically relevant? *Eur. Heart J.* 2003;24:225-48.

[15] Undas A, Brummel-Ziedins KE, Mann KG. Statins and blood coagulation. *Arterioscler Thromb. Vasc. Biol.* 2005;25:287-94.

[16] Di Sciascio G, Patti G, Pasceri V, Gaspardone A, Colonna G, Montinaro A. Efficacy of atorvastatin reload in patients on chronic statin therapy undergoing percutaneous coronary intervention: results of the ARMYDA-RECAPTURE (Atorvastatin for Reduction of Myocardial Damage During Angioplasty) Randomized Trial. *J. Am. Coll. Cardiol.* 2009;54:558-65.

[17] Schouten O, Boersma E, Hoeks SE et al., Fluvastatin and perioperative events in patients undergoing vascular surgery. *N. Engl. J. Med.* 2009;361:980-9.

[18] Chan WW, Wong GT, Irwin MG. Perioperative statin therapy. *Expert opinion on pharmacotherapy* 2013;14:831-42.

[19] Mannacio VA, Iorio D, De Amicis V, Di Lello F, Musumeci F. Effect of rosuvastatin pretreatment on myocardial damage after coronary surgery: a randomized trial. *J. Thorac. Cardiovasc. Surg.* 2008;136:1541-8.

[20] Patti G, Chello M, Candura D et al., Randomized trial of atorvastatin for reduction of postoperative atrial fibrillation in patients undergoing cardiac surgery: results of the ARMYDA-3 (Atorvastatin for Reduction of MYocardial Dysrhythmia After cardiac surgery) study. *Circulation* 2006;114:1455-61.

[21] Ali IS, Buth KJ. Preoperative statin use and outcomes following cardiac surgery. *Int. J. Cardiol.* 2005;103:12-8.

[22] Christenson JT. Preoperative lipid-control with simvastatin reduces the risk of postoperative thrombocytosis and thrombotic complications following CABG. *Eur. J. Cardiothorac. Surg.* 1999;15:394-9; discussion 99-400.

[23] Coleman CI, Lucek DM, Hammond J, White CM. Preoperative statins and infectious complications following cardiac surgery. *Curr. Med. Res. Opin.* 2007;23:1783-90.

[24] Subramaniam K, Koch CG, Bashour A et al., Preoperative statin intake and morbid events after isolated coronary artery bypass grafting. *J. Clin. Anesth* 2008;20:4-11.

[25] Strandberg TE, Pyorala K, Cook TJ et al., Mortality and incidence of cancer during 10-year follow-up of the Scandinavian Simvastatin Survival Study (4S). *Lancet* 2004;364:771-7.

[26] Christenson JT. Preoperative lipid control with simvastatin protects coronary artery bypass grafts from obstructive graft disease. *Am. J. Cardiol.* 2001;88:896-9, A8.

[27] Thielmann M, Neuhauser M, Marr A et al., Lipid-lowering effect of preoperative statin therapy on postoperative major adverse cardiac events after coronary artery bypass surgery. *J. Thorac. Cardiovasc. Surg.* 2007;134:1143-9.

[28] Kulik A, Voisine P, Mathieu P et al., Statin therapy and saphenous vein graft disease after coronary bypass surgery: analysis from the CASCADE randomized trial. *Ann. Thorac. Surg.* 2011;92:1284-90; discussion 90-1.

[29] Eagle KA, Guyton RA, Davidoff R et al., ACC/AHA 2004 guideline update for coronary artery bypass graft surgery: a report of the American College of Cardiology/American Heart Association Task Force on Practice Guidelines (Committee to Update the 1999 Guidelines for Coronary Artery Bypass Graft Surgery). *Circulation* 2004;110:e340-437.

[30] Quin JA, Hattler B, Bishawi M et al., Impact of lipid-lowering medications and low-density lipoprotein levels on 1-year clinical outcomes after coronary artery bypass grafting. *Journal of the American College of Surgeons* 2013;217:452-60.

[31] Pan W, Pintar T, Anton J, Lee VV, Vaughn WK, Collard CD. Statins are associated with a reduced incidence of perioperative mortality after coronary artery bypass graft surgery. *Circulation* 2004;110:II45-9.

[32] Magovern JA, Moraca RJ, Bailey SH et al., Preoperative statin is associated with decreased operative mortality in high risk coronary artery bypass patients. *Journal of cardiothoracic surgery* 2010;5:8.

[33] Aboyans V, Labrousse L, Lacroix P et al., Predictive factors of stroke in patients undergoing coronary bypass grafting: statins are protective. *Eur. J. Cardiothorac. Surg.* 2006;30:300-4.

[34] Liakopoulos OJ, Choi YH, Kuhn EW et al., Statins for prevention of atrial fibrillation after cardiac surgery: a systematic literature review. *J. Thorac. Cardiovasc. Surg.* 2009;138:678-86 e1.

[35] Winchester DE, Wen X, Xie L, Bavry AA. Evidence of pre-procedural statin therapy a meta-analysis of randomized trials. *J. Am. Coll. Cardiol.* 2010;56:1099-109.

[36] Kuhn EW, Liakopoulos OJ, Borys MJ et al., Statins improve surgical ablation outcomes for atrial fibrillation in patients undergoing concomitant cardiac surgery. *Interact Cardiovasc. Thorac. Surg.* 2010.

[37] Tabata M, Khalpey Z, Pirundini PA, Byrne ML, Cohn LH, Rawn JD. Renoprotective effect of preoperative statins in coronary artery bypass grafting. *Am. J. Cardiol.* 2007;100:442-4.

[38] Singh I, Rajagopalan S, Srinivasan A et al., Preoperative statin therapy is associated with lower requirement of renal replacement therapy in patients undergoing cardiac surgery: a meta-analysis of observational studies. *Interact Cardiovasc. Thorac. Surg.* 2013;17:345-52.

[39] Layton JB, Kshirsagar AV, Simpson RJ, Jr. et al., Effect of statin use on acute kidney injury risk following coronary artery bypass grafting. *Am. J. Cardiol.* 2013;111:823-8.

[40] Liakopoulos OJ, Choi YH, Haldenwang PL et al., Impact of preoperative statin therapy on adverse postoperative outcomes in patients undergoing cardiac surgery: a meta-analysis of over 30,000 patients. *Eur. Heart J.* 2008;29:1548-59.

[41] Kuhn EW, Liakopoulos OJ, Stange S et al., Preoperative statin therapy in cardiac surgery: a meta-analysis of 90,000 patients. *Eur. J. Cardiothorac. Surg.* 2014;45:17-26; discussion 26.

[42] Kuhn EW, Liakopoulos OJ, Stange S et al., Meta-analysis of patients taking statins before revascularization and aortic valve surgery. *Ann. Thorac. Surg.* 2013;96:1508-16.

[43] Liakopoulos OJ, Kuhn EW, Slottosch I, Wassmer G, Wahlers T. Preoperative statin therapy for patients undergoing cardiac surgery. *Cochrane Database Syst. Rev.* 2012;4:CD008493.

[44] Powell BD, Bybee KA, Valeti U et al., Influence of preoperative lipid-lowering therapy on postoperative outcome in patients undergoing coronary artery bypass grafting. *Am. J. Cardiol.* 2007;99:785-9.

[45] Mithani S, Kuskowski M, Slinin Y, Ishani A, McFalls E, Adabag S. Dose-dependent effect of statins on the incidence of acute kidney injury after cardiac surgery. *Ann. Thorac. Surg.* 2011;91:520-5.

[46] Thanassoulis G, Campbell CY, Owens DS et al., Genetic associations with valvular calcification and aortic stenosis. *N. Engl. J. Med.* 2013;368:503-12.

[47] Pohle K, Maffert R, Ropers D et al., Progression of aortic valve calcification: association with coronary atherosclerosis and cardiovascular risk factors. *Circulation* 2001;104:1927-32.

[48] Farivar RS, Cohn LH. Hypercholesterolemia is a risk factor for bioprosthetic valve calcification and explantation. *J Thorac. Cardiovasc. Surg.* 2003;126:969-75.

[49] Antonini-Canterin F, Leiballi E, Enache R et al., Hydroxymethylglutaryl coenzyme-a reductase inhibitors delay the progression of rheumatic aortic valve stenosis a long-term echocardiographic study. *J. Am. Coll. Cardiol.* 2009;53:1874-9.

[50] Takagi H, Kawai N, Umemoto T. Do statins delay the progression of aortic stenosis? *J. Thorac. Cardiovasc. Surg.* 2009;137:e6-9.

[51] Kulik A, Masters RG, Bedard P et al., Postoperative lipid-lowering therapy and bioprosthesis structural valve deterioration: justification for a randomised trial? *Eur J Cardiothorac. Surg.* 2010;37:139-44.

[52] Parolari A, Tremoli E, Cavallotti L et al., Do statins improve outcomes and delay the progression of non-rheumatic calcific aortic stenosis? *Heart* 2011.

[53] Vaduganathan M, Stone NJ, Andrei AC et al., Midterm benefits of preoperative statin therapy in patients undergoing isolated valve surgery. *Ann. Thorac. Surg.* 2012;93:1881-7.

[54] Gilmanov D, Bevilacqua S, Mazzone A, Glauber M. Do statins slow the process of calcification of aortic tissue valves? *Interact Cardiovasc. Thorac. Surg.* 2010;11:297-301.

[55] Paraskevas KI, Mikhailidis DP. Statins may not prevent structural valve degeneration of aortic bioprosthetic valves, but should probably be prescribed to patients undergoing heart valve surgery nonetheless. *Interact Cardiovasc. Thorac. Surg.* 2009;11:302.

[56] Fedoruk LM, Wang H, Conaway MR, Kron IL, Johnston KC. Statin therapy improves outcomes after valvular heart surgery. *Ann. Thorac. Surg.* 2008;85:1521-5; discussion 25-6.

[57] Tabata M, Khalpey Z, Cohn LH, Chen FY, Bolman RM, 3rd, Rawn JD. Effect of preoperative statins in patients without coronary artery disease who undergo cardiac surgery. *J. Thorac. Cardiovasc. Surg.* 2008;136:1510-3.

[58] Pullan M, Chalmers J, Mediratta N, Shaw M, McShane J, Poullis M. Statins and long-term survival after isolated valve surgery: the importance of valve type, position and procedure. *Eur. J. Cardiothorac. Surg.* 2014;45:419-24; discussion 24-5.

[59] Chacko J, Harling L, Ashrafian H, Athanasiou T. Can statins improve outcomes after isolated cardiac valve surgery? A systematic literature review. *Clinical cardiology* 2013;36:448-55.

[60] Thiago L, Tsuji S, Atallah A, Puga M, Gios A, Valente O. Statins for aortic valve stenosis. *Cochrane Summaries.* DOI: 10.1002/14651858.CD009571.

[61] Vahanian A, Alfieri O, Andreotti F et al., Guidelines on the management of valvular heart disease (version 2012). *Eur. Heart J.* 2012;33:2451-96.

[62] Weng TC, Yang YH, Lin SJ, Tai SH. A systematic review and meta-analysis on the therapeutic equivalence of statins. *Journal of clinical pharmacy and therapeutics* 2010;35:139-51.

[63] Tran YB, Frial T, Miller PS. Statin's cost-effectiveness: a Canadian analysis of commonly prescribed generic and brand name statins. *Can. J. Clin. Pharmacol.* 2007;14:e205-14.

[64] Ohsfeldt RL, Gandhi SK, Fox KM, Stacy TA, McKenney JM. Effectiveness and cost-effectiveness of rosuvastatin, atorvastatin, and simvastatin among high-risk patients in usual clinical practice. *Am. J. Manag. Care* 2006;12:S412-23.

[65] Conway AM, Musleh G. Which is the best statin for the postoperative coronary artery bypass graft patient? *Eur. J. Cardiothorac. Surg.* 2009;36:628-32.

[66] Zhou Q, Liao JK. Pleiotropic effects of statins. - Basic research and clinical perspectives. *Circ. J.* 2010;74:818-26.

[67] The effect of aggressive lowering of low-density lipoprotein cholesterol levels and low-dose anticoagulation on obstructive changes in saphenous-vein coronary-artery bypass

grafts. The Post Coronary Artery Bypass Graft Trial Investigators. *N. Engl. J. Med.* 1997;336:153-62.

[68] Cannon CP, Braunwald E, McCabe CH et al., Intensive versus moderate lipid lowering with statins after acute coronary syndromes. *N. Engl. J. Med.* 2004;350:1495-504.

[69] Kang S, Liu Y, Liu XB. Effects of aggressive statin therapy on patients with coronary saphenous vein bypass grafts: a systematic review and meta-analysis of randomized, controlled trials. *Clinical therapeutics* 2013;35:1125-36.

[70] Armitage J. The safety of statins in clinical practice. *Lancet* 2007;370:1781-90.

[71] Brown WV. Safety of statins. *Curr. Opin. Lipidol.* 2008;19:558-62.

[72] Pasternak RC, Smith SC, Jr., Bairey-Merz CN, Grundy SM, Cleeman JI, Lenfant C. ACC/AHA/NHLBI clinical advisory on the use and safety of statins. *J. Am. Coll. Cardiol.* 2002;40:567-72.

[73] Law M, Rudnicka AR. Statin safety: a systematic review. *Am. J. Cardiol.* 2006;97:52C-60C.

[74] Thompson PD, Clarkson P, Karas RH. Statin-associated myopathy. *Jama* 2003;289:1681-90.

[75] Kulik A, Levin R, Ruel M, Mesana TG, Solomon DH, Choudhry NK. Patterns and predictors of statin use after coronary artery bypass graft surgery. *J. Thorac. Cardiovasc. Surg.* 2007;134:932-8.

[76] Laufs U, Wassmann S, Hilgers S, Ribaudo N, Bohm M, Nickenig G. Rapid effects on vascular function after initiation and withdrawal of atorvastatin in healthy, normocholesterolemic men. *Am. J. Cardiol.* 2001;88:1306-7.

[77] Heeschen C, Hamm CW, Laufs U, Snapinn S, Bohm M, White HD. Withdrawal of statins increases event rates in patients with acute coronary syndromes. *Circulation* 2002;105:1446-52.

[78] Collard CD, Body SC, Shernan SK, Wang S, Mangano DT. Preoperative statin therapy is associated with reduced cardiac mortality after coronary artery bypass graft surgery. *J. Thorac. Cardiovasc. Surg.* 2006;132:392-400.

[79] Molnar AO, Parikh CR, Coca SG et al., Association between preoperative statin use and acute kidney injury biomarkers in cardiac surgical procedures. *Ann. Thorac. Surg.* 2014;97:2081-7.

[80] Mensah K, Mocanu MM, Yellon DM. Failure to protect the myocardium against ischemia/reperfusion injury after chronic atorvastatin treatment is recaptured by acute atorvastatin treatment: a potential role for phosphatase and tensin homolog deleted on chromosome ten? *J. Am. Coll. Cardiol.* 2005;45:1287-91.

[81] Sardella G, Lucisano L, Mancone M et al., Comparison of high reloading ROsuvastatin and Atorvastatin pretreatment in patients undergoing elective PCI to reduce the incidence of MyocArdial periprocedural necrosis. The ROMA II trial. *Int. J. Cardiol.* 2013;168:3715-20.

[82] Briguori C, Visconti G, Focaccio A et al., Novel approaches for preventing or limiting events (Naples) II trial: impact of a single high loading dose of atorvastatin on periprocedural myocardial infarction. *J. Am. Coll. Cardiol.* 2009;54:2157-63.

[83] Sardella G, Conti G, Donahue M et al., Rosuvastatin pretreatment in patients undergoing elective PCI to reduce the incidence of myocardial periprocedural necrosis: the ROMA trial. Catheterization and cardiovascular interventions : *official journal of the Society for Cardiac Angiography & Interventions* 2013;81:E36-43.

[84] Zhang F, Dong L, Ge J. Effect of statins pretreatment on periprocedural myocardial infarction in patients undergoing percutaneous coronary intervention: a meta-analysis. *Annals of medicine* 2010;42:171-7.

In: Statins
Editor: Eric R. Travers

ISBN: 978-1-63463-057-3

Chapter 6

THE ROLE OF STATIN THERAPY IN CHILDREN

Karen King, Alan Macken, Michael B. O'Neill and Clodagh S. O'Gorman
University of Limerick, Limerick, Ireland

ABSTRACT

Atherosclerosis is a disease that begins in childhood. Evidence of fatty streaks, the earliest precursor of atherosclerotic lesions, has been found in the coronary arteries of children as young as two years of age. Hypercholesterolemia is a risk factor for coronary artery disease. Hypercholesterolemia can be either primary, when it is characteristic of the main disease, or secondary when it occurs as a result of either a disease process or drug treatment.

Given the risk of vascular disease, including myocardial infarction (MI), cerebrovascular accidents (CVA, also known as strokes), peripheral vascular disease (PVD), and ruptured aortic aneurysm, any or all of which may follow atherosclerosis, it is important to prevent or slow the early development of atherosclerotic lesions. This prevention necessitates the control of key risk factors such hypercholesterolemia, dyslipidemia, hypertension etc. However, at what point this prevention ought to occur, and in what form, is uncertain.

This uncertainty stems from the fact that using pharmacological primary prevention in the paediatric population is controversial. In an adult patient the course of action is clear. Hypercholesterolemia warrants the initiation of a statin. Statins, also known as hydroxymethylglutaryl Co-enzyme A inhibitors (or HMG-CoA inhibitors) act by altering cholesterol metabolism. In considering the paediatric population, the clinical course of vascular disease and the effect of altering this clinical course,are less certain. Questions of safety, efficacy and ethics abound.The use of statins in the paediatric population will be examined in this chapter.

ABBREVIATIONS

AAP, American Academy of Pediatrics; AHA, American Heart Association; ApoA1, apolipoprotein A-1; ApoB, apolipoprotein B; BMI, body mass index; BP, blood pressure;

CABG, coronary artery bypass graft; CHILD 1, Cardiovascular Health Integrated Lifestyle Diet 1; CIMT, carotid intima media thickness; CT, computed tomography; CVA, cerebrovascular accident; FCH, familial combined hyperlipidemia; FH, familial hypercholesterolemia; FMD, flow-mediated dilation; FSH, follicle stimulating hormone; HDLc, high-density lipoprotein cholesterol; HeFH, heterozygous familial hypercholesterolemia; HMG-CoA, 3-hydroxy-3-methylglutaryl-coenzyme A; HoFH, homozygous familial hypercholesterolemia; IMT, intima media thickness; LDLc, low-density lipoprotein cholesterol; LH, luteinising hormone; MI, myocardial infarction; NHLBI, National Heart, Lung and Blood Institute; NICE, National Institute for Clinical Excellence; Non-HDL-C, non high-density lipoprotein cholesterol; OCP, oral contraceptive pill; PAT, peripheral arterial tonometry; P-Day, Pathobiological Determinants of Atherosclerosis in Youth Study; PVD, peripheral vascular disease; PWV, pulse wave velocity; RCT, randomized controlled trial; TC, total cholesterol; TG, triglycerides; VLDL, very-low-density lipoprotein

Introduction

Atherosclerosis is a disease that begins in childhood. [1-3] Evidence of fatty streaks, the earliest precursor of atherosclerotic lesions, has been found in the coronary arteries of children as young as two years of age. [4] Hypercholesterolemia is a risk factor for coronary artery disease. Hypercholesterolemia can be either primary, when it is characteristic of the main disease, or secondary when it occurs as a result of either a disease process or drug treatment.

Given the risk of vascular disease, including myocardial infarction (MI), cerebrovascular accidents (CVA, also known as strokes), peripheral vascular disease (PVD), and ruptured aortic aneurysm, any or all of which may follow atherosclerosis, it is important to prevent or slow the early development of atherosclerotic lesions. This prevention necessitates the control of key risk factors such hypercholesterolemia, dyslipidemia, hypertension etc. However, at what point this prevention ought to occur, and in what form, is uncertain.

This uncertainty stems from the fact that using pharmacological primary prevention in the paediatric population is controversial. In an adult patient the course of action is clear. Hypercholesterolemia warrants the initiation of a statin. [5] Statins, also known as hydroxymethylglutaryl Co-enzyme A inhibitors (or HMG-CoA inhibitors) act by altering cholesterol metabolism. In considering the paediatric population, the clinical course of vascular disease and the effect of altering this clinical course,are less certain. Questions of safety, efficacy and ethics abound.

The use of statins in the paediatric population will be examined in this chapter.

Atherosclerosis in Childhood

Atherosclerosis is a complex process in which lipids and inflammatory mediators cause the formation of fatty streaks which progress to plaque formation. The plaque is at risk of rupture and thrombus formation which increases the risk of myocardial infarction (MI) and ischaemic stroke.

Atherosclerosis has its origins in childhood. [1-3] This was first asserted in 1961 by Holman who claimed atherosclerosis was a 'pediatric problem'. [6] Several studies since then validate this claim, including the P-Day Study (Pathobiological Determinants of Atherosclerosis in Youth) [2] and the Bogalusa Heart Study [3]. In the P-Day study the subjects were 15-34 year olds who died unexpectedly from trauma, homicide or suicide. [7] Post-mortem studies revealed that cardiovascular risk factors such as hypercholesterolemia and smoking were associated with the size of fatty streaks and plaques in youth, being therefore, important determinants of early atherosclerosis in adolescents and young adults. [7] The Bogalusa Heart Study examined the coronary arteries and the aortas of 35 autopsied subjects, whose mean age at death was 18 years, and found that fatty streaks were positively associated with low-density lipoprotein cholesterol (LDL-C) and negatively associated with high-density lipoprotein cholesterol (HDL-C). [3] Fatty streaks, the earliest precursor of atherosclerosis, were found in the coronary arteries of children as young as two years of age. [1] In the Bogalusa study, the prevalence of fatty streaks and fibrous plaques were 50% and 8% respectively during childhood, and 69% and 85% respectively, during young adulthood. (1) These Bogalusa study results confirm that atherosclerosis begins during childhood and progresses during adulthood.

Risk factors for atherosclerosis in childhood include obesity, hypertension, dyslipidemia, family history of cardiovascular disease, smoking and hyperglycaemia. [8] Atherosclerosis in a young person is commonly found in the presence of elevated total and LDL cholesterol, elevated BMI, and systolic and diastolic hypertension. [1, 2] However, children in whom the atherosclerotic process has already begun are usually asymptomatic. [9] The Muscatine Study demonstrated that increased total cholesterol levels in childhood were associated with increased carotid intimal medial thickness (CIMT) in adults aged 33-42 years of age. [10] Intimal medial thickness is a surrogate marker of the atherosclerotic process. However, the severity of atherosclerosis correlates with the duration of hypercholesterolemia, therefore early initiation of a statin in a child with FH (familial hypercholesterolemia) may be beneficial in preventing atherosclerosis. [11]

It is necessary to measure atherosclerosis in children by non-invasive means, thus surrogate markers for atherosclerosis have been developed. Two markers of atherosclerosis are endothelial dysfunction, which can be measured by flow-mediated dilation (FMD), and thickening of the vessel walls, measurable by intimal medial thickness (IMT). IMT in the carotid arteries is predictive of MI, stroke and aneurysm. [12] Increased IMT is found in children with FH and in children with a parent with a history of premature cardiovascular disease. [13] Other non-invasive measures of atherosclerosis include pulse wave velocity (PWV) which estimates arterial stiffness, computed tomography (CT) which quantifies calcium deposits in the coronary arteries, and magnetic resonance imaging (MRI) which measures atheromatous plaques. [14] Of these, CT is not ideal for use in children due to the risk of exposure to ionizing radiation. MRI allows examination of the cardiovascular structures and plaques without radiation exposure.

The above surrogate measures of atherosclerosis are not frequently suitable for point of care testing, usually requiring dedicated expensive equipment and a dedicated laboratory or space and trained personnel. Increasingly, efforts are being made to develop point of care tests. One example is the use of peripheral arterial tonometry (PAT, © Itamar Medical, Israel) to measure endothelial dysfunction, one of the early and potentially reversible steps in the natural history of atherosclerosis.

Physiological Role of Cholesterol

Cholesterol is a lipid present in the cell membranes of tissues throughout the body. Cholesterol has many physiological functions, including transmembrane signalling, central nervous system myelin formation, synaptogenesis and neuronal plasticity. [15] Cholesterol is the base upon which the body's steroid hormones are formed – growth hormone and sex steroids require steroids for production. Thus, cholesterol is of vital importance if the body is to function correctly, including, for intellectual development, growth and puberty, of profound importance to normal progress through childhood. However, not all cholesterols are equal. Cholesterol can be subdivided into low-density lipoprotein cholesterol (LDL-C) and high-density lipoprotein cholesterol (HDL-C). Excess LDL-C contributes to atherosclerosis [16, 17] whereas HDL-C is cardio-protective. [18] An imbalance in these two types of cholesterol may lead to atherosclerosis.

Hyperlipidemia in Childhood

Hyperlipidemia may be primary, when it occurs as a main feature of the primary disease causing hyperlipidemia, or secondary, when it occurs as a consequence of a related disease, disorder, or treatment. [19]

Primary Hyperlipidemia

Primary hyperlipidemia occurs in children with a genetic predisposition; conditions include HeFH, HoFH, familial hypertriglyceridemia, familial combined hyperlipidemia (FCH), and dysbetalipoproteinemia. FH and FCH are the most common in paediatric practice [20] with HeFH being much more common than HoFH and HoFH affecting younger children than HeFH. Of these, FH forms the body of research into childhood primary dyslipidemia.

FH is characterized by increased total cholesterol (TC) and increased LDL-C, while triglycerides (TG) and HDL-C are typically normal. [20] FH also has an inflammatory component, in addition to dyslipidemia. [21] FH comprises HeFH and HoFH. HeFH is by far the most common of the two; its prevalence being 1 in 500 people. [22] HoFH has a prevalence of one per million people. [23] Both HeFH and HoFH are autosomal dominant. Mortality in FH is 100 fold greater between the ages of 20-39 years of age than in the normal population. [24]

HoFH is caused by mutations to both LDL receptor alleles, and results in markedly elevated plasma LDL-C present from birth, cutaneous or tendinous xanthomas, and cardiovascular disease early in childhood. [24] Severe FH is so rare that untreated carriers rarely survive past their second decade of life. [24] Total cholesterol concentrations in HoFH range between 18.1-31 mmol/L. [23] HoFH is treated with high-dose statins, LDL-C apheresis, and even liver transplantation.

HeFH is characterized by total cholesterol 6.98-12.93mmol/L [22] and LDL-C in excess of 5.5mmol/L [25] Total cholesterol and LDL-C in HeFH have been stated to be twice the normal level. [26, 27] This dyslipidemia causes premature cardiovascular disease, with 50% of men and 25% of women developing a cardiovascular event by the age of 50 years. [20] Due to this high level of risk, those with HeFH are candidates for the early initiation of statin therapy. Unlike HoFH, patients with HeFH do not usually exhibit clinical signs of hypercholesterolemia in childhood or adolescence. Children with HeFH have thicker carotid and aortic IMT, a subclinical measurement of atherosclerosis. [28, 29] Studies have demonstrated that adolescents with HeFH have significant arterial wall thickening and that the rate of progression is greater than in those without HeFH. [9, 30]

Secondary Hyperlipidemia

Secondary hyperlipidemia, i.e., hyperlipidemia which occurs as a result of a disease, disorder or treatment, has increased in recent years. Causes of secondary hyperlipidemia in childhood include: obesity, diabetes mellitus, chronic kidney disease, hypothyroidism, liver failure and connective tissue disease. [31, 19] Drugs which cause a secondary hyperlipidemia include glucocorticoids, retinoids, beta-blockers, and anti-retroviral therapies. [19]

In recent years there has been a dramatic rise in secondary dyslipidemia related to childhood obesity. In US epidemiological studies, childhood obesity affects between 20% [32] to 30% [20] of the population. The dyslipidemia associated with obesity is characterised by hypertriglyceridemia. [19, 32, 33] There is a strong association between childhood obesity and the metabolic syndrome (dyslipidemia, hypertension and insulin resistance), all of which leads to atherosclerosis. [32] It is established that childhood obesity, and indeed excess weight that is still in the normal range, is associated with the risk of cardiovascular disease in adulthood. [15]

Obesity-related dyslipidemia is best treated in the first instance by lifestyle changes such as low-fat diet and exercise. [34]

GUIDELINES

The most recent guidelines relating to childhood hyperlipidemia and the risk of cardiovascular disease were released by the National Cholesterol Education Program Expert Panel in 2012. [35]

The guidelines refer to primordial prevention (the prevention of risk factors developing) and primary prevention (recognition and management of those children in whom identified risk factors are already present). [35]

The guidelines stress the early identification of children with dyslipidemia using universal screening, and the importance of assessing serum lipid profiles. To this end, acceptable, borderline and high values for each of the cholesterol types, have been compiled. [35]

A positive family history refers to a cardiovascular event, such as myocardial infarction (MI), angina, stroke, coronary artery bypass graft (CABG), stent or angioplasty, in a first degree relative below the age of 55 years if male, and below the age of 65 years if female. [35] If LDL-C elevation persists at ≥130mg/dL (3.36mmol/L), referral to a lipid specialist for addition of second lipid lowering therapy is required. High level risk factors include: hypertension requiring drug therapy (BP ≥ 99th centile + 5 mmHg), current cigarette smoker, BMI ≥ 97th centile, presence of high risk conditions such as diabetes mellitus, chronic kidney disease and postorthotopic heart transplant. Moderate level risk factors include hypertension not requiring drug therapy, BMI ≥ 95th centile, < 97th centile, HDL-C < 40 mg/dL (1.03mmol/L), and the presence of moderate risk conditions such as Kawasaki disease, SLE, HIV and nephrotic syndrome. [35]

The initiation of pharmacological therapy should be based on the average of results from at least two fasting lipid profiles obtained at least 2 weeks but no more than 3 months apart. [35] The goal of LDL-lowering therapy in childhood and adolescence is LDL-C below the 95th centile (≤ 130 mg/dL or 3.36mmol/L). The guidelines advise that in children <10 years old, statin therapy should be limited to those with a severe primary hyperlipidemia, a high-risk condition such as post-cardiac transplantation, or evidence of cardiovascular disease, and should be initiated by a lipid specialist. However, for children aged 8-9 years old, whose LDL-C remains persistently >190mg/dL (4.9mmol/L) after a trial of lifestyle management, and in the presence of a positive family history of premature cardiovascular events, or at least one high level risk factor, or at least two moderate level risk factors, statin therapy ought to be considered. [35]

Plasma Lipids Value Ranges for Children and Adolescents			
Category	Acceptable	Borderline	High
TC	<170mg/dL (4.39mmol/L)	170-199 (4.39-5.14mmol/L)	≥ 200 (5.17mmol/L)
LDL-C	<110mg/dL (2.84mmol/L)	110-129mg/dL (2.84mmol/L-3.33mmol/L)	≥130 (3.36mmol/L)
Non-HDL-C	<120mg/dL (3.10mmol/L)	120-144mg/dL (3.10-3.72mmol/L)	≥145mg/dL (3.74mmol/L)
ApoB	<90mg/dL	90-109mg/dL	≥110mg/dL
TG			
0-9 years	<75mg/dL (0.84mmol/L)	75-99mg/dL (0.84-1.11mmol/L)	≥100mg/dL (1.12mmol/L)
10-19 years	<90mg/dL (1.01mmol/L)	90-129mg/dL (1.01-1.45mmol/L)	≥130mg/dL (1.46mmol/L)
HDL-C	>45mg/dL (1.16mmol/L)	40-45mg/dL (1.03-1.16mmol/L)	<40mg/dL (1.03mmol/L)
ApoA-1	>120mg/dL	115-120mg/dL	<115mg/dL

Adapted from: Expert Panel on Integrated Guidelines for Cardiovascular Health and Risk Reduction in Children and Adolescents. NHLBI 2012 [35].

Conversion mg/dL to mmol/L: Cholesterol is mg/dL x 0.0259 = mmol/L, Triglycerides is mg/dL x 0.0113.

Recommendations for Lipid Screening	
Age	Recommendation
Birth-2 years	No lipid screening
2-8 years	No routine lipid screening However, measure fasting lipid profile x2 if: Parent, grandparent, aunt, uncle or sibling with MI, angina, stroke, CABG, stent at <55 years in males, <65 years in females. Parent with TC ≥ 240 mg/dL or known dyslipidemia Child has diabetes, hypertension, BMI ≥ 95th%ile or smokes cigarettes Child has a moderate- or high-risk medical condition
9-11 years	Universal lipid screening recommended Non-fasting lipid profile: calculate non-HDL-C Non-HDL-C ≥ 145 mg/dL, HDL < 40 mg/dL→FLP × 2. Fasting lipid profile: LDL-C ≥ 130 mg/dL, non-HDL-C ≥ 145 mg/dL HDL-C < 40 mg/dL, TG ≥ 100 mg/dL if < 10 years; ≥ 130 mg/dL if ≥ 10 years→repeat fasting lipid profile after 2 weeks but within 3 months
12-16 years	No routine screening However, measure fasting lipid profile x2 if new knowledge of: • Parent, grandparent, aunt/uncle or sibling with MI, angina, stroke, CABG/stent/angioplasty, sudden death at < 55 years in males, < 65 years in females • Parent with TC ≥ 240 mg/dL or known dyslipidemia • Patient has diabetes, hypertension, BMI ≥ 85th%ile or smokes cigarettes • Patient has a moderate- or high-risk medical condition
17-21 years	Universal screening once in this time period

Adapted from: Expert Panel on Integrated Guidelines for Cardiovascular Health and Risk Reduction in Children and Adolescents. NHLBI 2012 [35].

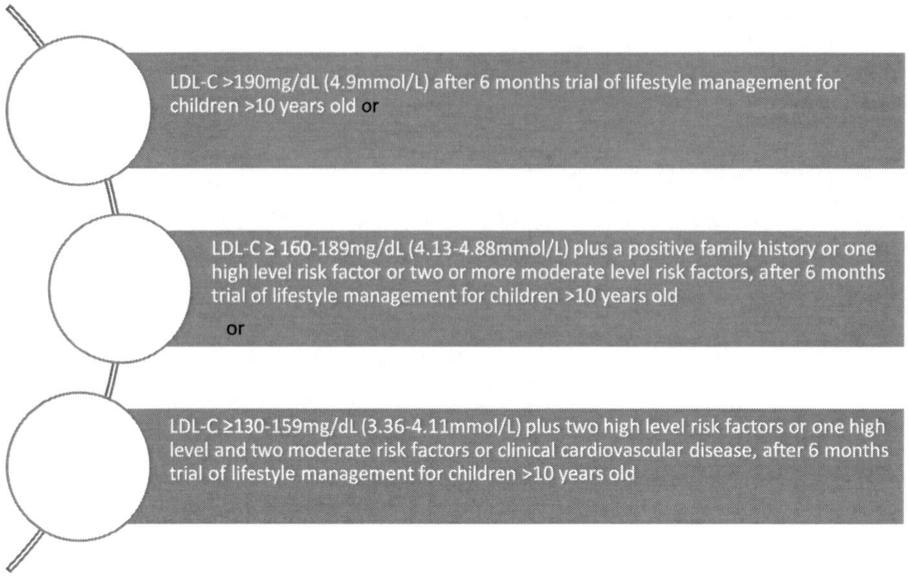

Adapted from: Expert Panel on Integrated Guidelines for Cardiovascular Health and Risk Reduction in Children and Adolescents. NHLBI 2012 [35].

Figure 1. When to Initiate Statin Therapy Based on LDL-C.

SCREENING FOR HYPERLIPIDEMIA IN CHILDHOOD

Universal Screening for Hyperlipidemia

The National Cholesterol Education Program Expert Panel have recommended universal screening of children aged 9-11 years old and again at 17-21 years old with a non-fasting lipid screen in order to identify those with hyperlipidemia. [35] Previously, targeted screening of those children at increased risk of cardiovascular disease was recommended. [36] However, some studies demonstrated that the AAP screening criteria lacked sensitivity. For example, in one such study dyslipidemia requiring pharmacologic treatment was more common among children who did not meet screening criteria than among those who did. [37] In another study of 678 children the sensitivity of the 2008 AAP screening guidelines was found to be 54-66% sensitive in identifying children with dyslipidemia. [38] Universal screening of children aged 9-11 years will overcome this issue. Targeted screening may lack sensitivity due to the factors used to decide whether a child was at increased cardiovascular risk i.e., family history, and parental serum cholesterol level. Family history may be unknown in some cases, whereas parental cholesterol may not have been checked. [14] However universal screening is not without its issues; there is a concern that universal screening will carry a heavy economic burden, and may cause unnecessary parental anxiety. [39]

An ideal screening test is valid, sensitive, specific, simple and safe. It must also be acceptable to the population that it is intended to screen. [40] Screening children for dyslipidemia, whether targeted or universal,is controversial, with some authors asserting that there are no studies demonstrating that treatment of dyslipidemias in childhood will prevent cardiovascular events later in life. [20] Also, universal screening will reveal children with dyslipidemia due to modifiable lifestyle factors; which many feel shouldn't be treated pharmacologically. However, there are studies which demonstrate that screening for and treating hyperlipidemia early in life delays progression of atherosclerosis. [11, 41] One additional important aspect of screening is to rule out secondary causes of dyslipidemia e.g., diabetes mellitus, hypothyroidism and renal failure. [14] Certainly, conditions such as FH confer an increased risk of cardiovascular disease, and since the atherosclerotic process begins early in life, on balance, many authors concur and the expert consensus [35] is, that early universal screening is justified. However, a recent survey of family medicine practitioners, paediatricians and general practitioners (n=548) confirmed that while 74% of respondents believed that lipid screening and treatment would reduce future cardiovascular risk, 34% performed no screening, 50% screened selectively, and only 16% performed universal screening. [42] The reasons cited for failing to screen were uneasiness addressing lipid disorders (43%), and unfamiliarity with screening guidelines (31%). Of interest, 57% of respondents were opposed to the use of lipid-lowering medication in children. [42]

Interpreting Cholesterol Assays in Children

Cholesterol levels are age and maturation dependent; therefore it is important to screen for hypercholesterolemia at the optimal time in childhood. [43] Total cholesterol levels are lower in the prenatal and early postnatal period, and both the total cholesterol and LDL-C begin to rise rapidly from the first week after birth before levelling at the age of two years. [44] Levels then remain stable until puberty, when LDL-C decreases by approximately 15%. [45] Thus, the National Cholesterol Education Program Expert Panel has designated the age range 9-11 years as the optimal period to assess lipids in childhood. [35] This age range (9-11 years) avoids confounding the cholesterol results because of pubertal lipid instability, while also being the best reflection of adult lipid levels. [14] NICE (National Institute for Clinical Excellence) recommends screening before the age of 10 years because after this point LDL-C variation is too great. [46]

When interpreting cholesterol assays one must consider gender and ethnicity also. Females have higher total cholesterol, LDL-C and HDL-C than males. [43] Ethnicity also complicates the interpretation of cholesterol assays in children, with black children having higher HDL-C, lower triglycerides, and higher total cholesterol than white and Hispanic children. [47, 48]

Treatment Options for Paediatric Dyslipidemia: Diet

Dietary modification and the introduction of exercise must be the cornerstone of paediatric dyslipidemias, whether or not pharmacological therapy must also be instituted. Dietary changes instituted in childhood are more successful if the entire family adheres to the new diet. [19]

Particularly in paediatric medicine, family-based therapy is essential to effect dietary and lifestyle changes. The Cardiovascular Health Integrated Lifestyle Diet (CHILD 1) is the first stage in dietary change for children with dyslipidemia, excess weight and obesity and risk factor clustering. [35] CHILD 1 is also the recommended diet for children with a positive family history of premature cardiovascular disease, dyslipidemia, obesity, primary hypertension, diabetes, or exposure to smoking in the home. [35] The diet recommends that in normal children and in children with hypercholesterolemia, intake of total fat can be safely limited to 30% of total calories, saturated fat intake limited to 7-10% of calories, and dietary cholesterol limited to 300 mg/d (7.75mmol/L). [35] The diet also encourages healthy eating habits such as breakfast every day, eating meals as a family, and limiting fast food meals. [35] In children <1 year old dietary fat ought not to be restricted as fats are important in infancy for brain and cognitive development. [35]

A healthy diet ought to be recommended for all children with dyslipidemia regardless of the aetiology of their condition. However, children with secondary hyperlipidemia can be expected to benefit more from a healthy diet than can children with primary hyperlipidemia. In particular, children with HeFH and HoFH will inevitably require statin therapy in addition to lifestyle changes.

Notwithstanding, dietary and lifestyle changes in a family-based setting are the cornerstone of treatment of paediatric dyslipidaemias.

TREATMENT OPTIONS FOR PAEDIATRIC DYSLIPIDEMIA: STATINS

Statins: Method of Action

Statins, or 3-hydroxy-3-methyl coenzyme A (HMG-CoA) reductase inhibitors, inhibit HMG-CoA, the rate-limiting step in endogenous cholesterol synthesis. This results in decreased intracellular cholesterol levels, and in the up-regulation of LDL-C receptors, resulting in increased LDL-C clearance in the circulation.

Statins: Efficacy

Statins are efficient at reducing LDL-C in children with FH. The LDL-C reduction achieved by statins in children ranges from 21-39%, [49] which varies by dose and agent used. A Cochrane review conducted in 2010, of 897 children with FH, concluded that statins reduce LDL-C by an average of 30%. [50]

In addition to lowering LDL-C, statin therapy has been shown to improve the surrogate markers of atherosclerosis; flow-mediated dilation and intimal-medial thickness. In one study, after 28 weeks treatment with simvastatin, FMD improved by 4% in the children with HeFH, as compared to the healthy controls who received a placebo. [51] Other studies have demonstrated the effect of statins on carotid intimal-medial thickness, notably Wiegman et al whose study of 214 children with HeFH demonstrated that after two years of therapy with pravastatin, CIMT reduced by 2%, compared with a 1% reduction in the untreated control group. [9, 30]

A follow-up study demonstrated that early initiation of statin therapy resulted in smaller increases in CIMT, thus the authors concluded that early initiation of statin treatment delays the progression of CIMT in adolescents and young adults. [11]

Statins Side Effect Profile

In adults, the most common side effects associated with statins are increased hepatic transaminase levels, elevations in creatine kinase, rhabdomyolysis and potential teratogenicity. [4] These side effects may be seen in the paediatric population also. [14] For example, elevations in alanine aminotransferase and/or aspartate aminotransferase have been reported in 1%-5% of children who were treated with simvastatin or atorvastatin. [51, 52] However, adverse effects such as increased hepatic transaminase levels and myopathy, are rare in the paediatric population. [14] Most studies on the use of statins in children with FH report that the drugs were well tolerated by the treatment group. [22, 43]

Statins: Safety

Although statins are generally a safe drug when used by adults, there is some concern about their use in the paediatric population. Concerned parties point to the lack of long-term studies to evaluate the life-time effects of initiating statins during childhood; the longest controlled trial is only two years long. [30] Also at issue, is whether inhibiting cholesterol synthesis at critical periods during childhood development may have adverse consequences. The steroid hormones, adrenal and gonadal, depend on cholesterol for synthesis. Therefore, there is a concern that statin therapy during childhood and adolescence may affect cholesterol dependent production of steroid hormones in the gonads and adrenal glands. [4] Puberty may be affected by statin therapy, theoretically at least, because cholesterol is required for all the sex steroid hormones. [19] However, Wiegman et al found no evidence of puberty being affected in their randomized control trial of children with FH. [30] De Ferranti et al point out that starting statin therapy at eight years of age, when the brain and other organ systems are in a dynamic stage of development, may affect the central nervous system, immune function, hormones, energy metabolism, or other systems in unanticipated ways. [15] There are additional concerns regarding the use of statins in adolescent girls, with potential effects on pituitary hormones (luteinising hormone, LH, and follicle stimulating hormone, FSH), menstrual cycle length, and physical development. [54] However, in a 24 week study during which adolescent girls with FH were treated with Lovastatin, there were no adverse effects recorded. [54]

Several studies have demonstrated the safety of statins for use in childhood in the short term i.e., in periods less than two years. [11, 30, 51, 53-56] A meta-analysis of six studies (n=798; 12 to 104 weeks of treatment) evaluating the safety and effectiveness of statins in children with FH found no statistically significant increases in adverse events compared with placebo. [49] There were no growth issues, side effects, muscle effects or liver toxicity. [49] In a study which assessed the use of statins in 214 children with FH, there was no effect on growth, development, adrenal or gonadal hormones. [30] This study was subject to follow-up giving a total treatment length of 4.5 years; no serious laboratory adverse events were reported, and statin treatment had no untoward effects on sexual maturation. [11] A Cochrane review summarised that statins are not associated with clinically significant changes in growth, maturation, liver enzymes, serum creatine kinase or myopathy. [50] However, the Cochrane review did not speak to the long-term safety of statins when initiated in childhood, as the studies thus far have had a short duration, with all lasting less than two years.

Statins: Use in FH

The National Cholesterol Education Program Expert Panel advise statins as first line therapy for HeFH and HoFH, after initial measures such as diet and exercise. [35] However, the Panel acknowledge that dietary measures alone are unlikely to achieve sufficient LDL-C reduction in primary hyperlipidemia. [35] Consideration should be given to starting treatment at the age of 8 years or older but, in special cases, such as those with HoFH, treatment might need to be initiated at earlier ages. [14] The treatment goal of statin therapy in paediatric FH patients is a $\geq$ 50% reduction in LDL cholesterol or LDL cholesterol <130 mg/dL (3.36mmol/L). [14] More aggressive LDL cholesterol targets should be considered for those with additional CHD risk factors. The initiation of statin therapy in children should be carried out in consultation with, or by referral to, a lipid specialist. [35] In paediatric HoFH patients statin therapy should be initiated earlier than 8 years of age. Although statins may be effective in HoFH patients, most will require the addition of LDL apheresis, or liver transplantation. [14]

The use of statins in pre-pubertal children is only recommended in the most serious cases of primary hyperlipidemia. [57] The American Heart Association recommends commencing statins after the age of 10 years and Tanner II puberty in males, or after 10 years and the onset of menses in female patients. [58] Although several studies of statin treatment to date have not demonstrated any effect on puberty, [30, 54] it would be sensible to delay initiating statin treatment until the onset of puberty if possible in order to demonstrate that normal puberty can occur in that individual patient.

Statin use in children must be monitored for muscle and liver toxicity through assessment of hepatic transaminases and creatine kinase. [35] In addition, female adolescents receiving statin therapy must be counselled about the possible teratogenicity of the drug, and receive contraception advice if indicated. Although, O'Gorman et al advise caution when prescribing the oral contraceptive pill (OCP), as it is contraindicated in hypertriglyceridemia and may be pro-thrombotic in FH. [19]

Statins: Use in Secondary Hyperlipidemia

Obese children with the dyslipidemic phenotype of elevated triglycerides and low HLD-C currently comprise the majority of children with lipid abnormalities. [4] However, the majority of studies on the use of statins in the paediatric population have focused on children with HeFH. The data taken from those studies on children with primary hyperlipidemia may not be representative of the children with secondary hyperlipidemia, which has an entirely different aetiology. Thus, some authors advise caution in extrapolating information from these studies in order to treat secondary dyslipidemia. [4, 19] For example, O'Gorman et al point out that dietary changes may be of more benefit to children with obesity-related dyslipidemia than to those with primary hyperlipidemia, and that lower doses of statins may be required as a result. [19]

The National Cholesterol Education Program Expert Panel guidelines focus primarily on children with primary hyperlipidemia. Kennedy et al assert that because the majority of childhood dyslipidemias are now due to secondary hyperlipidemia, the guidelines no longer apply to the majority of at-risk children. [4] One author takes issue with using statins to treat childhood dyslipidemia caused by modifiable lifestyle factors, and poses the scenario of ever stronger adult drugs being used to treat childhood obesity and its complications e.g., beta blockers, diuretics, aspirin, and insulin. [15] Certainly, unless children with obesity-related secondary hyperlipidemia incorporate a healthy diet and exercise into their lives they will remain at risk of cardiovascular disease in adulthood regardless of statin therapy begun in childhood.

Treatment Options for Paediatric Dyslipidemia: Other Pharmacological Agents

Bile Acid Binding Sequestrants

Bile acid–binding sequestrants work by binding the cholesterol in bile acids in the intestinal lumen, which prevents its reuptake into the blood. Bile acid binding sequestrants were originally the first line agent for hypercholesterolemia but they were supplanted by statins.

The National Cholesterol Education Program Expert Panel guidelines now advise that bile acid binding sequestrants be used in combination with a statin for patients who fail to meet LDL-C target levels with either medication alone. [35] There is no increase in adverse effects when both are used together, while the efficacy of both agents in combination appears to be additive. [35] Bile acid binding sequestrants are not ideal for use in the paediatric population due to their side effect profile which includes gastrointestinal effects, namely abdominal pain nausea, and constipation. [4, 14, 19, 43]

Cholesterol Absorption Inhibitors

Ezetimibe, a cholesterol absorption inhibitor, is currently approved for the treatment of FH in children ≥10 years of age. [4] Ezetimibe selectively inhibits cholesterol at the intestinal brush border, but does not affect absorption of triglycerides or the fat-soluble vitamins. [19] Although Ezetimibe has been shown to decrease LDL-C by up to 20% [59], there is no evidence that it decreases cardiovascular disease. [4] The ENHANCE study, which trialled Ezetimibe and Simvastatin in combination versus Simvastatin alone in adults with FH, demonstrated that Ezetimibe failed to improve CIMT over a two years period, despite achieving reductions in LDL-C and C-reactive protein (CRP). [59] The National Cholesterol Education Program Expert Panel guidelines state that cholesterol absorption inhibitors must be instituted only in consultation with a lipid specialist. [35]

Niacin and Fibrates

Niacin, a hydrophilic B-complex vitamin, works by decreasing hepatic production of very low-density lipoprotein (VLDL). Due to its serious side effects, poor tolerance and lack of safety data in paediatric patients, niacin therapy is usually reserved for children with HoFH or elevated lipoprotein-A levels. [4] Side effects of niacin include flushing, impaired glucose tolerance, liver failure, hyperuricaemia, and myopathy. [19, 43] The National Cholesterol Education Program Expert Panel guidelines state that niacin must be instituted only in consultation with a lipid specialist. [35]

Fibrates work by inhibiting the synthesis and increasing the clearance of the VLDL apoprotein B, which then leads to a decrease in VLDL production. They also inhibit peripheral lipolysis and decrease hepatic extraction of free fatty acids, which reduces hepatic triglyceride production. [43]

Fibrates are useful for reducing triglycerides, and increasing HDL-C. Their effect on LDL-C is variable. [4] Their primary use in treating primary hypertriglyceridemia. The fibrates have a similar side effect profile to statins, with rhabdomyolysis and myopathy increasing in incidence when statins and fibrates are used in combination. [43] The National Cholesterol Education Program Expert Panel guidelines state that fibrates must be instituted only in consultation with a lipid specialist. [35]

CONCLUSION

There is clear evidence that atherosclerosis begins in childhood, with the deposition of cholesterol and the formation of fatty streaks in the carotid and coronary arteries. Hypercholesterolemia is a key factor in the atherosclerotic process. Atherosclerosis may result in thrombotic plaque rupture causing MI, CVA, peripheral vascular disease or aortic aneurysm rupture. Given the risk of these cardiovascular events occurring, it is of vital importance to control risk factors such as hyperlipidemia.

In order to diagnose and treat childhood hyperlipidemia, the National Cholesterol Education Program Expert Panel guidelines have recommended universal cholesterol screening for all children between the ages of 9-11 years. Once diagnosed, control of dyslipidemia in childhood must begin with lifestyle intervention including a healthy low-fat diet and exercise.

This may be followed by the initiation of pharmacological therapy, of which statins are first-line. However, the control of hyperlipidemia using statin therapy has been dogged by controversy. Most authors accept the necessity of the use of statins in treating children with primary hyperlipidemia, namely HeFH and HoFH. However, this consensus is absent on the issue of treating secondary hypercholesterolemia caused by modifiable lifestyle factors such as obesity.

There are concerns, mainly theoretical albeit important, that statin therapy may interfere with normal growth, development and puberty. There have been several short-term studies that demonstrate both the safety and efficacy of statins in the paediatric population. However, long-term follow-up is lacking in the paediatric population. With the recommendation for universal screening in childhood, and the possibility that more children with dyslipidemia will come to light as a result, it is time to conduct a randomized control trial on the safety and efficacy of statins to discover if there are any long-term effects to initiating statin treatment in childhood.

Ongoing studies are required in order to fully understand the indications, risks and benefits to the use of statins in childhood dyslipidemia.

REFERENCES

[1] Berenson, G. S.; Srinivasan, S. R.; Bao, W.; Newman, W. P.; Tracy, R. E.; Wattigney, W. A. Association between multiple cardiovascular risk factors and atherosclerosis in children and young adults. The Bogalusa Heart Study.*N. Engl. J. Med.*, 1998, 338, 1650–1656.

[2] McGill, H. C. Jr.; McMahan, C. A.; Zieske, A. W.; Sloop, G. D.; Walcott, J. V.; Troxclair, D. A.; Malcom, G. T.; Tracy, R. E.; Oalmann, M. C.; Strong, J. P. Associations of coronary heart disease risk factors with the intermediate lesion of atherosclerosis in youth: the Pathobiological Determinants of Atherosclerosis in Youth (PDAY) Research Group. *Arterioscler. Thromb.Vasc. Biol.*, 2000, 20(8), 1998-2004.

[3] Newman, W. P. 3rd; Freedman, D. S.; Voors, A. W.; Gard, P. D.; Srinivasan, S. R.; Cresanta, J. L.; et al. Relation of serum lipoprotein levels and systolic blood pressure to early atherosclerosis. The Bogalusa Heart Study. *N. Engl. J. Med.*, 1986, 314(3), 138–144.

[4] Kennedy, M. J.; Jellerson, K. D.; Snow, M. Z.; Zacchetti, M. L. Challenges in the Pharmacologic Management of Obesity and Secondary Dyslipidemia in Children and Adolescents.*Pediatr. Drugs*, 2013, 15, 335-342.

[5] Shepherd, J.; Cobbe, S. M.; Ford, I.; Isles, C. G.; Lorimer, A. R.; MacFarlane, P. W.; McKillop, J. H.; Packard, C. J. Prevention of coronary heart disease with pravastatin in men with hypercholesterolemia. West of Scotland Coronary Prevention Study Group. *N. Engl. J. Med.*, 1995, 333(20), 1301-1307.

[6] Holman, R. L. Atherosclerosis–a pediatric nutrition problem? *Am. J. Clin. Nutr.*, 1961, 9, 565–569.

[7] Relationship of atherosclerosis in young men to serum lipoprotein cholesterol concentrations and smoking. A preliminary report from the Pathobiological Determinants of Atherosclerosis in Youth (PDAY) Research Group. *JAMA*, 1990, 264(23), 3018–3024.

[8] Hong, Y. M. Atherosclerotic CVD Beginning in Childhood.*Korean Circ. J.*, 2010, 40(1), 1-9.

[9] Wiegman, A.; de Groot, E.; Hutten, B. A.; Rodenburg, J.; Gort, J.; Bakker, H. D.; Sijbrands, E. J.; Kastelein, J. J. Arterial intima-media thickness in children heterozygous for familial hypercholesterolaemia. *Lancet*, 2004, 363, 369-70.

[10] Davis, P. H.; Dawson, J. D.; Riley, W. A.; Lauer, R. M. Carotid intimal-medial thickness is related to cardiovascular risk factors measured from childhood through middle age: the Muscatine Study. *Circulation*, 2001, 104(23), 2815–2819.

[11] Rodenburg, J.; Vissers, M. N.; Wiegman, A.; van Trotsenburg, A. S.; van der Graaf, A.; de Groot, E.; Wijburg, F. A.; Kastelein, J. J.; Hutten, B. A. Statin treatment in children

with familial hypercholesterolemia: the younger, the better. *Circulation*,2007, 116, 664–668.

[12] Lorenz, M. W.; Markus, H. S.; Bots, M. L.; Rosvall, M.; Sitzer, M. Prediction of clinical cardiovascular events with carotid intima-media thickness-asystematic review and meta-analysis.*Circulation*, 2007, 115, 459-467.

[13] Ford, E. S.; Mokdad, A. H.; Ajani, U. A. Trends in risk factors for cardiovascular disease among children and adolescents in the United States. *Pediatrics*, 2004, 114(6), 1534–1544.

[14] Daniels, S. R.; Gidding, S. S.; de Ferranti, S. D. Pediatric aspects of familial hypercholesterolemias: recommendations from the National Lipid AssociationExpert Panel on Familial Hypercholesterolemia. *J. Clin. Lipidol.*, 2011, 5, S30-S37.

[15] De Ferranti, S.; Ludwig, D. S. Storm over statins-thecontroversy surrounding pharmacologic treatment of children. *N. Engl. J. Med.*, 2008, 359(13), 1309-1312.

[16] Hoogeveen, R. C.; Gaubatz, J. W.; Sun, W.; Dodge, R. C.; Crosby, J. R.; Jiang, J.; Couper, D.; Virani, S. S.; Kathiresan, S.; Boerwinkle, E.; Ballantyne, C. M. Small dense low-density lipoprotein-cholesterol concentrations predict risk for coronary heart disease-the Atherosclerosis Risk in Communities (ARIC) study. *Arterioscler. Thromb. Vasc. Biol.*, 2014, 34, 1069-1077.

[17] Krauss, R. M. All Low-Density Lipoprotein Particles Are Not Created Equal. *Arterioscler. Thromb. Vasc. Biol.*, 2014, 34, 959-961.

[18] Rye, K. A.; Barter, P. J. Cardioprotective functions of HDLs. *J. Lipid. Res.*, 2014, 55(2), 168-179.

[19] O'Gorman, C. S.; O'Neill, M. B.; Conwell, L. S. Considering statins for cholesterol-reduction in children if lifestyle and diet changes do not improve their health: a review of the risks and benefits. *Vasc. Health Risk Manag.*, 2010,7, 1-14.

[20] Peterson, A. L.; McBride, P. E. A Review of Guidelines for Dyslipidemia in Children and Adolescents. *WMJ*, 2012, 111(6), 271-281.

[21] Holven, K. B.; Narverud, I.; Lindvig, H. W.; Halvorsen, B.; Langslet, G.; Nenseter, M. S.; Ulven, S. M.; Ose, L.; Aukrust, P.; Retterstøl, K. Subjects with FH are characterized by an inflammatory phenotype despite long-term intensive cholesterol lowering treatment. *Atherosclerosis,* 2014, 233(2), 561-567.

[22] Belay, B.; Belamarich, P. F.; Tom-Revzon, C. The use of statins in pediatrics: knowledge base, limitations, and future directions. *Pediatrics*, 2007, 119(2), 370-380.

[23] Familial Hypercholesterolaemia: a report of a second WHO consultation. Geneva. Switzerland. WHO. 1998.

[24] Raal, F. J.; Pilcher, G. J.; Panz, V. R.; van Deventer, H. E.; Brice, B. C.; Blom, D. J.; Marais, A. D. Reduction in mortality in subjects with homozygous familial hypercholesterolemia associated with advances in lipid-lowering therapy. *Circulation*, 2011, 124(20), 2202-2207.

[25] Descamps, O. S.; Tenoutasse, S.; Stephenne, X.; Gies, I.; Beauloye, V.; Lebrethon, M. C.; De Beaufort, C.; De Waele, K.; Scheen, A.; Rietzschel, E.; Mangano, A.; Panier, J. P.; Ducobu, J.; Langlois, M.; Balligand, J. L.; Legat, P.; Blaton, V.; Muls, E.; Van Gaal, L.; Sokal, E.; Rooman, R.; Carpentier, Y.; De Backer, G.; Heller, F. R. Management of familial hypercholesterolemia in children and young adults: consensus paper developed by a panel of lipidologists, cardiologists, paediatricians, nutritionists,

gastroenterologists, general practitioners and a patient organization. *Atherosclerosis*, 2011, 218(2), 272-280.

[26] Soutar, A. K.; Naoumova, R. P. Mechanisms of disease: genetic causes of familial hypercholesterolemia. *Nat. Clin. Pract. Cardiovasc. Med.*, 2007, 4(4), 214-225.

[27] Goldstein, J. L.; Brown, M. S. The LDL Receptor. *Arterioscler. Thromb. Vasc. Biol.*, 2009, 29 (4), 431-438.

[28] Noto, N.; Okada, T.; Abe, Y.; Miyashita, M.; Kanamaru, H.; Karasawa, K.; Ayusawa, M.; Sumitomo, N.; Mugishima, H. Changes in the textural characteristics of intima-media complex in young patients with familial hypercholesterolemia: implication for visual inspection on B-Mode ultrasound. *J. Am. Soc. of Echocardiogr.*, 2011, 24(4), 438–443.

[29] Di Salvo, G.; D'Aiello, A. F.; Castaldi, B.; Fadel, B.; Limongelli, G.; D'Andrea, A.; Pergola, V.; Pacileo, G.; Del Giudice, E. M.; Perrone, L.; Calabrò, R.; Russo, M. G. Early left ventricular abnormalities in children with heterozygous familial hypercholesterolemia. *J. Am. Soc. of Echocardiogr.*, 2012, 25(10), 1075–1082.

[30] Wiegman, A.; Hutten, B. A.; de Groot, E.; Rodenburg, J.; Bakker, H. D.; Büller, H. R.; Sijbrands, E. J.; Kastelein, J. J. Efficacy and safety of statin therapy in children with familial hypercholesterolemia: a randomized controlled trial. *JAMA*, 2004, 292, 331–337.

[31] EspinheiraMdo, C.; Vasconcelos, C.; Medeiros, A. M.; Alves, A. C;. Bourbon, M.; Guerra, A. Hypercholesterolemia-a disease with expression since childhood. *Rev. Port. Cardiol.*, 2013, 32(5), 379-386.

[32] Roger, V. L.; Go, A. S.; Lloyd-Jones, D. M.; et al. Executive summary: heart disease and stroke statistics-2012 update: a report from the American Heart Association. *Circulation*, 2012, 125(1), 188–97.

[33] Manlhiot, C.; Larsson, P.; Gurofsky, R. C.; Smith. R. W.; Fillingham, C.; Clarizia, N. A.; Chahal, N.; *Clarke*, J. T.; McCrindle, B. W. Spectrum and management of hypertriglyceridemia among children in clinical practice. *Pediatrics*, 2009, 123(2), 458-465.

[34] Ho, M.; Garnett, S. P.; Baur, L. A.; Burrows, T.; Stewart, L.; Neve, M.; Collins, C. Impact of dietary and exercise interventions on weight change and metabolic outcomes in obese children and adolescents: a systematic review and meta-analysis of randomized trials. *JAMA Pediatr.*, 2013, 167(8), 759-768.

[35] Expert Panel on Integrated Guidelines for Cardiovascular Health and Risk Reduction in Children and Adolescent. NHLBI 2012.

[36] Haney, E. M.; Huffman, L. H.; Bougatsos, C.; Freeman, M.; Steiner, R. D.; Nelson, H. D. Screening and treatment for lipid disorders in children and adolescents:systematic evidence review for the US Preventive Services Task Force. *Pediatrics*, 2007, 120(1), 189-214.

[37] Ritchie, S. K.; Murphy, E. C.; Ice, C.; Cottrell, L. A.; Minor, V.; Elliott, E.; Neal, W. Universal versus targeted blood cholesterol screening among youth: the CARDIAC project. *Pediatrics*, 2010, 126(2), 260-265.

[38] Eissa, M. A.; Wen, E.; Mihalopoulos, N. L.; Grunbaum, J. A.; Labarthe, D. R. Evaluation of AAP guidelines for cholesterol screening in youth: Project Heart Beat! *Am. J. Prev. Med.*, 2009, 37(1), S71-S77.

[39] De Ferranti, S. D.; Daniels, S. R.; Gillman, M.; Vernacchio, L.; Plutzky, J.; Baker A. L. NHLBI Integrated Guidelines on Cardiovascular Disease Risk Reduction: can we clarify the controversy about cholesterol screening and treatment in childhood? *Clin. Chem.*, 2012, 58(12), 1626-1630.

[40] Wilson, J. M. G.; Jungner, G. Principles and Practice of Screening for Disease. Geneva, Switzerland: World Health Organization; 1968.

[41] McGill, H. C. Jr.; McMahan, C. A.; Gidding, S. S. Preventing heart disease in the 21st century: implications of the Pathobiological Determinants of Atherosclerosis in Youth (PDAY) study. *Circulation*, 2008, 117(9), 1216-1227.

[42] Dixon, D. B.; Kornblum, A. P.; Steffen, L. M.; Zhou, X.; Steinberger, J. Implementation of lipid screening guidelines in children by primary pediatric providers. *J. Pediatr.*, 2014, 164(3), 572-576.

[43] Daniels, S. R.; Greer, F. R. Lipid Screening and Cardiovascular Health in Childhood. *Pediatrics*, 2008, 122(1), 198-208.

[44] Myśliwiec, M.; Walczak, M.; Małecka-Tendera, E.; Dobrzańska, A.; Cybulska, B.; et al. Management of familial hypercholesterolemia in children and adolescents. Position paper of the Polish Lipid Expert Forum. *J. Clin. Lipidol.*, 2014, 8(2), 173-180.

[45] Jolliffe, C. J.; Janssen, I. Distribution of lipoproteins by age and gender in adolescents. *Circulation*, 2006, 114, 1056-1062.

[46] Wierzbicki, A. S.; Humphries, S. E.; Minhas, R.; Familial hypercholesterolemia: summary of NICE guideline. *BMJ*, 2008, 337.

[47] Labarthe, D. R.; Dai, S.; Fulton, J. Cholesterol screening in children: insights from Project Heart Beat! and NHANES III. *Prog. Pediatr. Cardiol.*, 2003, 17(2), 169–178.

[48] Bradley, C. B.; Harrell, J. S.; McMurray, R. G.; Bangdiwala, S. I., Frauman, A. C.; Webb, J. P. Prevalence of high cholesterol, high blood pressure, and smoking among elementary school children in North Carolina. *N. C. Med. J.*, 1997, 58(5), 362–367.

[49] Avis, H. J.; Vissers, M. N.; Stein, E. A.; Wijburg, F. A.; Trip, M. D.; Kastelein, J. J.; Hutten, B. A. Asystematicreviewandmeta- analysis of statin therapy in children with familial hypercholesterolemia. *Arterioscler. Thromb.Vasc. Biol.*, 2007, 27, 1803–1810.

[50] Vuorio, A.; Kuoppala, J.; Kovanen, P. T.; Humphries, S. E.; Tonstad, S.; Wiegman, A.; Drogari, E. Statins for children with familial hypercholesterolemia. *Cochrane Database Syst. Rev.*, 2014 July 23;7:CD006401. doi: 10.1002/14651858.

[51] De Jongh, S.; Lilien, M. R.;op'tRoodt, J.; Stroes, E. S. G.; Bakker, H. D.; Kastelein, J. J. P. Early statin therapy restores endothelial function in children with familial hypercholesterolemia. *J. Am. Coll. Cardiol.*, 2002, 40, 2117–2121.

[52] McCrindle, B. W.; Ose, L.; Marais, A. D. Efficacy and safety of atorvastatin in children and adolescents with familial hypercholesterolemia or severe hyperlipidemia: a multicenter, ran- domized, placebo-controlled trial. *J. Pediatr.*, 2003, 142, 74–80.

[53] Carreau, V.; Girardet, J. P.; Bruckert, E. Long-term follow-up of statin treatment in a cohort of children with familial hypercholesterolemia. Efficacy and tolerability. *Pediatr. Drugs*, 2011, 13, 267–75.

[54] Clauss, S. B.; Holmes, K. W.; Hopkins, P.; Stein, E.; Cho, M.; Tate, A.; Johnson-Levonas, A. O.; Kwiterovich, P. O. Efficacy and safety of lovastatin therapy in adolescent girls with heterozygous familial hypercholesterolemia. *Pediatrics*, 2005, 116, 682–688.

[55] Knipscheer, H. C.; Boelen, C. C.; Kastelein, J. J.; van Diermen, D. E.; Groenemeijer, B. E.; van den Ende, A.; Büller, H. R.; Bakker, H. D. Short-term efficacy and safety of pravastatin in 72 children with familial hypercholesterolemia. *Pediatr. Res.*, 1996, 39, 867–871.

[56] Gandelman, K.; Glue, P.; Laskey, R.; Jones, J.; LaBadie, R.; Ose, L. An eight-week trial investigating the efficacy and tolerability of atorvastatin for children and adolescents with heterozygous familial hypercholesterolemia. *Pediatr. Cardiol.*, 2011, 32(4), 433-441.

[57] Vuorio, A.; Docherty, K. F.; Humphries, S. E.; Kuoppala, J.; Kovanen, P. T. Statin treatment of children with familial hypercholesterolemia – Trying to balance incomplete evidence of long-term safety and clinical accountability: Are we approaching a consensus? *Atherosclerosis*, 2013, 226(2), 315-320.

[58] McCrindle, B. W. Summary of the American Heart Association's scientific statement on drug therapy of high-risk lipid abnormalities in children and adolescents. *Arterioscler. Thromb. Vasc. Biol.*, 2007, 27(5), 982-985.

[59] Kastelein, J. J.; Akdim, F.; Stroes, E. S.; Zwinderman, A. H.; Bots, M. L.; Stalenhoef, A. F.;Visseren, F. L.; Sijbrands, E. J.; Trip, M. D.; Stein, E. A.; Gaudet, D.; Duivenvoorden, R.; Veltri, E. P.; Marais, A. D.; de Groot, E. Simvastatin with or without ezetimibe in familial hypercholesterolemia. *N. Engl. J. Med.*, 2008, 358(14), 1431–1443.

In: Statins
Editor: Eric R. Travers

ISBN: 978-1-63463-057-3

Chapter 7

STATINS AND PORTAL HYPERTENSION

Gonzalo Ramírez[1], Jimmy Briceño[1] and Armando Rojas[1,*]
[1]Biomedical Research Labs, Medicine Faculty,
Catholic University of Maule, Talca, Chile

ABSTRACT

Portal hypertension is a common clinical consequence of chronic liver disease that is associated with significant morbidity and mortality. Newly described pathophysiological mechanisms has opened new perspectives for therapeutic approaches, where statins may represent an attractive option to reduce portal pressure by targeting multiple molecular pathways such as endothelial dysfunction, oxidative stress, prostanoids production, angiogenesis and HSC activation. In this work we described how statins may correct hemodynamic abnormalities in portal circulation of cirrhotic patients and also summarize some promising results humans and animals in studies.

Keywords: Liver cirrhosis, statins, portal hypertension, hepatic stellate cell, intrahepatic vascular resistance, vascular endothelium, nitric oxide

INTRODUCTION

Portal hypertension is a hemodynamic abnormality characterized by an increase in portal venous pressure generating clinical complications such as ascites, hepatic encephalopathy and variceal bleeding [1].

These complications involve a high risk of disability and a reduced life expectancy. The results derived from several prognosis studies are not very encouraging, due to the high mortality of this clinical entity [2].

The current therapeutic use of statins is mainly based on the inhibition of 3-hydroxy-3-methyl-glutaryl-CoA (HMG-CoA) reductase, the rate-limiting enzyme in cholesterol synthesis and the subsequent increasing of low-density lipoprotein (LDL) receptors in the

[*] E-mail: arojasr@ucm.cl, Phone: 56-71-203134.

liver [3] and thus preventing cardiovascular events. These cardiovascular protective effects also include pleiotropic actions on vascular endothelium [4]which in turn, may represent a new therapeutic approach aimed to reduce portal pressure.

PATHOPHYSIOLOGY OF PORTAL HYPERTENSION

The syndrome of portal hypertension is defined as a pathological increase of portal venous pressure above normal values (6mmHg), reaching levels of 10 to 12 mmHg and thus generating significant hemodynamic changes that lead to the dreaded complications of this disease [5]

Increased vascular resistance to portal blood flow is the primary factor in causing portal hypertension. The cirrhotic process results in a significant alteration of hepatic angioarchitecture evidenced by the development of liver fibrosis, established septal portal-central anastomosis, as well as arterializations and capillarization of sinusoids. The formation of these "feeding vessels", derived from the hepatic artery,are produced as a consequence of the reduced portal flow. It is widely accepted that these processes are irreversible in nature, and they represent a point of no return, based on the capacity of generating increased portal pressure in cirrhosis [6, 7].

In recent years, it has become clear that another important factor in the development of portal hypertension is the active contraction of cellular elements, in both sinusoidal and extra-sinusoidal levels, including smooth muscle cells of the intrahepatic vasculature, hepatic stellate cells (HSC) [8, 9] as well as liver myofibroblasts, which may compress the regenerating nodules or venous shunt within the fibrous septum. These mechanisms create a dynamic and reversible process of intrahepatic resistance, which account 40% of total vascular resistance in cirrhosis of the liver [5].

Endothelial Dysfunction

In various pathological conditions there is an impairment of endothelium-dependent vasodilation. This state, known as "endothelial dysfunction", has been mainly ascribed to a decreased bioavailability of nitric oxide (NO) [10] and an increased prostanoid production leading to vasoconstriction [5].

In cirrhotic livers, endothelial dysfunction results in an impaired vasodilator response to acetylcholine and production of nitric oxide (NO) by endothelial nitric oxide synthase (eNOS). This dysfunctional state generates a loss of vascular accommodation to the increased flow caused by portal post-prandial hyperemia which, in turn, contributes to the progressive dilatation of porto-systemic collaterals and the development of varicose veins [11, 12].

Endothelial cells are the first line of defense protecting the liver from injury [13], therefore they are vulnerable to various types of liver injury. The type of endothelial dysfunction at the inthehepatic/sinusoidal microcirculation in the development of cirrhosis and portal hypertension is due to hypoactive endothelial cells [14].

The major hepatic endothelial cells are liver sinusoidal endothelial cells (LSECs), comprising ~98% of the total number of endothelial cells found in the non-parenchymal cell population of the liver [15]. Therefore, the endothelial dysfunction observed in the intrahepatic circulation is apparently due to LSECs, because LSECs have effects on liver functions such as blood clearance, vascular tone, immunity, hepatocyte growth and angiogenesis/sinusoidal remodeling [15, 16, 17]. These physiological impairment facilitate the development of cirrhosis and portal hypertension.

Bioavailability of NO

NO activates guanylate cyclase and increases guanosine 3′:5′-cyclic monophosphate levels (cGMP) which generates relaxation of the vascular wall. The main source of vascular NO is ascribed to eNOS [5]. A decreased production of NO is observed in cirrhosis-associated sinusoidal endothelial dysfunction, and it has been postulated as the most important factor in the increased hepatic vascular tone in cirrhosis patients [11, 12, 18, 19]. The molecular mechanisms responsible for the reduced NO production has been mainly ascribed to alterations at post-translational regulation level, particularly to decreased Akt-dependent eNOS phosphorylation [11]. Of note, Akt Ser/Thr kinase activity has been reported to be decreased in cirrhotic livers, which in turn, reduced eNOS activation [20].

In the context of post-translational regulation of eNOS, caveolin-1 is over-expressed in cirrhotic livers [18]. Caveolin-1 is an integral membrane protein, being the main component of caveolae and thus allowing a fine regulation of physiological responses, including activation and trafficking of eNOS [21, 22]. Caveolin-1 scaffolding domain (CSD) inhibits eNOS activity by reducing the electrons flow from the reductase domain to the oxygenase domain of eNOS and therefore decreases cellular NO production [23, 24]. The mechanisms involved in the increased expression of caveolin-1 reported in cirrhotic livers is still unknown, although it is likely to be related to intrahepatic cholesterol levels [25], considering that binding capacity of caveolin-1 to cholesterol [18]. In fact, Thabut et al [26] report that decreased HDL levels in cirrhotic rats lead to an increase in serum endotoxin LPS levels. As a result, the increased endotoxin level facilitates cavelin-1´s association with eNOS and decreases phosphorylation of Akt, thereby decreasing eNOS activity in cirrhotic livers [26].

The RhoA/Rho-kinase system at vascular level is linked to the regulation of both expression and activity of eNOS. When activated, this intracellular signaling pathway results in an impairment of both mRNA stability and phosphorylation-mediated eNOS activation [27, 28].

Oxidative Stress

The presence of oxidative stress has been reported in many pathophysiological conditions that cause chronic liver disease [29]. This condition is caused by a marked imbalance between reactive oxygen species (ROS) producing enzymatic systems (xanthine oxidase, nicotinamide adenine dinucleotide phosphate (NADPH) oxidase, and cyclooxigenases (COXs) and a decrease in ROS-detoxifying enzymes, such as superoxide dismutase, and thus producing a net increase of ROS. Of note, superoxide anion (O2-), which is also able to react with NO, produces a marked reduction on NO bioavailability, and thus increasing vascular tone [30]. The decrease in superoxide dismutase (SOD) activity is partly due to a decrease in the expression of Copper/Zinc superoxide dismutase (CuZnSOD) and Manganese superoxide dismutase (MnSOD) isoforms, but not the extracellular superoxide dismutase (EcSOD) [29].

A major determinant of oxidative stress in cirrhotic liver is the NADPH oxidase complex, which is expressed in both Kupffer and HSC cells. NADPH oxidases, also known as NOX enzymes, constitute the main enzymatic source of vascular O2-. Two main components of the catalytic subunit of this enzymatic system, p47 phox and Rac-1 are up-regulated by angiotensin-II; at both gene expression and post-transcriptional levels; increasing NADPH oxidase activity and the subsequent production of O2- and H2O2 as well as hydroxyethyl radicals [29, 31, 32].

One consequence of the increased superoxide production is dealt with the oxidation of tetrahydrobiopterin (BH4), a cofactor of eNOS. This process is known be linked to NOS uncoupling, a dysfunctional enzymatic state where eNOS is unable to transfer electrons to L-arginine, and thus favoring the production of superoxide rather than NO [5, 31, 32].

BH4 deficiency may be also raised by a reduction on either the expression or the activity of cyclohydrolase guanosine-5`-triphosphate, the limiting enzyme in BH4 synthesis, which is associated with decreased activity of NOS and NO availability [6].

At present, a compelling body of evidence suggests that ROS play an important role in liver fibrosis. in particular to impairs eNOS activity in at least three ways [33]: (1) increasing association of eNOS with caveolin-1; (2) inhibiting endothelin-1 (ET-1) induced NOS phosphorylation; (3) increasing dissociation of eNOS from endothelin receptos B (ETRb). In addition to this, oxidative stress has a pro-fibrogenic effect that is mediated in part by the activation and the phenotypic switch of HSC in response to liver tissue injury. Depending on the extent of damage caused by oxidative stress it may, in addition to fibrosis, lead to cell death by necrosis and apoptosis [29, 32, 34].

Vasoconstrictor Prostanoid Production

Endothelial dysfunction is also linked to an increased production of the cyclooxygenase-mediated vasoconstrictor prostanoid thromboxane A2 TXA_2. At present, it is widely accepted that TXA_2 plays a major role in endothelial dysfunction [35]. Of note, indomethacin, a well-known inhibitor of COX-1, markedlyreduced portal hypertension in patients with cirrhosis [5, 35].

Intrahepatic Microcirculation Sensitivity to Vasoconstrictors

Activation of RhoA/Rho-kinase signaling pathway contributes to an increased intrahepatic resistance with a marked sensitivity to vasoconstrictor stimuli [36]. Of note, geranylgeranyl pyrophosphate (GGPP), a byproduct of the synthesis of endogenous cholesterol, is a key element in the activation of the RhoA/Rho-kinase pathway [27, 28].

Kruppel-Like Factor 2, Gene Expression and LSECs

Kruppel-like factor 2 (KLF2) is a transcriptional factor expressed in endothelium, lung, and lymphocytes [37], conferring vasoprotection inducing the expression of vasodilator, antithrombotic, and anti-inflammatory genes, including eNOS and thrombomodulin [38]. Furthermore, KLF2 expression in LSECs inhibits oxidative stress-mediated cell injury and apoptosis, through a NO-independent antioxidant mechanism, namely KLF2-dependent induction of the cytoprotective enzyme heme oxygenase-1 (HO-1), the rate-limiting enzyme in the catabolism of heme, in endothelial cells. HO-1 products activate antiapoptotic [39], anti-inflammatory [40] and antioxidant signaling pathways [41, 42, 43]. By these characteristics, KLF2 is considered an essential nuclear factor in maintaining a functional endothelial phenotype. [44].

Shear-stress is the most potent know inducer of KLF2 expression [29, 30, 45], finding increased its expression in cirrhotic livers [45]. Nevertheless, there is not an increased in eNOS levels in cirrhotic livers, changes in the stability of eNOS mRNA may play a role in the final level [14].

Role of Hepatic Stellate Cells (HSC)

A growing body of evidences has supported the role of HSC in the pathophysiology of portal hypertension. Its location in the space of Disse allows a close interaction with both hepatocytes and sinusoidal endothelial cells. Their spatial arrangement and extent cover the entire microcirculation networks of sinusoids.In fact, recent data have demonstrated that LSECs and HSC regulate their phenotypes in a paracrine manner [46]. Paracrine communication and matrix-cell interactions in the sinusoidal niche are keyregulators of cellular phenotype and functional status. The LSECs-HSC cross-talk has been proposed as a means of regulation both LSECs and HSC activation. Local NO production by differentiated LSECs promotes HSC quiescence, and activation of the VEGF-NO pathway in hepatocytes and HSCs maintains LSECs in a quiescent differentiated state [47]. Therefore, disruption of paracrine communication propagates fibrosis and endothelial dysfuncton in the cirrhotic liver [48]. Another feature of HSC, is that contains cytoplasmic lipid droplets with a diameter of 1-2 μm, which are important reservoirs of retinyl esters and therefore have a fundamental role in the metabolism of retinoids. [49]

Because of HSC are oriented around the periphery of the sinusoids and in close interaction with endothelium, they have even been considered as analogs of perivascular cells or pericytes [49, 50].

Morphological studies have showed that during a progressive liver injury, HSC are activated and underwent a transitional phenotypic switch to α-smooth muscle actin-positive myofibroblast-like cells, which have been described in the fibrous septum, and around sinusoids and terminal venules in cirrhotic livers [51, 52, 53].

In this activation step angiotensin II, in addition to other factors produced by Kupffer cells and hepatocytes, triggers the over-production of many extracellular matrix components, such as collagen, heparan sulfate, chondroitin sulfate, proteoglycans, and laminin among others.

Obviously, this over-expression of extracellular matrix components plays a major role in liver fibrosis [50, 54-58].

Endothelin-1 is the most powerful vasoactive molecule that induces contraction of activated HSC. This agonist is markedly elevated in patients with portal hypertension and produces a profound effect on HSC contractile function, considering that this cell type has the greater number of receptors for endothelin-1 than of any other liver cells. The magnitude of the contraction force generated in HSC has been shown to be sufficient to modulate sinusoidal blood flow, increasing vascular resistance and thus increasing portal pressure [8, 59, 60, 61].

The mechanism by which endothelin-1 induces contraction of the HSC is controversial. Although previous studies highlighted the importance of signaling triggered by Ca^{2+} to activate the light-chain myosin kinase and the subsequent phosphorylation of light-chain myosin [51, 61, 62, 63, 64]; current knowledge indicates that Ca^{2+} -mediated signaling has a minor role in regulating the force of contraction of HSC. An elevation above physiological thresholds of Ca^{2+}, triggered by a Ca^{2+}ionofore, induces a minimal increase in the force of contraction. In contrast, treatment with calcium chelators does not have any effect on endothelin-1-induced HSC contraction [65, 66].

At present, signaling pathways mediated by Rho are considered as key elements in HSC contraction, and both RhoA and Rho-kinase are expressed in this cell type [67, 68]. The specific inhibition of RhoA causes a mismatch in the actin cytoskeleton of HSC, which in turn produce a diminished contractile force in HSC [67].

Endothelin in Portal Resistance

Endothelins are a family of vasoactive peptides of 21 amino acids homologous (ET-1, ET-2, ET-3), and their potent vasoconstrictor action are mediated by two receptors named A and B. The ET-A receptor has higher affinity to ET-1 and is involved in vasoconstriction. The ET-B receptor has similar affinity for ET-1 and ET-3. Activation of ET-B receptor on endothelial cells promotes a vasodilation mediated by NO and prostacyclin. In contrast, endothelins promote vasoconstriction in smooth muscle cells [3, 67].

Circulating plasma levels of ET-1 and ET-3 are elevated in patients with cirrhosis and their levels correlate with the severity of disease and portal pressure [68, 69]. Its production is regulated by mRNA transcript levels of PreproET-1, which is stimulated by vasopressor hormones such as epinephrine, angiotensin-II, vasopressin, mechanical stress and also by cytokines [70, 71, 72].

ET-1 plasma levels are also regulated by a clearance mechanism mediated by hepatic receptors. The liver is responsible for 85% of ET-1 clearance and this capacity is reported to be lowered by 50% in cirrhosis mainly due to the fibrosis in liver sinusoids. [73].

ET-1 binding sites have been identified in many cell types in the liver, as demonstrated for HSC, sinusoidal endothelial cells and endothelial cells from central portal vein. However, HSC has the greater density of such receptors [74, 75], and their activation trigger different processes such as fibrogenesis, cell proliferation and vasoregulation. Noteworthy, ET-1 is able to induce the expression of α-smooth muscle actin in HSC [76] thus promoting cell contraction [8, 51]. ET-1 also induces vasoconstriction in preterminal portal venules, causing a significant increase in portal pressure [69].

Toll-Like Receptor Signaling, Inflammation and Angiogenesis

The unique anatomical location and vascular supply of the liver lends itself to frequent exposure to intestinal bacteria and bacterial products, particularly in cirrhosis and portal hypertension, where studies showed that LPS-binding protein was increased in 42% of cirrhotic patients.Therefore the inmmunobiology of gut bacterial translocation generates a downstream innate inflammatory responses and play a role in processes such as hepatic fibrogenesis [48, 77, 78].

Downstream signals following bacterial translocation are numerous, but among others, the activation of TLR on parenchymal and non-parenchymal cells is one of these [48]. Kupffer cells are the primary cells that respond to pathogen-associated molecular pattern adopting a proinflammatory phenotype through TLR-mediated signaling, producing cytokines such as TNF-α, IL-1, IL-6 and IL-12 [48].

LSECs express many types of Toll-like receptors (TLRs) [17, 21]. In particular TLR4, characterized by being a receptor of endotoxin and regulate angiogenic responses [17]. Several animal studies support the importance of TLR4 in liver fibrosis. Interestingly, when TLR4-mutant mice loss TLR4 function, they diminish tubulogenesis, an indicator of angiogenic capacity of vascular cells, in response to the bacterial endotoxin, lipopolysaccharide (LPS), and have less liver fibrosis than wild type [17, 79, 80]. Given that angiogenesis is postulated to contribute to portal hypertension by enhancing fibrogenesis [16, 23], these result suggest that LSECs after the exposition to LPS, mediate angiogenesis through the TLR4/MyD88 signaling pathway resulting in fibrosis and portal hypertension. [14]

THE POTENTIAL OF STATINS IN PORTAL HYPERTENSION

The pleiotropic actions of statins have many potential targets on the vasculature, including molecular targets involved in the development of portal hypertension. Of note, studies in cirrhotic rats by bile duct ligation (BDL), and statin administration demonstrated that atorvastatin caused a significant decrease in portal pressure, through a decrease in hepatic vascular resistance [27],and increased eNOS in livers of cirrhotic BDL rats [27].Others studies in Cirrhotic rats (by CCl4), show that simvastatin attenuated the increase of portal pressure caused by volume expansion and increased ENOS expression [81]. Together with this, simvastatin reduces portal-systemic collateral vascular resistance and portal pressure in portal hypertensive rats [82].These results suggested that statin improved flow-mediated hepatic relaxation (and thereby, hepatic endothelial function) by enhancing the availability of NO at the intrahepatic circulation. However, in other studies in cirrotics rats treated with statins, the portal pressure was not modified [83-85].

Studies also has been made in human; in 2004 Zafra et al carried out a study with 30 patients with cirrhosis and concluded that Simvastatin administration increases the hepatosplanchnic output of nitric oxide products and decreases hepatic resistance in patients with cirrhosis, However, the decrease in hepatic resistance achieved by simvastatin was not associated with any decrease in portal pressure (bearing in mind that insufficient NO production seems to be the major factor involved in increased hepatic resistance in cirrhosis) [86]

Moreover, in 2009 Abraldes et al. conducted a double-blind randomized controlled trial (59 patients) and demonstrated that simvastatin administration significantly decreases portal pressure and improves liver function in cirrhotic patients with portal hypertension and no reported significant changes in arterial pressure and systemic vascular resistance, that suggestive to simvastatin behaves a true selective vasodilator [87]

Statins display a myriad of beneficial actions on multiple molecular pathways in vasculature that may be considered as potential targets to reverse or improve the impaired hepatic vascular tone (figure 1).

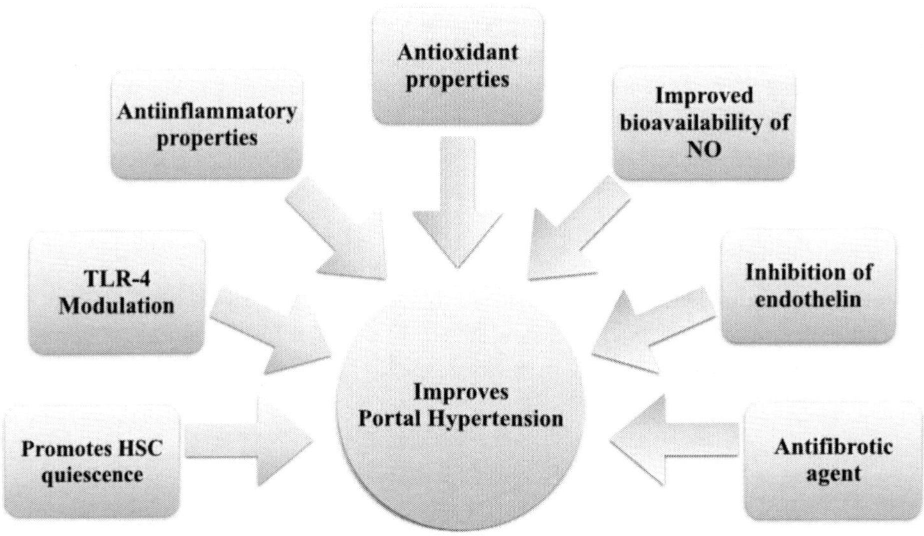

Figure 1. The figure demonstrates the variety of beneficial effects of statins in subjects with portal hypertension.

Improving the Bioavailability of NO

Inhibition of HMG-CoA reductase blocks the production of cholesterol and also reduces the production of their intermediaries, including isoprenoids like farnesylpyrophosphate (FPP) and geranylgeranylpyrophosphate (GGPP). These isoprenoids are involved in the post-transcriptional modification and intracellular trafficking of a series of membrane proteins including GTP-binding protein Ras, an a number of Ras-like proteins such as Rho, Rac, Rab, Ral, Rap [4, 34, 88]. Members of the Ras and Rho GTPase family are major substrates for post-transcriptional modification by prenylation. Based on the ability of statins to inhibit isoprenylation of Rac, Ras and Rho, they favor the accumulation of the corresponding inactive forms in the cytoplasm [34, 88, 89].Ras translocation from the cytoplasm to the plasma membrane is dependent on farnesylation, whereas Rho translocation is dependent on geranylgeranylation [89, 90].

Rho/ROCK adversely affect the stability of eNOS mRNA and they reduce eNOS phosphorylation through inhibition of Akt signaling in human endothelial cells. Activation of

Akt kinase is a key element in posttranslational activation of eNOS(eNOS is also a substrate of Akt and is phosphorylated at Ser 1177/1179) [4, 90, 95]. Statins, as inhibitors of Rho kinase pathway, favor the activation of phosphatidyl inositol kinase and the subsequent activation of eNOS via Akt [96, 97]. Statins have been shown to rapidly promote the activation of Akt in endothelial cells leading to eNOS phosphorylation and increased NO production [90, 95-98]. In cirrhotic rats, simvastatin increased Akt activity [81].

Statins are also known to negatively regulate both the expression of caveolin-1, and its interaction with eNOS [98, 99, 100]. Noteworthy. in endothelial cells, statins (atorvastatin) promoted the interaction between Heat-shock protein 90 (Hsp90) and eNOS [98, 100]. Hsp90 is a molecular chaperone that facilitates long-term activation of eNOS, by phosphorylation of eNOS on Ser1177, depend on the ability of hsp90 to recruit Akt in the eNOS [98],results in an increase in eNOS activity [98, 100, 101].

Tetrahydrobiopterin (BH4) is a key co-factor regulating the eNOS activity. It prevents the uncoupling and production of superoxide instead of NO. Of note, statins increase the cellular biopterin through inducing GTP cyclohydrolase I (GTPCH) gene expression, which is the limiting enzyme in de novo synthesis of BH4. [102, 103]. Atorvastatin increase vascular BH4 bioavailability, indicating an effect on That BH4 biosynthesis in vivo Occurs [103].

The induction of the transcription factor KLF2 in endothelial cells conferred a highly vasoprotective phenotype [8, 37]. KLF2 expression can be stimulated by blood flow-derived shear stress, like in cirrhotic patients and by exogenous administration of small molecules, including statins and resveratrol [104, 105], being simvastatin the most effective one, followed by mevastatin, upregulating KLF2 expression just after 6h of simvastatin administration and reaching a maximum peak at 24h of treatment, enhancing the KLF2-derived vasoprotective phenotype induction by shear stress, exhibitied a significant upregulation of KLF2 expression and the target gene of eNOS [44]

Inhibition of the Expression of ET-1

oxLDL is a potent agonist triggering the production and release of ET-1 from endothelial cells. Statins can reduce the levels of ox-LDL [4]. Statins are also able to inhibit gene expression of pre-pro ET-1. This inhibition appears to be mediated by the inactivation of Rho proteins [106, 107].

Antioxidant Properties

Statins can inhibit isoprenylation of Rac, and produce accumulation of the inactive forms in the cytoplasm. Rac is a member of the small Rho GTPase subfamily, their signaling pathway is involved in reactive oxygen species (ROS) generation, among others [88, 108].Inhibition of Rac1 protein, has important consequences on NADPH oxidase catalytic activity, and thus decreasing the production of superoxide [31, 88, 109].

O2- from NADPH oxidase may oxidize and degrade BH4, thereby leading to eNOS uncoupling [88, 110]. A recent study showed that patients receiving statins (atorvastatin) had a significantly lower arterial O2- generation and improved vascular NO bioavailability. [103].

A growing body of experimental evidence supports that activation of angiotensin II type-1 (AT1)receptor by angiotensin-II in vascular cells is one of the major mechanisms to stimulate the ROS production. In this context, statins negatively regulate AT1 receptor gene expression and consequently the production of ROS [31, 109, 88, 111]. Furthermore, statins also up-regulate the activity of antioxidant enzymes such as catalase and paraoxonase [31].

Of note, statins are also able to increase NO bioavailability by regulation of ROS production [34, 88, 103].

Furthermore, a novel cholesterol and NO-independent antioxidant mechanism with statins has been described, namely KLF2-dependent induction of the cytoprotective enzyme HO-1 [43]. The regulation of HO-1 expression by statins remains to be fully understood, because the effect of atorvastatin on HO-1 expression is indirect.Nevertheless the protective rol of statins against ROS generation and H2O2-induce cell death is well known, although the role of HO-1 and the end-products of heme breakdown by HO-1 (bile pigments, CO and iron) as a powerful antioxidant was confirmed by HO-1 siRNA, which reversed statin protection, exposing endothelial cells to oxidant-induced injury [43, 112].

Interestingly, statins induced a rapid increase in KLF2 mRNA levels, whereas KLF2 siRNA abrogated statins-mediated upregulation of HO-1 and cytoprotection against H2O2-induced cell death. The precise relationship between KLF2 and the transcription factors implicated in the regulation of HO-1, which include NF-E2-related factor-2(NrF2), heat shock factor1, NF-kB, Sp-1 and AP-1, remains to be determined [112].

Effects on Hepatic Stellate Cells

HSC are largely responsible for intrahepatic vascular tone. Animal studies have shown that chronic treatment with statins, particularly atorvastatin, inhibited the translocation to the membrane of myofibroblastic HSC and thereby disruption of RhoA/Rho-kinase signaling in cirrhotic liver of rats [27, 113]. These signaling pathways are involved in vasoconstrictor mechanisms. By inhibiting these pathways, statins significantly decrease HSC contraction ability which, in turn, produces a decrease in intrahepatic vascular tone [27, 113].

The mayor fibrogenic cells in the liver are hepatic myofibroblasts, mainly deriving from HSC [114, 115], in vitro estudies shows that statins (atorvastatin) attenuates activation of quiescent HSC and inhibits proliferation of myofibroblastic HSC, and decreased cytokine and collagen production [113]. In rats models of hepatic fibrosis, atorvastatin demonstrated a decreased in profibrotic cytokines [114, 116], and significantly attenuated fibrosis and HSC activation [115, 116], Statin can be an effective antifibrotic agent in hepatic fibrosis.

Statins induces activated HSC apoptosis thought activating mitochondrial apoptotic signals, statins also activates protein kinase C (PKC) in these cells. The combination of statins with a PKC inhibitor enhances statins-induced activated HSC apoptosis and leads to a reduction of hepatic fibrosis in animal models. The induction of activated HSC apoptosis might be the most important mode of action of the antifibrotic effects of statins, because activated HSC apoptosis is essential for the fibrosis reversibility. Nevertheless, activated HSC apoptosis by statins may be interrupted by PKC activation, which can be induced by statin treatment itself [115].

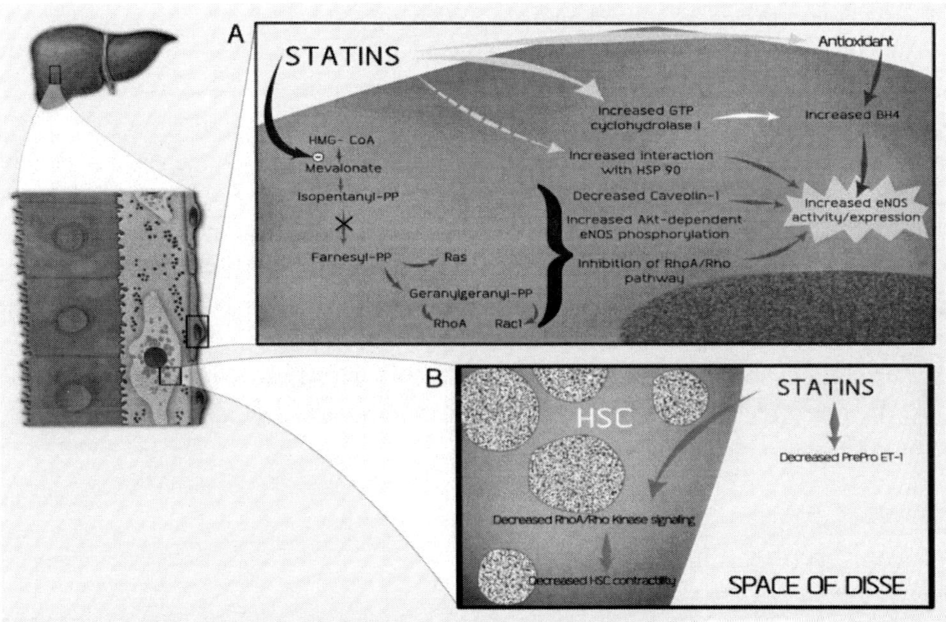

Figure 2. Statins promote vasodilation at portal circulation through different mechanisms in both endothelial and hepatic stellate cells (HSCs). Panel A. Statins actions on endothelial cells from hepatic vasculature are depicted in Panel A. By blocking cholesterol synthesis, the availability of key activators of Rho kinase pathway are also reduced, which may then favor the AkT-dependent activation of endothelial nitric oxide synthase (eNOS). In addition, statins also down-regulate caveolin-1 expression, display direct antioxidant effects, increase guanosine triphosphate (GTP) cyclohydrolase I and promote the interaction with heat-shock protein 90 (Hsp90). In Panel B are depicted the actions on HSCs, including the inhibition of pre-pro endothelin-1 (ET-1) gene expression, as well as a decrease in HSCs contractility by interfering with RhoA/Rho kinase signaling.

Although a study from Moreno *et al* failed to show an effect of atorvastatin on HSC activation [117], recent studies suggest that statin administration to cirrhotic animals reduces HSC activation, and liver fibrosis [116]. Moreover, recent data have demonstrated that LSECs and HSC regulate their phenotypes in a paracrine manner [118, 119], Marrone *et al.* demonstrate that LSECs vasoprotective phenotype improvement due to simvastatin-dependent KLF2 upregulation is necessary to paracrinally ameliorate HSC phenotype. In fact, co-culture experiments have shown that induction of endothelial KLF2 programs by simvastatin results in HSC de-activation, which is mediated at least in part via a KLF2-NO-cGMP dependent mechanism [44].

Antiinflammatory Properties

At present, the anti-inflammatory actions of statins have also been demonstrated in different experimental models of liver injury, both *in vivo* and *in vitro* and studies in rat hepatocytes treated with pro-inflammatory cytokine, showed that pitavastatin treatment resulted in up-regulation of iNOS in these inflammatory liver, followed by increased NO production [120, 4, 121, 113, 122].

One of the most relevant anti-inflammatory properties ascribed to statins is dealt with the reduction of monocyte adhesion to vascular endothelium. Many adhesion molecules involved in this process are induced by proinflammatory cytokines such as TNF-α and IL-1. Of note, TNF-α plasma levels are reported to be increased in patients with liver diseases [58, 123].

Both simvastatin and atorvastatin are able to reduce TNF-α-induced expression of vascular cell adhesion molecule 1 (VCAM-1) and Intercellular Adhesion Molecule-1 (ICAM-1) via a NF-kB-dependent mechanism, resulting in a decrease in actin polymerization after inactivation of RhoA [124, 125]. Another reported mechanism is the binding capacity of statins to the leukocyte integrin leukocyte function–associated antigen 1 (LFA-1), and thus interfering with the binding to ICAM-1 [126, 127].

Statins are also reported to attenuate inflammatory events induced by angiotensin-II in the liver, by down-regulating the AT1 receptor expression and the subsequent reduction of angiotensin II-induced NF-kβ activation [31, 125].

Toll-Like Receptor 4 Modulation

In this context, Methe *et al.* demonstrated a dose dependent of simvastatin or atorvastatin decrease TLR4 mRNA and protein expression in CD14+ human monocytes incubated in vitro and they had a similar effect in vivo, in 12 normocholesterolemic healthy volunteers [128]. The mechanism of action could include the Ras family and the phosphoinositide 3-kinase/protein kinase Akt-pathway.

Hodgkinson and Yee demonstrated that statins has an additive inhibitory effect on TLR4-mediated response to LPS, in term of NFkB activation and cytokine production [129]. Nevertheless, mechanism remains to be determined

Conclusion

One of the recognized mechanisms involved in increased intrahepatic vascular resistance is endothelial dysfunction. At present, many factors are involved in this dysfunctional state in cirrhotic livers such as, the activation RhoA/Rho-kinase pathway, a decreased Akt-mediated eNOS phosphorylation, the over-expression of caveolin-1, the presence of oxidative stress, as well as the oxidation of BH4. In this very complex context, the pharmacological activities of statins, beyond their hypocholesterolemic actions, may represent new insights to modulate the above mentioned factors thus increasing NO bioavailability (figure 2). Furthermore, statins are also able to modulate HSC contractile functions, promotes HSC quiescence, inhibit both ET-1 expression and release, in addition to their antioxidant, antifibrotic and anti-inflammatory properties.

Based on the pharmacological properties ascribed to this highly pleiotropic drug family, it is necessary to conduct clinical trials to assess the long-term effects of statin use in portal hypertension and to evaluate the association with currently used drugs.

Declaration of Interest

The authors are not aware of any affiliation, funding or financial holdings that might be perceived as affecting the objectivity of this review.

References

[1] Cichoz-Lach H., Celiński K., Słomka M., *et al.* Pathophysiology of portal hypertension. *J. Physiol. Pharmacol.*, 2008 Aug.;59 Suppl. 2:231-8.).

[2] Sorensen H., Thulstrup A. M., Mellemkjar L., et al. Long-term survival and cause-specific mortality in patients with cirrhosis of the liver: a nationwide cohort study in Denmark. *J. Clin. Epidemiol.*, 2003;56: 88-93.

[3] Istvan E. S., Deisenhofer J. Structural mechanism for statin inhibitionof HMG-CoA reductase. *Science,* 2001; 292: 1160 – 1164.

[4] Athyros V. G., Kakafika A. I., Tziomalos K., Karagiannis A., Mikhailidis D. P. Pleiotropic effects of statins--clinical evidence. *Curr. Pharm. Des.*, 2009;15:479-89.

[5] Rodriguez-Vilarrupla A., Fernandez M., Bosch J., *et al.* Current concept on the pathophysiology of portal hypertension. *Ann. Hepatol.*, 2007; 6: 28-36.

[6] Bosch J., Abraldes J., Fernandez M., *et al.*Hepatic endothelial dysfunction and abnormal angiogenesis: New target in the treatment of portal hypertension. *J. Hepatol.,* 2010;23: 558-67.

[7] Shibayama Y., Nakata K. Significance of septal fibrosis for disturbance of hepatic circulation. *Liver,* 1992; 12: 22-25.

[8] Kawada N., Tran-Thi T., Klein H., *et al.* The contraction of hepatic stellate cells stimulated with vasoactive substances. Possible involvement of endothelin 1 and nitric oxide in the regulation of the sinusoidal tonus. *Eur. J. Biochem.,* 1993; 213: 815-23.

[9] Zhang J., Pegoli W., Clemens M. Endothelin-1 induces direct constriction of hepatic sinusoids. *Am. J. Physiol.*, 1994; 266: 624-32.

[10] Harrison D. Cellular and molecular mechanisms of endothelial cell dysfunction. *J. Clin. Invest.*, 1997; 100: 2153-7.

[11] Gupta T. K., Toruner M., Chung M. K., *et al.* Endothelial dysfunction and decreased production of nitric oxide in the intrahepatic microcirculation of cirrhotic rats. *Hepatology,* 1998; 28: 926-31.

[12] Bellis L., Berzigotti A., Abraldes J., *et al.* Low doses of isosorbide mononitrate attenuate the postprandial increase in portal pressure in patients with cirrhosis. *Hepatology,* 2003; 37:378-84.

[13] Iwakiri Y., Groszmann R. J. Vascular endothelial dysfunction in cirrhosis. *J. Hepatol.,* 2007; 46: 927-34.

[14] Iwakiri Y. Endothelial dysfunction in the regulation of cirrhosis and portal hypertension. *Liver International*, 2012; 199-213.

[15] Ding B. S., Nolan D. J., Butler J. M., *et al.* Inductive angiocrine signals from sinusoidal endothelium are required for liver regeneration. *Nature,* 2010; 468: 310-5.

[16] Thabut D., Shah V. Intrahepatic angiogenesis and sinusoidal remodeling in chronic liver disease: new targets for the treatment of portal hypertension? *J. Hepatol.*, 2010; 53: 976-80.

[17] Jagavelu K., Routray C., Shergill U., *et al.* Endothelial cell toll-like receptor 4 regulates fibrosis-associated angiogenesis in the liver. *Hepatology,* 2010; 52: 590-601.

[18] Shah V., Toruner M., Haddad F., *et al.* Impaired Endothelial nitric oxide synthase activity associated with enhanced caveolin binding in experimental cirrhosis in the rat. *Gastroenterology*, 1999; 117: 1222-28.

[19] Rockey D., Chung J. Reduced nitric oxide production by endothelial cells in cirrhotic rat liver: Endothelial dysfunction in portal hypertension. *Gastroenterology*, 1998; 114: 344-51.

[20] Morales-Ruiz M. Cejudo-Martin P., Fernández-Varo G., *et al* Transduction of the liver with activated akt normalizes portal pressure in cirrhosis. *Gastroenterology*, 2003;125: 522-31.

[21] Minshall R., Sessa W., Stan R. Caveolin regulation of endothelial function. *Am. J. Physiol. Lung Cell Mol. Physiol.*, 2003; 285: 1179-83.

[22] Isshiki M., Ying Y., Fujita T., *et al.* A molecular sensor detects signal transduction from caveolae in living cells. *J. Biol. Chem.*, 2002; 277: 43389-98.

[23] Ghosh S., Gachhui R., Crooks C., *et al.* Interaction between caveolin-1 and the reductase domain of endothelial nitric-oxide synthase. Consequences for catalysis. *J. Biol. Chem.*, 1998 ;273: 22267-71.

[24] Gratton J. P., Bernatchez P., Sessa W. Caveolae and caveolins in the cardiovascular system. *Circ. Res.*, 2004; 94: 1408-17.

[25] Bist A., Fielding P., Fielding C. Two sterol regulatory element-like sequences mediate up-regulation of caveolin gene transcription in response to low density lipoprotein free cholesterol. *Cell Biology*, 1997; 94: 10693-8.

[26] Thabut D., Tazi K. A., Bonnefont-Rousselot D., *et al.* High-density lipoprotein administration attenuates liver proinflammatory response, restores liver endothelial nitric oxide synthase activity, and lowers portal pressure in cirrhotic rats. *Hepatology,* 2007; 46: 1893-906.

[27] Trebicka J., Hennenberg M., Laleman W., *et al.* Atorvastatin lowers portal pressure in cirrhotic rats by inhibition of RhoA/Rho-kinase and activation of endothelial nitric oxide synthase. *Hepatology,* 2007; 45: 242-53.

[28] Rikitake Y., Liao J. Rho GTPases, statins, and nitric oxide. Circ Res 2005; 97: 1232-5.

[29] Parola M, Robina G. Oxidative stress-related molecules and liver fibrosis. *Journal of Hepatology,* 2001; 35: 297-06.

[30] Heistad D. D. Oxidative Stress and Vascular Disease: 2005 Duff Lecture. *Arterioscler. Thromb Vasc. Biol.,* 2006; 26: 689-95.

[31] Rojas A., Figueroa H., Morales M. A., *et al.* Facing Up the ROS labyrinth – Where to go?. *Curr. Vasc. Pharmacol.*, 2006; 4: 277-89.

[32] De Minics S., Brenner D. NOX in liver fibrosis. *Arch. Biochem. Biophys.*, 2007; 462: 266-77.

[33] Karaa A., Kamoun W. S., Clemens M. G. Oxidative stress disrupts nitric oxide synthase activation in liver endothelial cells. *Free Radic. Biol. Med.*, 2005; 39: 1320-31.

[34] Adam O., Laufs U. Antioxidative effects of statins. *Arch. Toxicol.*, 2008; 82: 885-92.

[35] Graupera M., García-Pagán J., Parés M., *et al* Cyclooxygenase-1 inhibition corrects endothelial dysfunction in cirrhotic rat livers. *J. Hepatol.*, 2003; 39: 515-24.
[36] Zhou Q., Hennenberg M., Trebicka J., *et al.* Intrahepatic upregulation of RhoA and Rho-kinase signaling contributes to increased hepatic vascular resistance in rats with secondary biliary cirrhosis. *Gut,* 2006; 55: 1296-05.
[37] Atkins G. B., Jain M. K. Role of Kruppel-like transcription factors in endothelial biology. *Circ. Res.*, 2007; 100: 1686-1695.
[38] SenBanerjee S., Lin Z., Atkins G. B., Greif D. M., Rao R. M., Kumar A., *et al.* KLF2 is a novel transcriptional regulator of endothelial proinflammatory activation. *J. Exp. Med.*, 2004; 199:1305-1315.
[39] Brouard S., Otterbein L. E. Anrather J., Tobiasch E., Bach F. H., Choi A. M., Soares M. P. Carbon monoxide generated by heme oxygenase 1 suppresses endothelial cell apoptosis. *J. Exp. Med.*, 2000; 192: 1015-26.
[40] Otterbein Le, Zuckerbraun B. S., Haga M., Liu F., Song R., *et al.* Carbon monoxide suppresses arteriosclerotic lesions associated with chronic graft rejection and with balloon injury. *Nat. Med.,* 2003; 9: 183-90.
[41] Brunt K. R., Fenrich K. K., Kiani G., Tse M. Y., Pang S. C., *et al.* Protection of human vascular smooth muscle cells from H2O2-induced apoptosis through functional codependence between HO-1 and AKT. *Arterioscler. Thromb Vasc. Biol.,* 2006; 26: 2027-34.
[42] Dai G., Vaughn S., Zhang Y., Wang E. T., Garcia-Cardena G., Gimbrone Jr. M. A. Biomechanical forces in aterosclerosis-resistant vascular regions regulate endotelial redox balance via phosphoinositol 3-kinase/akt-dependent activation of Nrf2. *Circ. Res.*, 2007; 101: 723-733.
[43] Ali F., Hamdulay S., Kinderlerer A., Boyle J., Lidington E. Statin-mediated cytoprotection of human vascular endothelial cells: a role for Kruppel-like factor 2-dependent induction of heme oxygenase-1. *Journal of Thrombosis and Haemosotasis*, 5: 2537-2546.
[44] Marrone G., Russo L., Rosado E., Hide D., Garcia-Cardeña G., *et al.* The transcription factor KLF2 mediates hepatic endotelial protection and paracrine endotelial-stellate cell deactivation induced by statins. *Journal of Hepatology*, 2013; 58: 98-103.
[45] Gracia-Sancho J., Russo L., Garcia-Caldero H., *et al.* Endothelial expression of transcription factor Kruppel-like factor 2 and its vasoprotective target genes in the normal and cirrhotic rat liver. *Gut,* 2011; 60: 517-24.
[46] Deleve L. D., Wang X., Gui Y. Sinusoidal endothelial cells prevent rat stellate cell activation and promote reversion to quiescence. *Hepatology,* 2008; 48: 920-930.
[47] DeLeve L. D., Wang X., Hu L., McCuskey M. K., McCuskey R. S. Rat liver sinusoidal endothelial cell phenotype is maintained by paracrine and autocrine regulation. *Am. J. Physiol. Gastrointest. Liver Physiol.*, 2004; 287: G757-763.
[48] Mehta G., Gustot T., Mookerjee R., Garcia J., Fallon M. Inflammation and portal hypertension- The undiscovered Country. *Journal of Hepatology*, 2014.
[49] Marra F. Pinzani M. Role of hepatic stellate cells in the pathogenesis of portal hypertension. *Nefrología,* 2002; 22 Suppl. 5: 34-40.
[50] Friedman S. L. The cellular basis of hepatic fibrosis. *N. Engl. J. Med.*, 1993; 328: 1828-35.

[51] Pinzani M., Failli P., Ruocco C., *et al.* Fat-storing cells as liver-specific paricytes. Spatial dynamics of agonist-stimulated intracellular calcium transients. *J. Clin. Invest.*, 1992; 90: 642-6.

[52] Nakano M., Worner T. M., Lieber C. S. Perivenular fibrosis in alcoholic liver injury: ultrastructure and histological progression. *Gastroenterology*, 1982; 83: 777-85.

[53] Rockey C., Weisiger R. Endothelin induces contractility of stellate cells from normal and cirrhotic rat liver: Implications for regulation of portal pressure and resistance. *Hepatology*, 1996 ;24: 233-40.

[54] Friedman S. L., Roll F. J., Boyles J., *et al.* Hepatic lipocytes: the principal collagen producing cells of normal rat liver. *Proc. Natl. Acad. Sci. U S A,* 1985; 82: 8681-5.

[55] Loreal O., Clement B., Schuppan D., *et al.* Distribution and cellular origin of collagen VI during development and in cirrhosis. *Gastroenterology,* 1992; 102: 980-7.

[56] Maher J. J., Friedman S. L., Roll F. J., *et al.* Inmunolocalization of laminin in normal rat liver and biosynthesis of laminin by hepatic lipocytes in primary culture. *Gastroenterology,* 1988; 94: 1053-152.

[57] Rockey D. The cellular pathogenesis of portal hypertension: Stellate cell contractility, endothelin, and nitric oxide. *Hepatology,* 1997; 25: 2-5.

[58] Yin M., Wheele M. D., Kono H., *et al.* Essential role of tumor necrosis factor alpha in alcohol-induced liver injury in mice. *Gastroenterology,* 1999; 177: 942-52.

[59] Thimgan M., Yee H. Quantitation of rat hepatic stellate cell contraction: Stellate cells contribution to sinusoidal resistance. *Am. J. Physiol.,* 1999; 277: 137-43.

[60] Stephenson K., Harvey S. A., Mustafa S. B., *et al.*Endothelin association with the cultured rat Kupffer cell: characterization and regulation. *Hepatology,* 1995; 22: 896-05.

[61] Housset C., Rockey D. C., Bissell D. M. Endothelin receptors in rat liver: lipocytes as a contractile target for endothelin 1. *Proc. Natl. Acad. Sci. U S A*, 1993; 90: 9266-70.

[62] Reynaert H., Thompson Mg., Thomas T., *et al.* Hepatic stellate cells: role in microcirculation and pathophysiology of portal hypertension. *Gut,* 2002; 50: 571-81.

[63] Bataller R., Nicolas J. M., Ginees P., *et al.* Contraction of human hepatic stellate cells activated in culture: a role of voltage-operated calcium channels. *J. Hepatol.,* 1998; 29: 398-08.

[64] Saab S., Tam S., Tran B. N., *et al.* Myosin mediates contractile force generation by hepatic stellate cells in response to endothelin-1. *J. Biomed. Sci.,* 2002; 9: 607-12.

[65] Soon R., Yee H. Stellate cell contraction: Role, regulation, and potential therapeutic target. *Clin. Liver Dis.,* 2008; 12: 791-03.

[66] Melton Ac., Datta A., Yee H. F. Jr. Ca+2 independent contractile force generation by rat hepatic stellate cells in response to endothelin-1. *Am. J. Physiol. Gastrointest. Liver Physiol.,* 2006; 290: 7-13.

[67] Yee H. F. Rho directs activation-associated changes in rat hepatic stellate cell morphology via regulation of the actin cytoskeleton. *Hepatology,* 1998; 28: 843-50.

[68] Kawada N., Seki S., Kuroki T., *et al.*ROCK inhibitor Y-27632 attenuates stellate cell contraction and portal pressure increase induced by endothelin-1. *Biochem. Biophys. Res. Commun.,* 1999; 266: 296-300.

[69] Kamath P., Carpenter H., Loyd R., *et al.* Hepatic localization of endothelin-1 in patients with idiopathic portal hypertension and cirrhosis of the liver. *Liver Transpl.*, 2000; 6: 596-02.

[70] Moller S., Gulberg V., Henriksen J. H., *et al.*Endothelin-1 and endothelin-3 in cirrhosis: relations to systemic and splanchnic haemodynamics. *J. Hepatol.*, 1995; 23: 135-44.
[71] Moore K., Wendon J., Frazer M., *et al.* Plasma endothelin inmunoreactivity in liver disease and the hepatorenal syndrome. *N. Engl. J. Med.*, 1992; 327: 1774-8.
[72] Malek A. M., Greene A. L., Inzumo S. Regulation of endothelin 1 gene by fluid shear stress is transcriptionally mediated and independent of protein kinase C and cAMP. *Proc. Natl. Acad. Sci. U S A,* 1993; 90: 5999-03.
[73] Tran Duc A. T., Schwab A. J., Simard A., *et al.*Reduction in hepatic endothelin-1 clearance in cirrhosis. *Clinical Science*, 2003; 105: 227-34.
[74] Gondo K., Ueno T., Sakamoto M., *et al.*The endothelin-1 binding site in rat liver tissue: light and electro-microscopic autoradiographic studies. *Gastroenterology,* 1993; 104: 1745-9.
[75] Housset C., Rocket D. C., Bissell D. M. Endothelin receptors in rat liver: lipocytes as a contractile target for endothelin 1. *Porc. Natl. Acad. Sci. U S A*, 1993:90: 9266-70.
[76] Rockey D. C., Fouassier L., Chung J., *et al.* Cellular localization of endothelin-1 and increased production in liver injury in the rat: potential for autocrine and paracrine effects on stellate cells. *Hepatology*, 1998; 27: 472-80.
[77] Wiest R., Garcia-Tsao G. Bacterial translocation (BT) in cirrhosis. *Hepatology,* 2005; 41: 422-433.
[78] Neugebauer H., Hartmann P., Krenn S., Gluck T., Scholmerich J., *et al.* Bacterial translocation increases phagocytic activity of polymorphonuclear leucocytes in portal hypertension: priming independent of liver cirrhosis. *Liver Int.,* 2008; 28:1149-1157.
[79] Zhu Q., Zou L., Jagavelu K., Simonwtto D. A., Huebert R. C., *et al.* Intestinal decontamination inhibits TLR4 dependent fibronectin-mediated cross-talk between stellate cells and endotelial cells in liver fibrosis in mice. *J. Hepatol.*, 2012; 56: 893-899.
[80] Seki E., De Minicis S., Osterreicher C. H., Kluwe J., Osawa Y., *et al.* TLR4 enhances TGF-beta signaling and hepatic fibrosis. *Nat. Med.,* 2007; 13:1324-1332.
[81] Abraldes J., Rodríguez-Vilarrupla A., Graupera M., *et al.* Simvastatin treatment improves liver sinusoidal endothelial dysfunction in CCl4 cirrhotic rats. *J. Hepatol.,* 2007; 46: 1040-6.
[82] Huang H., Wang S., Lee J., Chen Y., Lee F., *et al.* Simvastatin effects on portal-systemic collaterals of portal hypertensive rats. *Journal of Gastroenterology and Hepatology*, 2010; 25: 1401–1409.
[83] Oberti F., Pilette C., Rifflet H., Maïga M. Y., Moreau A., *et al.* Effects of simvastatin, pentoxifylline and spironolactone on hepatic fibrosis and portal hypertension in rats with bile duct ligation. *J. Hepatol.*, 1997; 26(6):1363-71.
[84] Shirin H., Sharvit E., Aeed H., Gavish D., Bruck R. Atorvastatin and rosuvastatin do not prevent thioacetamide induced liver cirrhosis in rats. Haim Shirin. *World J. Gastroenterol.*, 2013 14; 19(2): 241-248.
[85] Chang C. C. 1., Wang S. S., Huang H. C., Lee J. Y., Lee F. Y., *et al.* Pravastatin administration does not induce detrimental effects on hemodynamics and collaterals of portal hypertensive rats. *J. Gastroenterol. Hepatol.*, 2010; 25(8):1394-400.
[86] Zafra C., Abraldes J., Turnes J., Berzigotti A., Fernandez M., *et al.* Simvastatin Enhances Hepatic Nitric Oxide Production and Decreases the Hepatic Vascular Tone in Patients With Cirrhosis. *Gastroenterology,* 2004;126:749–755.

[87] Abraldes J., Albillos A., Bañares R., *et al.* Simvastatin lowers portal pressure in patients with cirrosis and portal hypertension: a randomized controlled trial. *Gastroenterology,* 2009; 136: 1651-8.

[88] Oliver Adam, Ulrich Laufs. Rac1-Mediated Effects of HMG-CoA Reductase Inhibitors (Statins) in Cardiovascular Disease. *Antioxidants and Redox signaling*, 2014; 20 (8).

[89] Hermida N., Balligand J. L. Low-Density Lipoprotein-Cholesterol-Induced Endothelial Dysfunction and Oxidative Stress: The Role of Statins. *Antioxidants and Redox signaling,* 2014; 20(8): 1216 – 1237.

[90] Sawada N., Liao J. K. Rho/Rho-Associated Coiled-Coil Forming Kinase Pathway as Therapeutic Targets for Statins in Atherosclerosis. *Antioxidants and Redox signaling,* 2014; 20(8): 1251-1267.

[91] Antoniades C., Channon C. Statins: Pleiotropic Regulators of Cardiovascular Redox State. *Antioxidants and Redox signaling*, 2014; 20(8): 1195-1197.

[92] Rikitake Y., Liao J. K. Rho GTPases, Statins, and Nitric Oxide. *Circ. Res.,* 2005; 97: 1232-5.

[93] Margaritis M., Channon K. M., Antoniades C. Statins as Regulators of Redox State in the Vascular Endothelium: Beyond Lipid Lowering. *Antioxidants and Redox signaling,* 2014; 20(8): 1198- 1215.

[94] Laufs U., La Fata V., Plutzky J., *et al.*Upregulation of endothelial nitric oxide synthase by HMG CoA reductase inhibitors. *Circulation*, 1998; 97: 1129-35.

[95] Kureishi Y., Luo Z., Shiojima I., Bialik A., Fulton D., *et al.* The HMG-CoA reductase inhibitor simvastatin activates the protein kinase Akt and promotes angiogenesis in normocholesterolemic animals. *Nat. Med.,* 2000; 6(9): 1004–1010.

[96] Wolfrum S., Dendorfer A., Rikitake Y., *et al.* Inhibition of Rho-kinase leads to rapid activation of phosphatidylinositol 3-kinase/protein kinase akt and cardiovascular protection. *Arterioscler. Thromb Vasc. Biol.*, 2004; 24:1842-47.

[97] Ota H., Eto M., Kano M. R., Kahyo T., Setou M., *et al.* Induction of Endothelial Nitric Oxide Synthase, SIRT1, and Catalase by Statins Inhibits Endothelial Senescence Through the Akt Pathway. *Arterioscler. Thromb. Vasc. Biol.*, 2010;30:2205-2211.

[98] Brouet A., Sonveaux P., Dessy C., Moniotte S., Balligand J. L., Olivier Feron. Hsp90 and Caveolin Are Key Targets for the Proangiogenic Nitric Oxide-Mediated Effects of Statins. *Circ. Res.,* 2001;89:866-873.

[99] Arora R., Hare D. L., Zulli A. Simvastatin Reduces Endothelial NOS: Caveolin-1 Ratio but not the Phosphorylation Status of Enos In Vivo. *Journal of atherosclerosis and thrombosis*, 2012; 19(8): 705-11.

[100] Feron O., Dessy C., Desager J. P., *et al.* Hydroxy-methylglutaryl-coenzyme a reductase inhibition promotes endothelial nitric oxide synthase activation through a decrease in caveolin abundance. *Circulation,* 2001;103: 113-8.

[101] Garcia-Cardena G., Fan R., Shah V., *et al.* Dynamic activation of endothelial nitric oxide synthase by Hsp90. *Nature,* 1998; 392: 821– 4.

[102] Hattori Y., Nakanishi N., Akimoto S., *et al.* HMG-CoA Reductase inhibitor increases GTP cyclohydrolase i mRNA and tetrahydrobiopterin in vascular endothelial cells. *Arterioscler. Thromb. Vasc. Biol.,* 2003; 23: 176-82.

[103] Antoniades C., Bakogiannis C., Leeson P., Guzik T. J., Zhang M. H., *et al.* Rapid, Direct Effects of Statin Treatment on Arterial Redox State and Nitric Oxide

Bioavailability in Human Atherosclerosis via Tetrahydrobiopterin-Mediated Endothelial Nitric Oxide Synthase Coupling. *Circulation,* 2011;124:335-345.

[104] Parmar K. M., Nambudiri V., Dai G., Larman H. B., Gimbrone r M. A., Garcia Cardena G. Statins exert endotelial atheroprotective effects via the KLF2 transcription factor. *J. Biol. Chem.,* 2005; 280: 26714-26719.

[105] Sen-Baneree S., Mir S., Lin Z., Hamik A., Atkins G. B., Das H., *et al.* Kruppel-like factor 2 as a novel mediator of statin effects in endothelial cells. *Circulation,* 2005; 112: 720-726.

[106] Hernández-Perera O., Pérez D., Navarro J., *et al.* Effects of the 3-Hydroxy-3-methylglutaryl-CoA reductase inhibitors, atorvastatin and simvastatin, on the expression of endothelin-1 and endothelial nitric oxide synthase in vascular endothelial cells. *J. Clin. Invest.*, 1998; 101(12): 2711-9.

[107] Hernández O., Pérez D., Soria E., *et al.* Involvement of Rho GTPases in the transcriptional inhibition of preproendothelin-1 gene expression by simvastatin in vascular endothelial cells. *Circ. Res.,* 2000; 29: 616-22.

[108] Zhou Q. and Liao J. K. Statins and cardiovascular diseases: from cholesterol lowering to pleiotropy. *Curr. Pharm. Des.*, 2009;15(5):467-78.

[109] Wassman S., Laufs U., Baumer A. T., *et al.* Inhibition of geranylgeranylation reduces angiotensin ii mediated free radical production in vascular smooth muscle cells: involvement of angiotensin AT1 receptor expression and RAC1 GTPase. *Mol. Pharmacol.*, 2001; 59: 646-54.

[110] Verhaar M. C., Westerweel P. E., van Zonneveld A. J., Rabelink T. J. Free radical production by dysfunctional eNOS. *Heart,* 2004; 90(5):494-5.

[111] Wassmann S., Laufs U., Baumer A. T., Muller K., Ahlbory K., *et al.* HMGCoA reductase inhibitors improve endothelial dysfunction in normocholesterolemic hypertension via reduced production of reactive oxygen species. *Hypertension,* 2001; 37(6):1450-7.

[112] Ryter S. W., Alam J., Choi A. M. Heme oxygenase-1/carbon monoxide: from basic science to therapeutic applications. *Physiol. Rev.,* 2006; 86: 583-650.

[113] Klein S., Klosel J., Schierwagen R., Korner C., Granzow M., *et al.* Atorvastatin inhibits proliferation and apoptosis, but induces senescence in hepatic myofibroblasts and thereby attenuates hepatic fibrosis in rats. *Laboratory Investigation*, (2012) 92, 1440–1450.

[114] Schierwagen R., Leeming D. J., Klein S., Granzow M., Nielsen M. J., *et al.* Serum markers of the extracellular matrix remodeling reflect antifibrotic therapy in bile-duct ligated rats. *Frontiers in physiology*, 2013; 4(195). 1-9.

[115] Yang J., Yoon J. H., Bang Y. J., Lee S. H., Lee S. M., *et al.* Synergistic antifibrotic efficacy of statin and protein kinase C inhibitor in hepatic fibrosis. *Am. J. Physiol. Gastrointest. Liver Physiol.*, 2010; 298: G126–G132.

[116] Trebicka J., Hennenberg M., Odenthal M., Shir K., Klein S., *et al.* Atorvastatin attenuates hepatic fibrosis in rats after bile duct ligation via decreased turnover of hepatic stellate cells. *Journal of Hepatology*, 2010; 53:. 702–712.

[117] Moreno M., Ramalho L. N., Sancho-Bru P., Ruiz-Ortega M., Ramalho F., Abraldes J. G., *et al.* Atorvastatin attenuates angiotensin II-induced inflammatory actions in the liver. *Am. J. Physiol. Gastrointest. Liver Physiol.*, 2009; 296: G147-156.

[118] Deleve L. D., Wang X., Gui Y. Sinusoidal endothelial cells prevent rat stellate cell activation and promote reversion to quiescence. *Hepatology*, 2008; 48: 920-930.

[119] Xie G., Wang X., Wang L., Wang L., Atkinson R. D., *et al.* Role of differentiation of liver sinusoidal endothelial cells in progression and regression of hepatic fibrosis in rats. *Gastroenterology,* 2012; 142: 918-927.

[120] Habara K., Hamada Y., Yamada M., Tokuhara K., Tanaka H., *et al.* Pitavastatin up-regulates the induction of iNOS through enhanced stabilization of its mRNA in pro-inflammatory cytokine-stimulated hepatocytes. *Nitric Oxide,* 18 (2008) 19–27.

[121] Yoshida M., Sawada T., Ishii H., *et al.* HMG-CoA reductase inhibitor modulates monocyte-endothelial cell interaction under physiological flow conditions in vitro involvement of rho gtpase-dependent mechanism. *Arterioscler. Thromb. Vasc. Biol.,* 2001;21:1165-71.

[122] Marrone G., Russo L., Rosado E., Hide D., Garcia-Cardena G., *et al.* The transcription factor KLF2 mediates hepatic endotelial protection and aracrine endotelial-stellate cell deactivation induced by statins. *J. Hepatol.*, 2012; 58:98-103.

[123] Lucey M., Mathurin P., Morgan T. Alcoholic hepatitis. *N. Engl. J. Med.,* 2009; 360: 2758-69.

[124] Zapolska-Downar D., Siennicka A., Kaczmarczyk M., et al. Simvastatin modulates TNF α-induced adhesion molecules expression in human endothelial cells. *Life Sci.,* 2004; 75: 1287-02.

[125] Moreno M., Ramalho L. N., Sancho-Bru P., *et al.* Atorvastatin attenuates angiotensin II-induced inflammatory actions in the liver. *Am. J. Physiol. Gastrointest. Liver Physiol.,* 2009; 296: 147-56.

[126] Weitz G., Welzenbach K., Brinkmann V., *et al.* Statins selectively inhibit leukocyte function antigen-1 by binding to a novel regulatory integrin site. *Nat. Med.,* 2001;7: 687-92.

[127] Greenwood J., Mason J. Satins and the vascular endothelial inflammatory response. *Trends Immunol.,* 2007; 28:88-98.

[128] Hu T., Chouinard M., Cox A. L., Sipes P., Marcelo M., *et al.* Farnesoid X receptor agonist reduces serum asymmetric dimethylarginine levels through hepatic dimethylarginine dimethylaminohydrolase-1 gene regulation. *J. Biol. Chem.,* 2006; 281: 39831-39838.

[129] Marrone G., Russo L., Rosado E., Hide D., Garcia-Cardena G., *et al.* The transcription factor KLF2 mediates hepatic endotelial protection and aracrine endotelial-stellate cell deactivation induced by statins. *J. Hepatol.*, 2012; 58:98-103.

In: Statins
Editor: Eric R. Travers

ISBN: 978-1-63463-057-3

Chapter 8

MOLECULAR MECHANISMS BEHIND THE BENEFICIAL EFFECTS OF STATINS IN OVARIAN CANCER

Mauricio A. Cuello, Sumie Kato and Lorena Abarzúa-Catalán
Division of Obstetrics and Gynecology
Faculty of Medicine, School of Medicine,
Pontificia Universidad Católica de Chile,
Santiago, Chile

ABSTRACT

Worldwide, epithelial ovarian cancer constitutes the most lethal gynecological malignancy. Annually, about 240.000 women are newly diagnosed and 150.000 die of this disease. Its lethality is mainly explained by a late diagnosis, at advanced stages, and by a transient response to available therapies. Thus, despite optimal surgical cytoreduction and a complete response to platinum-based chemotherapy, the majority of cases eventually relapses and dies of their disease determining a 5-year survival not exceeding 40%.

Current hypothesis for ovarian carcinogenesis establishes as a major determinant for malignant transformation of ovarian surface epithelium the chronic exposure to an inflammatory environment. Several conditions predispose to chronic inflammation, one of them the obesity. More importantly, recent studies confer a prognosis even worse to those ovarian cancer patients that are obese. A possible explanation for a more deleterious outcome in this subpopulation can be found in the presence of metabolic abnormalities and higher levels circulating of pro-inflammatory mediators. In fact, studies by our group and others show that alterations in lipid metabolism and the presence of higher levels of leptin, both conditions commonly found in the obese population, favor a pro-inflammatory environment that promotes cell growth, invasion, metastasis, and resistance to chemotherapeutic agents by the cancer cells.

Interestingly, some retrospective evidence suggests that patients receiving statins during their ovarian cancer treatment experience a better outcome than those not receiving them. Statins, HMGCoA reductase inhibitors, are usually prescribed to reduce cholesterol levels but they also possess pleiotropic effects that negatively influence ovarian carcinogenesis. By inhibiting the mevalonate pathway, statins would have a systemic effect, similar to that observed in atherosclerosis, reducing the inflammatory stimuli present in the tumor microenvironment and inhibiting the activation of multiple intracellular signaling cascades critical for metabolism, proliferation, cell death, migration, invasion, metastasis, and drug sensitivity of the ovarian cancer cell.

In the present chapter we summarize the current evidence on molecular mechanisms supporting the beneficial effect of statins in ovarian cancer. In particular, reasons to maintain statin use among those newly diagnosed ovarian cancer patients already taking this medication. Furthermore, reasons to consider this drug in the design of future clinical trials in the treatment of epithelial ovarian cancer.

Obesity-Induced Chronic Inflammation a 'Driving Force' for Epithelial Ovarian Cancer Development

Epithelial ovarian cancer remains the most lethal of gynecologic malignancies. Annually, approximately 240000 women are diagnosed with ovarian cancer and about 150000 women die from this disease [1]. A number of factors contribute to this outcome, including a late diagnosis, the absence of highly curative chemotherapies and the high degree of molecular heterogeneity among ovarian cancers [2]. In total, the overall cure rate for newly diagnosed ovarian cancer in women is less than 40% across all stages [3,4].

Several groups have attempted to identify modifiable factors contributing to ovarian carcinogenesis that can be targeted for new therapeutic strategies. Potential modifiable risk factors that have already been explored include diet, exercise, cigarette smoking, alcohol intake and obesity. For most of these factors, the evidence is conflicting or inconsistent and does not support an association with ovarian cancer risk [5]. However, accumulating evidence has begun to support the role of obesity in ovarian carcinogenesis. In this respect, two epidemiological studies established an association between ovarian cancer and body mass index, a strong marker for obesity [6] [7]. Consistent with these findings, our group has shown a 20% increase in ovarian cancer age-adjusted mortality rate among Chilean women, a population where the obesity prevalence has strikingly risen above 30% in recent decades [8,9].

How obesity contributes to ovarian carcinogenesis and influences its behavior is not fully understood. For ovarian cancer, one potential explanation that has been proposed is the 'inflammation theory'. This hypothesis contends that chronic exposure of the ovarian epithelium to inflammatory stimuli triggers malignant transformation and subsequently favors more aggressive behavior of cancer cells [10]. Obesity is characterized by accumulated adipose tissue deposits and a state of chronic low-grade inflammation. In this activated state, adipocytes and inflammatory cells secrete adipokines and several inflammatory cytokines that have been associated with tumor progression and metastasis in other epithelial cancers, including breast, colon and prostate cancer [11].

Two adipokines abnormally secreted among obese women are leptin and adiponectin. Typically, serum leptin levels are elevated in obese patients, while adiponectin levels are decreased [12]. Leptin is a peptide hormone that plays a major role in regulating energy intake and expenditure processes, including appetite and metabolism. Leptin acts through its receptor (Ob-R), which is encoded by the *ob* gene [13]. Ob-Rb is the predominant, fully functional isoform, responsible for the biological actions of leptin [14]. This isoform has been identified in several epithelial cancers including thyroid cancer, hepatocellular carcinoma, breast cancer and colon cancer [15]. Upon leptin binding to Ob-Rb, there is concomitant activation of the JAK/STAT, MAPK and PI3K/AKT signaling leading to cell proliferation and migration. [16-20]. Recent studies have suggested that higher circulating levels of leptin, higher leptin receptor expression by the tumor and a high leptin to adiponectin (L:A) ratio all correlate with a worseoutcome in several epithelial cancers, including ovarian cancer [21,22]. Little is known regarding leptin's effects on ovarian cancer cells. *In vitro* studies performed in BG-1, SKOV3 and OVCAR-3 cancer cells have shown that leptin stimulates cell growth and inhibits apoptosis. [17,23]. In this respect, we have recently shown that leptin can also act as a regulator of the metastatic process promoting cell migration and cell invasion of ovarian cancer cells. Upon leptin binding, the leptin/Ob-Rb complex recruits and activates different kinase cascades including the PI3/AKT and RhoA/ROCK signaling pathways that are critical for cell migration [24]. Others authors have also shown that leptin could foster drug resistance in other cancers through activation of Ob-Rb receptor and downstream PI3/AKT pathway [25].

Role of Statins in Cancer

Statins are 3-hydroxy-3-methylglutaryl coenzyme (HMG-CoA) reductase inhibitors commonly prescribed to patients with dyslipidemia, most of them with overweight or obesity, to reduce low-density lipoproteins (LDL), cholesterol and triglycerides and to raise high-density lipoproteins (HDL). The main goal of this indication is the primary and secondary prevention of cardiovascular diseases [26].

Beyond its preventive role for cardiovascular diseases, different epidemiological and molecular studies have supported a potential benefit of using statins for different cancers including breast, colon, and prostate carcinoma, among others [27-37]. The benefit is related not only in reducing cancer risk but also in contributing to cancer therapeutics [38].

From a preventive perspective, statins have been associated with a significant reduction in the risk of developing different cancers based mainly in observational studies [37,38]. In this respect, a recent epidemiological study conducted in Danish population upon the relationship between statin use (prior to cancer diagnosis) and cancer-related mortality has shown that patients using statins prior to cancer diagnosis were 15% less likely to die from any cause or cancer specifically [39]. These findings have opened the window to a possible role of statins in cancer prevention.

From a therapeutic view, statins have also shown synergistic cytotoxicity with different anti-cancerous reagents (mainly chemotherapeutic drugs) currently used for treatment of different cancers both *in vitro* and *in vivo* models [38,40].

To understand how statins can influence the natural history of cancer is necessary shortly review the current cancer model. According to this model, carcinogenesis is viewed as a multistage process where the cells that become malignant acquired at least six biological capabilities that gave it advantages over its normal counterparts and allowed them to influence its surrounding microenvironment to contribute to tumor progression. These capabilities have been named as the hallmarks of cancer and include sustaining proliferative signaling, evading growth suppressors, resisting cell death, enabling replicative immortality, inducing angiogenesis, and activating invasion and metastasis. Behind these hallmarks, there are other two major characteristics. First, genomic instability that generates the genetic diversity expediting the acquisition of these capabilities, and secondly inflammation, which stimulates almost all hallmark functions [41].

Besides its cholesterol lowering effect, statins possess pleiotropic properties that explain their therapeutic benefit in several diseases were inflammation plays a major role, such as multiple sclerosis, rheumatoid arthritis [42]. Pre-clinical studies have shown that statins may exert anti-cancerous effects based on these properties, through both HMGCoA reductase-dependent and HMGCoA reductase-independent pathways [38,43,44]. As seen in figure 1, by inhibition of HMGCoA reductase and reducing mevalonate synthesis, statins prevent post-translational prenylation of the Rho/Ras small GTPases superfamily, which are mediators of key cellular processes such as cell growth, differentiation, survival, cell shape and cell movement [45-47].

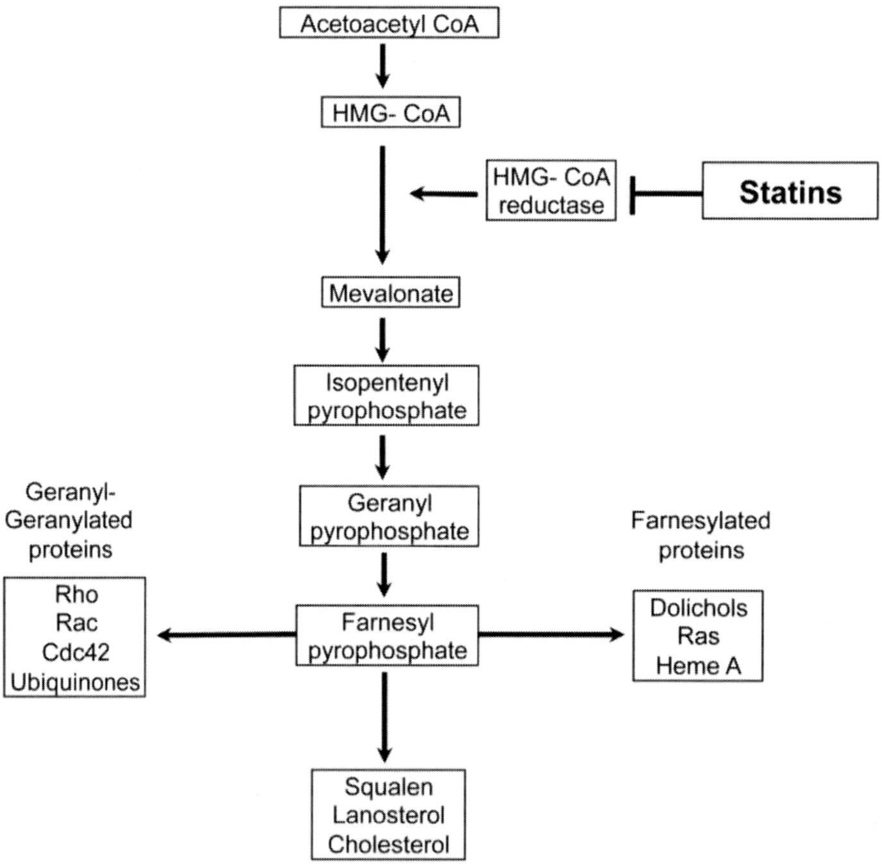

Figure 1. Pleiotropic effects of statins in the mevalonate synthesis pathway. Statins are HMGCoA reductase inhibitors that prevent mevalonate synthesis, a precursor of non-steroidal isoprenoids, which are lipid attachment molecules (prenylation) for downstream small GTPase family members such as Ras, Rho and Rac. By inhibiting prenylation, statins suppress the activation of these proteins.

Table 1. Explanatory molecular mechanisms for beneficial effect of statins in cancer. Statins exert different effects in cancer cells including anti-proliferative and pro-apoptotic effects, inhibition of cell migration, invasion and metastasis, inhibition of angiogenesis, inhibition of lipid raft/caveolae signaling, and inhibition of inflammation

Inhibition of cell proliferation (cell cycle arrest)	Inhibition of lipid raft/caveolae signaling
Ras, Rho Inhibition p21, p27 Stabilization Inhibition of IGF signaling ↓ Rb expression ↓ D1, D3, CDK4, CDK6 cyclin expression	Inhibition of EGF receptor signaling Inhibition of PI3K/Akt signaling pathway
Angiogenesis inhibition (high dose)	**Apoptosis induction**
Rho Inhibition, ↓eNOS ↓VEGF Inhibition of endothelial cell proliferation Blockage of adhesion to extracellular matrix	Caspase -3, -7, -8, -9 activation ↓Bcl-2, ↓Bcl-xL, ↓cIAP1, ↓c-Flip ↑Bax, ↑BMP
Inhibition of inflammation	**Inhibition of cell migration, invasion and metastasis**
↑ T reg lymphocytes (CD4+/CD25+) ↓Adhesion molecules (CD11b, ICAM-1, VCAM-1) PPAR activation ↓Expression of major histocompatibility complex II ↓IL-6, IL-8, IL1β, TNFα, MCP-1 secretion	Rho Inhibition ↓Matrix metalloproteinases (e.g. MMP-9) ↓EGF induced tumor invasion ↓Endothelial adhesion molecule expression (e.g. E-selectin)

Function of these family members depends on its cellular localization and its membrane attachment [47]. Such a condition is determined by the addition of the mevalonate-derived prenyl groups, farnesyl pyrophosphate and geranylgeranyl pyrophosphate [45,47]. Interestingly, many cancer cells from different origins show increased HMGCoA reductase activity, suggesting a metabolic dependence of this pathway to maintain its cancer hallmarks [43,48,49]. In fact, recent studies have shown that by inhibiting the enzyme activity and the prenylation of Ras and Rho GTPases, cancer cells experience cell death by induction of oxidative stress and apoptosis [38,43,50,51]. In addition, statins exert anti-proliferative, anti-angiogenic, and immunomodulatory effects (inhibition of inflammation), which may prevent tumor growth and dissemination [38,44,52]. In Table 1 are summarized the major molecular mechanisms underlying all these statin-mediated effects in cancer.

WHAT IS ALREADY KNOWN ABOUT STATINS EFFECTS IN EPITHELIAL OVARIAN CANCER?

As observed in other epithelial cancers, epidemiological and pre-clinical studies have begun to support the beneficial effect of statins in epithelial ovarian cancer both in prevention and therapeutics.

In this section we will review the current evidence, including the most relevant studies related to reduction of cancer risk and the explanatory molecular mechanisms for its therapeutic effect. We will also include some unpublished results of our group that support the beneficial effect of statins in epithelial ovarian cancer, specifically among obese women.

Statins and Ovarian Cancer Risk

Until 2012, most of the evidence in relation to the effects of statins on the risk of ovarian cancer came from epidemiological studies with methodological flaws that did not allow drawing conclusions [37,53]. Since then, two studies have been published that contribute to clarify the potential beneficial role of statins in reducing ovarian cancer risk.

The first one, a case-control study of newly diagnosed cases of gynecologic cancers and age/sex/clinic/ethnic-group matched population controls where the effect of statin use prior to and following the diagnosis was assessed. This study named CITOUS (The Haifa Cancer in the Ovary and Uterus Study), included 126 pairs of women with ovarian cancer and their matched controls. The main finding of this study was a significant reduction in ovarian cancer risk (OR=0,56; 95% CI, 0,33-0,94) among statin users for more than one year prior to diagnosis [54].

More recently, Liu et al conducted a meta-analysis to evaluate the effects of statins on the risk of gynecologic cancers. They included a total of 14 (4 randomized controlled trials, 5 cohorts, and 5 case-control) studies, involving 12904 gynecologic cancer cases. Pooled results indicated a non-significant decrease of total gynecologic cancer risk among statin users. However, a stratified analysis across cancer site revealed a protective effect of statins on ovarian cancer (RR=0,79; 95% CI, 0,64-0,98). Furthermore, long-term use (> 5 years use) had an obvious decrease on the risk of ovarian cancer (RR=0,48; 95% CI, 0,28-080) [55].

Thus, based on current evidence, it seems that statin use could have a preventive role reducing ovarian cancer risk in long-term statin users as seen in other epithelial cancers [37,38]. These findings justify the design of randomized controlled trials where the protective role of statins in cancer risk could be assessed in a prospective cohort.

Molecular Mechanisms Behind Therapeutic Effect of Statins in Ovarian Cancer

An intriguing retrospective study conducted by Elmore et al demonstrated that advanced ovarian cancer patients who were taking statins experienced improved median progression-free and overall survival compared with those not taking statins. A multivariate analysis identified statin use as an independent positive prognostic factor, after controlling for age, stage, grade and suboptimal cytoreduction [56]. Recently, this finding has been reaffirmed by CITOUS study where women who used statins only after diagnosis of cancer had a significantly better survival (log rank test, p=0,0021, age adjusted HR=0,47, 0,26-0,85) [54].

How statins contribute to a better survival can be explained by molecular mechanisms that involve impairing different cancer hallmarks.

a) Effects in Cell Proliferation and Cell Survival

Our group has recently demonstrated that ovarian cancer cells show increased HMGCoA reductase expression compared to the normal counterparts [43]. Interestingly, Brennan et al have correlated this expression with better prognosis. A multivariate Cox regression analysis demonstrated that patients with tumors expressing HMGCoA reductase had a significantly prolonged recurrence free survival (RR=0,49; 95% CI, 0,25-0,93, p=0,03) independently of other prognostic factors such as residual disease, stage, and grade [57].

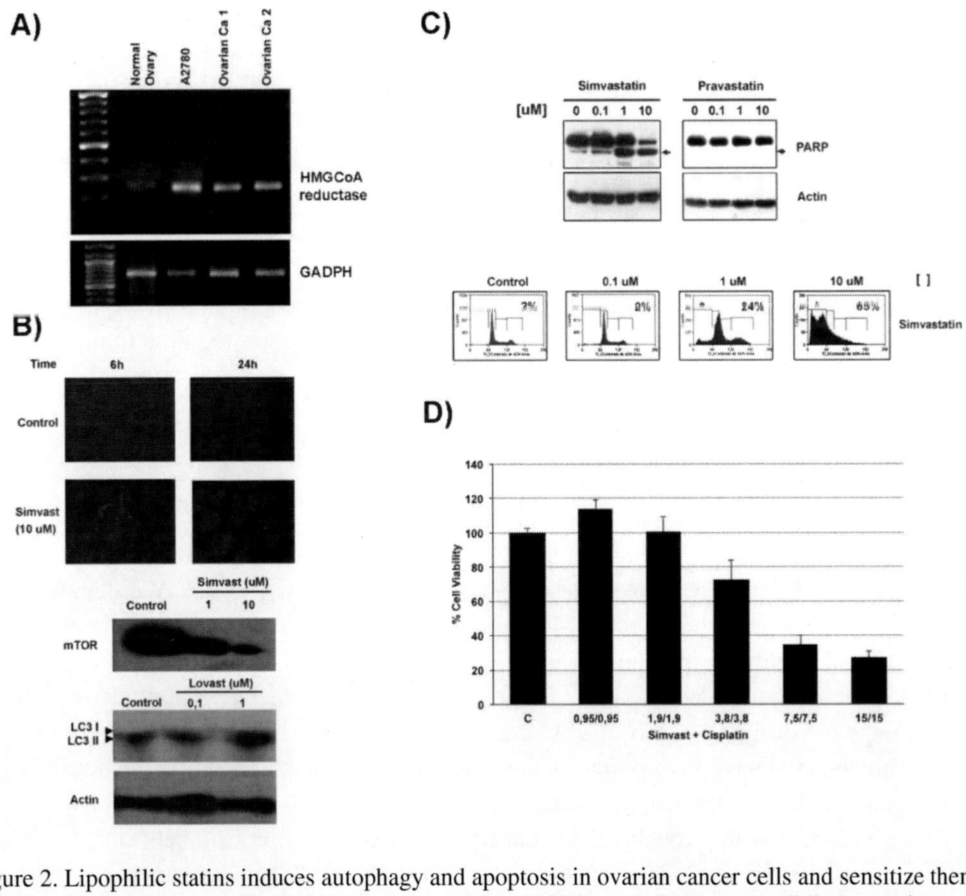

Figure 2. Lipophilic statins induces autophagy and apoptosis in ovarian cancer cells and sensitize them to chemotherapy in dose- and time- dependent manner. A) Either ovarian cancer cell lines or primary tissue cultures establishes from ascites of advanced ovarian cancer patients overexpress HMGCoA reductase compared to normal counterpart measured by RT-PCR. GADPH is shown as loading control; B) In the HMGCoA overexpressing A2780 ovarian cancer cell line, simvastatin and lovastatin induce autophagy in time- and dose-dependent manner, measured by immunocytochemistry (*upper panel*, using LC3 II autophagy marker, red color, 100X) and immunoblotting (*lower panel*, showing a reduction of mTOR expression and an increase in LC3II expression upon statin treatment. Actin is shown as loading control), respectively. C) Lipophilic statins (e.g., simvastatin) but not hydrophilic statins (e.g., pravastatin) induce cell death (apoptosis) in A2780 cells in dose-dependent manner measured by immunoblotting (by detecting the cleaved form of PARP) and flow cytometer (measuring the sub G1/Go fraction in the DNA histogram). D) Synergistic reduction in cell viability of A2780 cells with the combination of simvastatin and cisplatin, measured by colorimetric MTS assay.

We have also shown that lipophilic (e.g., simvastatin or lovastatin) but no hydrophilic (e.g., pravastatin) forms of statins in a concentration dependent manner induce cell arrest, autophagy and consequently cell death in ovarian cancer. These effects also depend on HMGCoA expression levels, since normal counterparts expressing lower levels are not affected as well as tumor expressing similar lower levels, suggesting a metabolic dependence in the mevalonate pathway for HMGCoA overexpressing ovarian cancers (figure 2).

The pro-apoptotic effect induced by statins is explained by activation of intrinsic and extrinsic apoptotic cascades in a cholesterol-independent manner [43]. We have also demonstrated that this effect depends on the inhibition of prenylation of the proteins regulating the cascade [43]. Confirming our findings, Liu et al have shown that both lovastatin and atorvastatin effectively induced apoptosis in ovarian cancer cells and suppressed anchorage-independent growth of these cells in soft agar. These authors also found out that these effects are related to increased expression of Cdc42 and Rac1, also members of small GTPase family, activation of Jun-N-terminal kinase (JNK) and induction of Bim, a pro-apoptotic protein, all induced by these statins [58]. More recently, Robinson et al have shown that simvastatin has conflicting effects in autophagy stimulating earlier stages (accumulation of LC3-II) and blocking late stages (accumulation p62 and loss of Rab7) that are related to autophagosome trafficking. These authors have also shown that longer incubation (up to 96 h) and higher doses of statins (up to 10 uM) are required to induced cell death [59].

b) Effects in Drug Sensitivity

Besides inducing cell death, others and we have shown that statins can sensitize ovarian cancer cells to different chemotherapies by several mechanisms [60-62]. We demonstrated both additive and synergistic effects of lovastatin and simvastatin when used in combination con cisplatin, doxorubicin, paclitaxel, and gemcitabine [44,63]. The synergism was mainly observed when statins were used before adding chemotherapy and combined to chemotherapeutic drugs to which ovarian cancer cells were relatively resistant. As observed by us, Robinson et al have shown that varying the order of drug addition and the dose ratio of the combination can dramatically influence the synergism [59].

Different mechanisms have been postulated to explain the synergism between statins and chemotherapy. The first explanation is the effect that statins and chemotherapeutic drugs have on apoptotic paths that converge in a final common pathway. Statins induce apoptosis by activation of the extrinsic (activation of caspase-8) and intrinsic (activation of caspase-9, cytochrome C release) pathways and chemotherapeutic drugs act mainly via the intrinsic pathway [43]. Another mechanism of sensitization involved the effect of statins in membrane pumps regulating the drug efflux out of the cancer cell and causing multidrug resistance (MDR) in recurrent ovarian cancers. This resistance mechanism implies an elevated drug efflux, which is often due to increased activity of the ATP-binding cassette (ABC) transporter *ABCB1* (previously named *MDR1*) gene that encodes P-glycoprotein [64]. Martirosyan et al demonstrated in A2780ADR cells, which overexpress P-glycoprotein, that these cells exposed to a combination of lovastatin and doxorubicin contained more intracellular doxorubicin than cells treated with doxorubicin alone. Lovastatin inhibited drug transport by blocking P-glycoprotein potentiating doxorubicin-mediated DNA damage and tumor cell apoptosis

[61,65]. More recent studies conducted by the same group have demonstrated that other lipophilic statins (rosuvastatin, fluvastatin and atorvastatin) interact differentially with this efflux pump with no direct bounding or the high affinity as seen with lovastatin [65]. Finally, our group has recently identified a new mechanism to explain drug sensitization involving drug uptake and intracellular drug activation. Indeed, we have shown both in sensitive and resistant ovarian cancer cell lines that simvastatin enhances gemcitabine cytotoxicity. Interestingly, the effect is limited to ovarian cancer cells with no effect in normal HOSE ovarian epithelial cells. The synergism observed with this combination is explained by increase in the expression of equilibrative nucleoside transporter 1 and 2 (hENT1, hENT2) and activity of hENT1 (Figure 3). Both nucleosides transporters are involved in nucleoside-analog uptake. We have also observed that the increase in transporter uptake is dependent on in inhibition of HMGCoA reductase activity since the supplementation of mevalonate almost completely abrogates the effect induced by the combination [63].

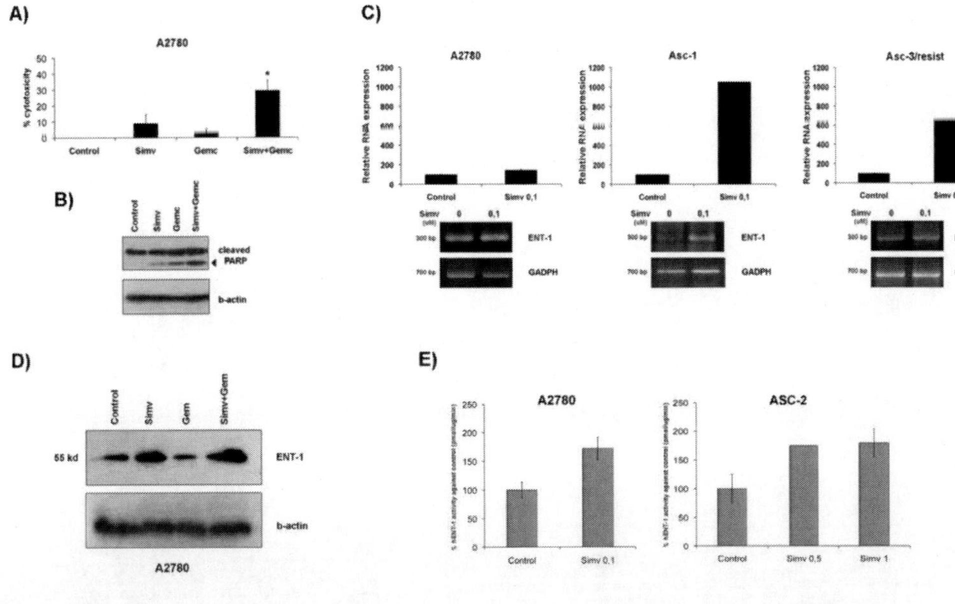

Figure 3. Simvastatin sensitizes ovarian cancer cells to gemcitabine by increasing expression and activity of human equilibrative nucleoside transporters. As seen in the figure, the combination of simvastatin (Simv) and gemcitabine (Gemc) significantly increases A) cell cytotoxicity (measured by colorimetric MTS assay) due to B) apoptosis (by detecting the cleaved form of PARP by immunoblotting) in A2780 cells compared to treatment with each reagent used alone. The increase in apoptosis observed in either A2780 cells or primary tissue cultures (Asc-1, Asc-2, Asc-3 resistant to cisplatin) is due to an increase in expression (measured by C) RT-PCR and D) immunoblotting) and activity of hENT1 transporter (measured by E) [^{3}H]-adenosine uptake assays).

c) Effects in Cell Migration and Invasion

Recently we began to explore the effects of statins in cell migration and invasion in ovarian cancer. As described for other epithelial cancers (e.g., colon cancer) we postulated that lipophilic statins could also affect cell migration and invasion, a key hallmark of cancer and a crucial step for progression of disease and the metastatic process [66,67]. We also hypothesized that statins could counteract the effect of different pro-inflammatory signals present in tumor microenvironment and induced by obesity (e.g., IL-6 and Leptin) [68,69]. Others and we have shown that these signals induced cell migration and invasion of ovarian cancer cells determining a more aggressive behavior of epithelial ovarian cancer and a poorer prognosis [23,70-73]. To address these hypotheses we stimulated ovarian cancer cells cultured in the presence or absence of statins directly with leptin or with conditioned medium harvested from cultures of other cell components (e.g., macrophages) present in the tumor microenvironment (and previously treated with leptin). Upon leptin or conditioned medium exposure, ovarian cancer cells (either cell lines or primary tissue cultures) significantly increase cell migration and invasion compared to control conditions measured by wound healing assays and matrigel Boyden chamber assays (Figure 4).

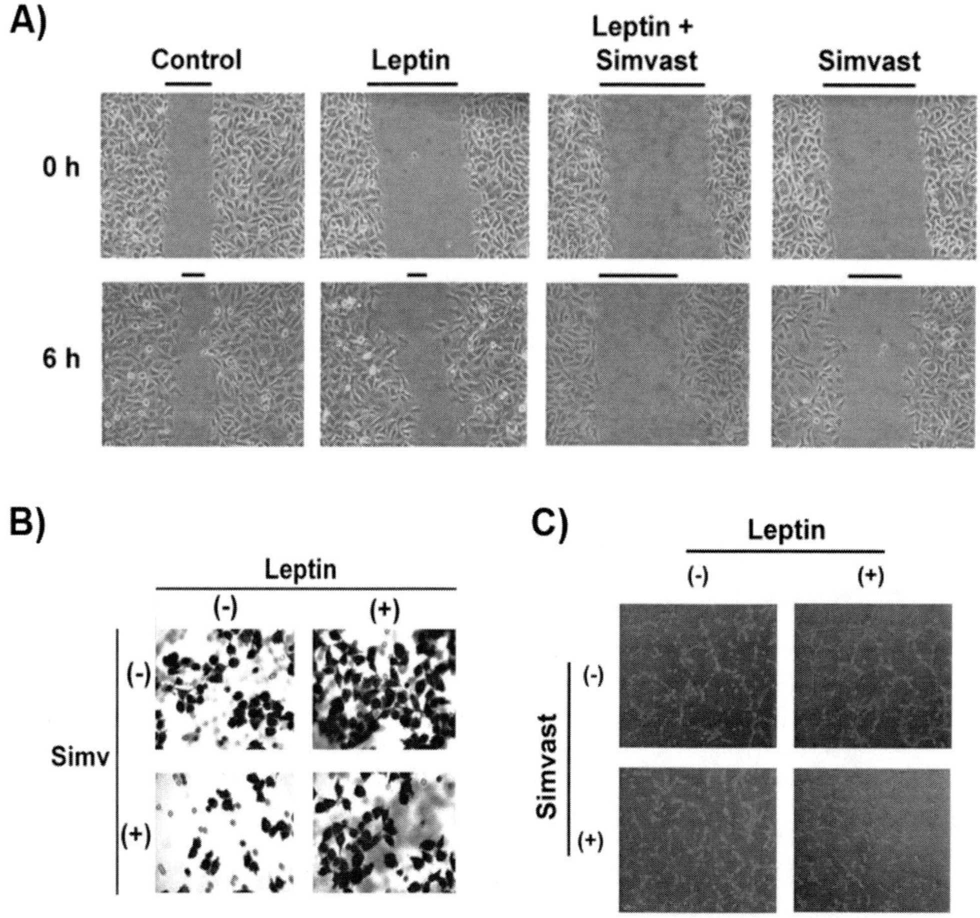

Figure 4. Simvastatin counteracts leptin-induced cell migration, invasion and angiogenesis. A) Simvastatin (Simv) at 1 uM decreases cell migration of SKOV3 cells either under control culturing conditions or upon leptin exposure (100 ng/ml), measured by wound healing assays. **B)** Similar effect is observed in the invasion of HEY cells in matrigel Boyden chamber assays. **C)** Additionally, Simvastatin inhibits leptin induced vessel-like formation by Ea.hy926 cells in matrigel angiogenesis assays.

Interestingly, simvastatin significantly reduces not only cell migration and invasion of cancer cells under control conditions but also under the different pro-inflammatory conditions [24]. To metastasize, a subset of ovarian cancer cells (cancer-initiating cells or cancer-metastasizing cells) present in the tumor must experience epithelial mesenchymal transition (EMT), a condition where EMT and stemness markers are expressed [41]. EMT is a reflex of cell plasticity and evolution that allow the cancer cells to detach from primary tumor, to survive while in transit and to adapt to the conditions offered by the new final environmental destination [74-81]. As we mentioned earlier, leptin acts as a pro-inflammatory cytokine activating different signaling pathways involved not only in cell proliferation but also in cell migration [82,83]. These pathways include activation of PI3/AKT pathway and downstream recruitment and activation of different members of the small GTPase family (RhoA). Leptin has also involved in the maintenance of an EMT or stemness phenotype in other epithelial cancers [82,84]. Preliminary results from our group suggest that simvastatin is capable to inhibit the PI3/AKT signaling pathway and the subsequent recruitment and activation of RhoA induced by leptin or the conditioned medium not only in ovarian cancer cells but also in the subset of cancer-initiating cells. By inhibiting prenylation of small GTPase family members, statins preclude lamellipodial, stress-fiber and new focal adhesion formation, all critical steps for cell migration [46,85]. In addition, statins would interfere with cancer cell plasticity and EMT modifying the expression of EMT and stemness markers that are required for the maintenance of the more invasive cancer cell phenotype [52].

d) Effects in Angiogenesis

Initially, the evidence connecting statins and angiogenesis was contradictory. Depending on the statin, the dose and the experimental model chosen to study their effect, both angiogenic and angiostatic responses were observed. To clarify this controversy, Khaidakov et al tested two different statins, rosuvastatin and simvastatin, in two different assay systems. In the matrigel angiogenesis assay, both statins enhanced vessel-like formation by human umbilical vein endothelial cells (HUVEC) compared to control conditions. In contrast, in the ex-vivo mouse aortic ring-sprouting assay, both statins virtually abolished new vessel formation. Both angiogenesis models differentiate in the compaction state of cells exposed to statins. In the matrigel angiogenesis assay, the cells are disperse while in the aortic ring-sprouting assay are in a compact monolayer. These authors demonstrated in HUVEC cells that statins through VE-cadherin stimulation modulate cell-cell adhesion and diminish the ability of cells to proliferate and migrate favoring aggregation and tube formation. Additionally, these authors postulated that the anti-atherosclerotic and anti-cancer effects of statins explained the inhibition of angiogenesis in the intact vessel [86]. In relation to cancer, most of studies have favored an anti-angiogenic effect of statins [38]. In this respect, we have recently carried out matrigel angiogenesis assay, using Ea.hy926 cells, to assess the effects of leptin and statins in angiogenesis.

As observed in figure 4, leptin induced vessel-like formation while statins did not. More importantly, simvastatin in a dose and time dependent manner inhibited leptin-induced angiogenesis in this model. To explain this anti-angiogenic effect, multiple mechanisms have been suggested including the inhibition of angiogenesis through down-regulation of pro-angiogenic factors, such as vascular endothelial growth factor, inhibition of endothelial cell proliferation and inhibition of adhesion to extracellular matrix by blocking intercellular adhesion molecules [38].

d) Effect in Immune-Modulation

Multiple pathways have been involved in the statin immune-modulation along with the regulation of genes encoding key molecules of the antigen presentation and immune regulation [87]. An additional mechanism involved the down-regulation of the nuclear factor-kappa-B (NF-κB) encoding the transcription of many immune genes such as MHC-1, chemokines, interferon-inducible protein-10, monocyte chemo-attractant protein 1 (MCP-1), and COX-2 [38]. It has been suggested that atorvastatin reduced these chemokines by inhibition of NF-κB activation [88]. Our group has recently started to study the effects of statins in the interactions between ovarian cancer cells and immune cells present in tumor microenvironment, particularly macrophages in ascites. Our data using models of THP-1 cells differentiated to TAM (tumor-associated macrophages) and ovarian cancer cells co-culture indicated that TAM could stimulate cancer cell proliferation and migration while statin would exert an inhibitory effect in this interaction.

Conclusion

Epithelial ovarian cancer remains as the deadliest gynecologic malignancy. Despite using extensive cytoreductive surgery to achieve optimal debulking and improving chemotherapeutic response with current schemes, many women will still die from their disease. Therefore is urgent to better understand ovarian carcinogenesis and finding better or alternative options to improve the poor survival. Based on the available knowledge, chronic inflammation seems to play a key role not only in the early events leading to cancer development in the normal ovarian epithelium but also at advanced stages of the disease where inflammation would participate regulating almost all hallmarks of cancer including among them genomic instability, cell proliferation and cell death, EMT and cell plasticity required to invade and metastasize, capabilities to evade immune system and to adapt to the conditions offered by the new home microenvironment, and acquiring drug resistance. Evidence also supports a role of obesity in maintaining a state of low chronic inflammation. Statins through its pleiotropic effects, by inhibiting mevalonate synthesis and the prenylation of small GTPase family members, counteract the effect of pro-inflammatory cytokines normally present at higher levels among obese women (e.g., IL-6 and Leptin), and acting as driving forces at different steps during ovarian carcinogenesis. Here we provide evidence favoring the use of statins not only as a potential preventing tool reducing risk of ovarian cancer but also as a therapeutic tool, potentially effective by themselves in ovarian cancers expressing higher levels of HMGCoA reductase activity and as a sensitizing tool for the low expressing cancers to current chemotherapeutic schemes. Particularly, lipophilic statins, prescribed at higher doses than those chosen to lower cholesterol levels, exert anti-proliferative and pro-apoptotic effects, modulate EMT and cell plasticity diminishing cell migration, invasion and angiogenesis, sensitize to chemotherapy, and reduce cancer cell capability to evade immune system. This evidence strongly support the option of maintaining statin use among those women diagnosed with ovarian cancer not only during their chemotherapy but also beyond ending their planned treatment. Statins are worldwide used and considered a safe medication with very low rate of adverse side effects. So far, no major adverse effects have been reported among ovarian cancer patients undergoing surgery and chemotherapy that it could contraindicate this option. Considering their safety and the current evidence favoring their benefit in cancer, statins might be also included in the design of future clinical trials for epithelial ovarian cancer as well as other cancers where they would have also shown benefit.

ACKNOWLEDGMENTS

The research included in this book chapter has been supported by Chilean Funds Fondecyt nº1120292 and 1080163 granted to Mauricio A. Cuello and Fondecyt nº3140335 granted to Lorena Abarzúa-Catalán.

REFERENCES

[1] Jemal A, Bray F, Center MM, Ferlay J, Ward E, Forman D. Global cancer statistics. *CA: a cancer journal for clinicians*. 2011; 61: 69-90.

[2] Hunn J, Rodriguez GC. Ovarian cancer: etiology, risk factors, and epidemiology. *Clinical obstetrics and gynecology*. 2012; 55: 3-23.

[3] Romero I, Bast RC, Jr. Minireview: human ovarian cancer: biology, current management, and paths to personalizing therapy. *Endocrinology*. 2012; 153: 1593-602.

[4] Berek JS, Crum C, Friedlander M. Cancer of the ovary, fallopian tube, and peritoneum. *International journal of gynaecology and obstetrics: the official organ of the International Federation of Gynaecology and Obstetrics*. 2012; 119 Suppl 2: S118-29.

[5] Hunn J, Rodriguez GC. Ovarian cancer: etiology, risk factors, and epidemiology. *Clinical obstetrics and gynecology*. 2012; 55: 3-23.

[6] Collaborative Group on Epidemiological Studies of Ovarian Cancer. Ovarian cancer and body size: individual participant meta-analysis including 25,157 women with ovarian cancer from 47 epidemiological studies. *PLoS medicine*. 2012; 9: e1001200.

[7] Protani MM, Nagle CM, Webb PM. Obesity and ovarian cancer survival: a systematic review and meta-analysis. *Cancer prevention research*. 2012; 5: 901-10.

[8] Donoso E, Cuello M. Mortalidad por cáncer en la mujer chilena. Análisis comparativo entre los años 1997 y 2003. *Revista Chilena de Obstetricia y Ginecología*. 2006; 71: 10-6.

[9] Cuello M. GES en cáncer de ovario epitelial: un avance sanitario necesario pero no exento de riesgos y dificultades futuras. *Rev Chil Obstet Ginecol*. 2013; 78: 161-6.

[10] Maccio A, Madeddu C. Inflammation and ovarian cancer. *Cytokine*. 2012; 58: 133-47.

[11] Nieman KM, Romero IL, Van Houten B, Lengyel E. Adipose tissue and adipocytes support tumorigenesis and metastasis. *Biochimica et biophysica acta*. 2013; 1831: 1533-41.

[12] van Kruijsdijk RC, van der Wall E, Visseren FL. Obesity and cancer: the role of dysfunctional adipose tissue. *Cancer Epidemiology, Biomarkers & Prevention*. 2009; 18: 2569-78.

[13] Gautron L, Elmquist JK. Sixteen years and counting: an update on leptin in energy balance. *The Journal of clinical investigation*. 2011; 121: 2087-93.

[14] Wauman J, Tavernier J. Leptin receptor signaling: pathways to leptin resistance. *Frontiers in bioscience*. 2011; 16: 2771-93.

[15] Dutta D, Ghosh S, Pandit K, Mukhopadhyay P, Chowdhury S. Leptin and cancer: Pathogenesis and modulation. *Indian journal of endocrinology and metabolism*. 2012; 16: S596-600.

[16] Chen C, Chang YC, Lan MS, Breslin M. Leptin stimulates ovarian cancer cell growth and inhibits apoptosis by increasing cyclin D1 and Mcl-1 expression via the activation of the MEK/ERK1/2 and PI3K/Akt signaling pathways. *International journal of oncology*. 2013; 42: 1113-9.

[17] Choi JH, Park SH, Leung PC, Choi KC. Expression of leptin receptors and potential effects of leptin on the cell growth and activation of mitogen-activated protein kinases in ovarian cancer cells. *The Journal of clinical endocrinology and metabolism*. 2005; 90: 207-10.

[18] Huang CY, Yu HS, Lai TY, Yeh YL, Su CC, Hsu HH, Tsai FJ, Tsai CH, Wu HC, Tang CH. Leptin increases motility and integrin up-regulation in human prostate cancer cells. *Journal of cellular physiology*. 2011; 226: 1274-82.

[19] Ratke J, Entschladen F, Niggemann B, Zanker KS, Lang K. Leptin stimulates the migration of colon carcinoma cells by multiple signaling pathways. *Endocrine-related cancer*. 2010; 17: 179-89.

[20] Vona-Davis L, Rose DP. Adipokines as endocrine, paracrine, and autocrine factors in breast cancer risk and progression. *Endocrine-related cancer*. 2007; 14: 189-206.

[21] Diaz ES, Karlan BY, Li AJ. Obesity-associated adipokines correlate with survival in epithelial ovarian cancer. *Gynecologic oncology*. 2013; 129: 353-7.

[22] Uddin S, Bu R, Ahmed M, Abubaker J, Al-Dayel F, Bavi P, Al-Kuraya KS. Overexpression of leptin receptor predicts an unfavorable outcome in Middle Eastern ovarian cancer. *Molecular cancer*. 2009; 8: 74.

[23] Ptak A, Kolaczkowska E, Gregoraszczuk EL. Leptin stimulation of cell cycle and inhibition of apoptosis gene and protein expression in OVCAR-3 ovarian cancer cells. *Endocrine*. 2013; 43: 394-403.

[24] Cuello M, Kato S, Diaz D, Vecchiola A, Branes J, Barriga MI, Gejman R, Owen GI. Simvastatin Inhibits Leptin-activated Signaling Pathways That Promote Migration and Invasiveness of Ovarian Cancer Cells. *European Journal of Cancer*. 2012; 48: s193-s4.

[25] Chi M, Chen J, Ye Y, Tseng HY, Lai F, Tay KH, Jin L, Guo ST, Jiang CC, Zhang XD. Adipocytes contribute to resistance of human melanoma cells to chemotherapy and targeted therapy. *Current medicinal chemistry*. 2014; 21: 1255-67.

[26] Pignone M, Phillips C, Mulrow C. Use of lipid lowering drugs for primary prevention of coronary heart disease: meta-analysis of randomised trials. *Bmj*. 2000; 321: 983-6.

[27] Hachem C, Morgan R, Johnson M, Kuebeler M, El-Serag H. Statins and the risk of colorectal carcinoma: a nested case-control study in veterans with diabetes. *The American journal of gastroenterology*. 2009; 104: 1241-8.

[28] Poynter JN, Gruber SB, Higgins PD, Almog R, Bonner JD, Rennert HS, Low M, Greenson JK, Rennert G. Statins and the risk of colorectal cancer. *The New England journal of medicine*. 2005; 352: 2184-92.
[29] Khurana V, Bejjanki HR, Caldito G, Owens MW. Statins reduce the risk of lung cancer in humans: a large case-control study of US veterans. *Chest*. 2007; 131: 1282-8.
[30] Bonovas S, Nikolopoulos G, Filioussi K, Peponi E, Bagos P, Sitaras NM. Can statin therapy reduce the risk of melanoma? A meta-analysis of randomized controlled trials. *European journal of epidemiology*. 2010; 25: 29-35.
[31] Bonovas S, Filioussi K, Sitaras NM. Statin use and the risk of prostate cancer: A metaanalysis of 6 randomized clinical trials and 13 observational studies. *International journal of cancer Journal international du cancer*. 2008; 123: 899-904.
[32] Bonovas S, Tsantes A, Drosos T, Sitaras NM. Cancer chemoprevention: a summary of the current evidence. *Anticancer research*. 2008; 28: 1857-66.
[33] Undela K, Srikanth V, Bansal D. Statin use and risk of breast cancer: a meta-analysis of observational studies. *Breast cancer research and treatment*. 2012; 135: 261-9.
[34] Bonovas S, Filioussi K, Tsantes A, Sitaras NM. Use of statins and risk of haematological malignancies: a meta-analysis of six randomized clinical trials and eight observational studies. *British journal of clinical pharmacology*. 2007; 64: 255 62.
[35] Bonovas S, Filioussi K, Tsavaris N, Sitaras NM. Use of statins and breast cancer: a meta-analysis of seven randomized clinical trials and nine observational studies. *Journal of clinical oncology : official journal of the American Society of Clinical Oncology*. 2005; 23: 8606-12.
[36] Lochhead P, Chan AT. Statins and colorectal cancer. *Clinical gastroenterology and hepatology : the official clinical practice journal of the American Gastroenterological Association*. 2013; 11: 109-18; quiz e13-4.
[37] Boudreau DM, Yu O, Johnson J. Statin use and cancer risk: a comprehensive review. *Expert Opin Drug Saf*. 2010; 9: 603-21.
[38] Vallianou NG, Kostantinou A, Kougias M, Kazazis C. Statins and cancer. *Anti-cancer agents in medicinal chemistry*. 2014; 14: 706-12.
[39] Nielsen SF, Nordestgaard BG, Bojesen SE. Statin use and reduced cancer-related mortality. *The New England journal of medicine*. 2012; 367: 1792-802.
[40] Wang CY, Shui HA, Chang TC. In vivo evidence of duality effects for lovastatin in a nude mouse cancer model. *International journal of cancer Journal international du cancer*. 2010; 126: 578-82.
[41] Hanahan D, Weinberg RA. Hallmarks of cancer: the next generation. *Cell*. 2011; 144: 646-74.
[42] Mihos CG, Santana O. Pleiotropic effects of the HMG-CoA reductase inhibitors. *International journal of general medicine*. 2011; 4: 261-71.
[43] Kato S, Smalley S, Sadarangani A, Chen-Lin K, Oliva B, Branes J, Carvajal J, Gejman R, Owen GI, Cuello M. Lipophilic but not hydrophilic statins selectively induce cell death in gynaecological cancers expressing high levels of HMGCoA reductase. *Journal of cellular and molecular medicine*. 2010; 14: 1180-93.
[44] Cuello FM, Kato CS, Diaz SD, Owen G. [Effects of statins in cancer]. *Revista medica de Chile*. 2013; 141: 227-36.
[45] Ridley AJ. Rho family proteins: coordinating cell responses. *Trends in cell biology*. 2001; 11: 471-7.

[46] Ridley AJ. Rho GTPases and cell migration. *Journal of cell science*. 2001; 114: 2713-22.

[47] Ridley AJ. Rho proteins: linking signaling with membrane trafficking. *Traffic*. 2001; 2: 303-10.

[48] Bengtsson E, Nerjovaj P, Wangefjord S, Nodin B, Eberhard J, Uhlen M, Borgquist S, Jirstrom K. HMG-CoA reductase expression in primary colorectal cancer correlates with favourable clinicopathological characteristics and an improved clinical outcome. *Diagnostic pathology*. 2014; 9: 78.

[49] Borgquist S, Jogi A, Ponten F, Ryden L, Brennan DJ, Jirstrom K. Prognostic impact of tumour-specific HMG-CoA reductase expression in primary breast cancer. *Breast cancer research : BCR*. 2008; 10: R79.

[50] Zhu Y, Casey PJ, Kumar AP, Pervaiz S. Deciphering the signaling networks underlying simvastatin-induced apoptosis in human cancer cells: evidence for non-canonical activation of RhoA and Rac1 GTPases. *Cell death & disease*. 2013; 4: e568.

[51] Benhar M, Dalyot I, Engelberg D, Levitzki A. Enhanced ROS production in oncogenically transformed cells potentiates c-Jun N-terminal kinase and p38 mitogen-activated protein kinase activation and sensitization to genotoxic stress. *Molecular and cellular biology*. 2001; 21: 6913-26.

[52] Gauthaman K, Fong CY, Bongso A. Statins, stem cells, and cancer. *J Cell Biochem*. 2009; 106: 975-83.

[53] Yu O, Boudreau DM, Buist DS, Miglioretti DL. Statin use and female reproductive organ cancer risk in a large population-based setting. *Cancer causes & control : CCC*. 2009; 20: 609-16.

[54] Lavie O, Pinchev M, Rennert HS, Segev Y, Rennert G. The effect of statins on risk and survival of gynecological malignancies. *Gynecol Oncol*. 2013; 130: 615-9.

[55] Liu Y, Qin A, Li T, Qin X, Li S. Effect of statin on risk of gynecologic cancers: a meta-analysis of observational studies and randomized controlled trials. *Gynecol Oncol*. 2014; 133: 647-55.

[56] Elmore RG, Ioffe Y, Scoles DR, Karlan BY, Li AJ. Impact of statin therapy on survival in epithelial ovarian cancer. *Gynecologic oncology*. 2008; 111: 102-5.

[57] Brennan DJ, Brandstedt J, Rexhepaj E, Foley M, Ponten F, Uhlen M, Gallagher WM, O'Connor DP, O'Herlihy C, Jirstrom K. Tumour-specific HMG-CoAR is an independent predictor of recurrence free survival in epithelial ovarian cancer. *BMC Cancer*. 2010; 10: 125.

[58] Liu H, Liang SL, Kumar S, Weyman CM, Liu W, Zhou A. Statins induce apoptosis in ovarian cancer cells through activation of JNK and enhancement of Bim expression. *Cancer chemotherapy and pharmacology*. 2009; 63: 997-1005.

[59] Robinson E, Nandi M, Wilkinson LL, Arrowsmith DM, Curtis AD, Richardson A. Preclinical evaluation of statins as a treatment for ovarian cancer. *Gynecol Oncol*. 2013; 129: 417-24.

[60] Goard CA, Mather RG, Vinepal B, Clendening JW, Martirosyan A, Boutros PC, Sharom FJ, Penn LZ. Differential interactions between statins and P-glycoprotein: implications for exploiting statins as anticancer agents. *International Journal of Cancer*. 2010; 127: 2936-48.

[61] Martirosyan A, Clendening JW, Goard CA, Penn LZ. Lovastatin induces apoptosis of ovarian cancer cells and synergizes with doxorubicin: potential therapeutic relevance. *BMC cancer*. 2010; 10: 103.

[62] Taylor-Harding B, Orsulic S, Karlan BY, Li AJ. Fluvastatin and cisplatin demonstrate synergistic cytotoxicity in epithelial ovarian cancer cells. *Gynecologic oncology*. 2010; 119: 549-56.

[63] Kato S, Leisewitz AV, Barriga MI, Branes J, Owen GI, Cuello M. Simvastatin increases expression and activity of human equilibrative nucleoside transporter 1 (HENT1) in ovarian cancer cells sensitizing to gemcitabine. Mechanisms and Models of Cancer. Cold Spring Harbor Laboratory: Cold Spring Harbor, 2010. p. 99.

[64] Agarwal R, Kaye SB. Ovarian cancer: strategies for overcoming resistance to chemotherapy. *Nature reviews Cancer*. 2003; 3: 502-16.

[65] Goard CA, Mather RG, Vinepal B, Clendening JW, Martirosyan A, Boutros PC, Sharom FJ, Penn LZ. Differential interactions between statins and P-glycoprotein: implications for exploiting statins as anticancer agents. *Int J Cancer*. 2010; 127: 2936-48.

[66] Al-Haidari AA, Syk I, Thorlacius H. HMG-CoA reductase regulates CCL17-induced colon cancer cell migration via geranylgeranylation and RhoA activation. *Biochemical and biophysical research communications*. 2014; 446: 68-72.

[67] Mehta N, Hordines J, Sykes D, Doerr RJ, Cohen SA. Low density lipoproteins and Lovastatin modulate the organ-specific transendothelial migration of primary and metastatic human colon adenocarcinoma cell lines in vitro. *Clinical & experimental metastasis*. 1998; 16: 587-94.

[68] Khan S, Shukla S, Sinha S, Meeran SM. Role of adipokines and cytokines in obesity-associated breast cancer: therapeutic targets. *Cytokine & growth factor reviews*. 2013; 24: 503-13.

[69] Howe LR, Subbaramaiah K, Hudis CA, Dannenberg AJ. Molecular pathways: adipose inflammation as a mediator of obesity-associated cancer. *Clinical cancer research : an official journal of the American Association for Cancer Research*. 2013; 19: 6074-83.

[70] Chen C, Chang YC, Lan MS, Breslin M. Leptin stimulates ovarian cancer cell growth and inhibits apoptosis by increasing cyclin D1 and Mcl-1 expression via the activation of the MEK/ERK1/2 and PI3K/Akt signaling pathways. *International journal of oncology*. 2013; 42: 1113-9.

[71] Choi JH, Park SH, Leung PC, Choi KC. Expression of leptin receptors and potential effects of leptin on the cell growth and activation of mitogen-activated protein kinases in ovarian cancer cells. *The Journal of clinical endocrinology and metabolism*. 2005; 90: 207-10.

[72] Diaz ES, Karlan BY, Li AJ. Obesity-associated adipokines correlate with survival in epithelial ovarian cancer. *Gynecologic oncology*. 2013; 129: 353-7.

[73] Uddin S, Bu R, Ahmed M, Abubaker J, Al-Dayel F, Bavi P, Al-Kuraya KS. Overexpression of leptin receptor predicts an unfavorable outcome in Middle Eastern ovarian cancer. *Molecular cancer*. 2009; 8: 74.

[74] Davidowitz RA, Selfors LM, Iwanicki MP, Elias KM, Karst A, Piao H, Ince TA, Drage MG, Dering J, Konecny GE, Matulonis U, Mills GB, Slamon DJ, Drapkin R, Brugge JS. Mesenchymal gene program-expressing ovarian cancer spheroids exhibit enhanced mesothelial clearance. *The Journal of clinical investigation*. 2014; 124: 2611-25.

[75] Davidson B, Trope CG, Reich R. Epithelial-mesenchymal transition in ovarian carcinoma. *Frontiers in oncology*. 2012; 2: 33.

[76] Elloul S, Vaksman O, Stavnes HT, Trope CG, Davidson B, Reich R. Mesenchymal-to-epithelial transition determinants as characteristics of ovarian carcinoma effusions. *Clinical & experimental metastasis*. 2010; 27: 161-72.

[77] Geiger TR, Peeper DS. Metastasis mechanisms. *Biochimica et biophysica acta*. 2009; 1796: 293-308.

[78] Lili LN, Matyunina LV, Walker LD, Wells SL, Benigno BB, McDonald JF. Molecular profiling supports the role of epithelial-to-mesenchymal transition (EMT) in ovarian cancer metastasis. *Journal of ovarian research*. 2013; 6: 49.

[79] Luo X, Dong Z, Chen Y, Yang L, Lai D. Enrichment of ovarian cancer stem-like cells is associated with epithelial to mesenchymal transition through an miRNA-activated AKT pathway. *Cell proliferation*. 2013; 46: 436-46.

[80] Nakayama K, Nakayama N, Katagiri H, Miyazaki K. Mechanisms of ovarian cancer metastasis: biochemical pathways. *International journal of molecular sciences*. 2012; 13: 11705-17.

[81] Vergara D, Merlot B, Lucot JP, Collinet P, Vinatier D, Fournier I, Salzet M. Epithelial-mesenchymal transition in ovarian cancer. *Cancer letters*. 2010; 291: 59-66.

[82] Yan D, Avtanski D, Saxena NK, Sharma D. Leptin-induced epithelial-mesenchymal transition in breast cancer cells requires beta-catenin activation via Akt/GSK3- and MTA1/Wnt1 protein-dependent pathways. *The Journal of biological chemistry*. 2012; 287: 8598-612.

[83] Ratke J, Entschladen F, Niggemann B, Zanker KS, Lang K. Leptin stimulates the migration of colon carcinoma cells by multiple signaling pathways. *Endocrine-related cancer*. 2010; 17: 179-89.

[84] Zheng Q, Banaszak L, Fracci S, Basali D, Dunlap SM, Hursting SD, Rich JN, Hjlemeland AB, Vasanji A, Berger NA, Lathia JD, Reizes O. Leptin receptor maintains cancer stem-like properties in triple negative breast cancer cells. *Endocrine-related cancer*. 2013; 20: 797-808.

[85] Horiuchi A, Kikuchi N, Osada R, Wang C, Hayashi A, Nikaido T, Konishi I. Overexpression of RhoA enhances peritoneal dissemination: RhoA suppression with Lovastatin may be useful for ovarian cancer. *Cancer science*. 2008; 99: 2532-9.

[86] Khaidakov M, Wang W, Khan JA, Kang BY, Hermonat PL, Mehta JL. Statins and angiogenesis: is it about connections? *Biochemical and biophysical research communications*. 2009; 387: 543-7.

[87] Novak A, Binnington B, Ngan B, Chadwick K, Fleshner N, Lingwood CA. Cholesterol masks membrane glycosphingolipid tumor-associated antigens to reduce their immunodetection in human cancer biopsies. *Glycobiology*. 2013; 23: 1230-9.

[88] Li J, Li JJ, He JG, Nan JL, Guo YL, Xiong CM. Atorvastatin decreases C-reactive protein-induced inflammatory response in pulmonary artery smooth muscle cells by inhibiting nuclear factor-kappaB pathway. *Cardiovascular therapeutics*. 2010; 28: 8-14.

In: Statins
Editor: Eric R. Travers
ISBN: 978-1-63463-057-3

Chapter 9

STATIN-INDUCED MYOPATHY

Marilita Falangola Accioly, Ph.D.[1] and Camila Ferreira Leite[2]
[1]Department of Applied Physical Therapy,
Federal University of Triângulo Mineiro, UFTM, Uberaba-MG, Brazil
[2]Postgraduate Program in Health Sciences,
Federal University of Triângulo Mineiro, UFTM, Uberaba-MG, Brazil

ABSTRACT

Inhibitors of 3-hydroxy- 3-methylglutaryl-coenzyme A reductase (HMG- CoA) or statins are important drugs used in the treatment of dyslipidemia by reducing the biosynthesis of cholesterol. In addition to the main effect of lowering blood cholesterol levels, they have pleiotropic effects of which can be highlighted: i) improvement of endothelial function through modulation of endothelial nitric oxide synthase (eNOS) activity and inhibition of endothelin; ii) anti-inflammatory effects resulting from the reduction of proinflammatory cell signaling, oxidative stress, interaction of leukocytes to endothelial cells, and platelet and tissue factor activation; iii) stabilization of atherosclerotic plaque; iv) reduction of osteoclast formation and stimulation of osteoblasts (antiosteoporotic effect); and v) immunomodulation. It is known that these effects are variable and are not common to all statins. Even so, given the potential of these drugs, statins are currently the most prescribed medicines worldwide, and generally are extremely well tolerated by patients. However, adverse effects with different magnitudes can be observed in muscles, with occurrences ranging from a mild myalgia to rhabdomyolysis, progressing to acute renal failure and even death. The statin-induced rhabdomyolysis is a rare event, and is estimated to occur in 0.3 per 100,000 patient years of exposure, with a mortality rate of 9%. Regarding muscular symptoms, myalgia is characterized by pain with or without muscle weakness, not accompanied by an increased in creatine phosphokinase (CPK) enzyme, contrasting to myositis, that leads to an increase of this enzyme associated with muscle symptoms. Conversely, rhabdomyolysis, in generally, is characterized by muscle symptoms and significant increases in CPK levels (generally greater than 10 times the normal upper limit), and elevated levels of creatinine, renal dysfunction, dark urine, and myoglobinuria. Therefore, monitoring CPK levels is recommended during treatment with statins, since it is known the occurrence of an increase in their levels with potential severe effects on muscles even in the absence of muscular symptomatology. On the other hand, the opposite also occurs with muscle manifestations even in the absence of elevated CPK. The mechanisms by which statins develops miotoxicity remains not fully understood. Among the hypotheses proposed, the blocked in cholesterol biosynthesis induced by statins can be a myotoxicity determinant since the reduction in cholesterol content of cell membranes of skeletal muscle could make them unstable. Another hypothesis considers the farnesyl pyrophosphate and geranylgeranyl pirosfofate decrease, which normally activate regulatory proteins binding to guanosine triphosphate (GTP), which promotes cell maintenance and growth while decreasing apoptosis. Lastly, the hypothesis of myopathy occurrence across the depletion of coenzyme Q10 (CoQ10) in mitochondria is also considered. In association with drug therapy in clinical practice, it is often recommended to dyslipidemic patients the practice of regular physical exercises, which are known to be the most effective and cheapest intervention in reducing morbidity and mortality from cardiovascular diseases. However, miotoxicity can negatively interfere with the exercise or, in the opposite direction, the exercises may, itself, potentiate the statin myotoxic effect.

INTRODUCTION

Inhibitors of 3-hydroxy 3-methylglutaryl Coenzyme A reductase (HMG-CoA) or statins are important drugs used for the management of dyslipidemia due their effectiveness in reducing the biosynthesis of cholesterol. They work by competitively inhibiting the enzyme necessary for conversion of HMG-CoA to mevalonate that is the rate-limiting step in the synthesis of cholesterol and other isoprenoids.

The finding of this class of drugs is relatively recent (late 70s and early 80s) [1] and statins were initially isolated from a culture of fungi such as *Penicillium citrinum*, *Aspergillus terreus* and *Nocardia autrophica*, which originated mevastatin, lovastatin and pravastatin, respectively. Subsequently, some structural modifications in lovastatin originated simvastatin. After, fluvastatin, atorvastatin, cerivastatin (now withdrawn from the market), rosuvastatin and pitavastatin were developed.

Although belonging to the same class of drugs, the statins molecules differ from each other regarding the absorption, the linkage with plasma proteins, the hepatic extraction, the plasma half-life, as well concerning the impact of diet over their systemic use. [2]

Thus, showed as lactones, lovastatin and simvastatin inhibit HMG-CoA only after hydrolysis in liver and, therefore, are considered prodrugs; the others, considered as active drugs, are presented in the active acid form and do not require processing. [3,4]

Statins are metabolized in the liver and their excretion occur by the intestinal (predominantly) and kidney route. [3] Most of the statins are metabolized by cytochrome P450 3A4. Differently, fluvastatin uses the P450 2C9 route and pravastatin, which is enzymatically transformed in the cytosol of hepatocytes, does not use the cytochrome enzymes. The absorption is intestinal, but there are differences regarding the percentage of absorption between the statins [2]

Besides the dyslipidemia-associated effects, pleiotropic effects are also attributed to statins, of which can be highlighted: 1) the improvement of endothelial function through modulating the activity of endothelial nitric oxide synthase (eNOS) and inhibition of endothelin; 2) the antiinflammatory effects resulting from the reduction of proinflammatory cell signaling, oxidative stress, interaction of leukocytes to endothelial cells and the decrease of tissue factor and platelet aggregation; 4) the stabilization of atherosclerotic plaque; 5) lower osteoclast formation and stimulation of the osteoblasts (anti-osteoporosis effect); and 6) immunomodulation. [5]

Thus, statins appear as a class of drugs useful in the prevention of coronary artery disease (CAD) and cerebrovascular accident, as well. The pleiotropic effects attributed to this class of drugs are variable and not common to all statins. Even so, given the potential of this drug, statins are currently the most prescribed drugs worldwide and generally are extremely well tolerated by most individuals. [5] The Heart Protection Study (HPS) indicated a 23% reduction in CAD events among 20,536 high-risk patients treated with 40 mg daily simvastatin for 5 years. [6]

Nevertheless, some adverse effects may be associated with the use of statins. The most serious of them can be seen in muscular level, presenting as mild myalgia that can advance to rhabdomyolysis with acute renal failure evolution and death. As a result, cerivastatin was withdrawn recently (2001) from the market following reports of rhabdomyolysis and death. It should be emphasized that the occurrence of harmful event is low, and the risk of rhabdomyolysis is 0.3 per 100,000 persons / year of exposure, and the mortality rate of 9%. This risk increases to almost 6.0 per 1000,000 people / year by combining statins with fibrates. [7,8]

Regarding muscular symptoms, myalgia is characterized by pain with or without muscle weakness, not accompanied by increased muscle creatine phosphokinase (CPK), unlike myositis, that leads to increase of this enzyme associated with muscle symptoms. Generally, rhabdomyolysis is characterized by muscular symptoms, with a significant increase in CPK levels (in general, greater than 10 times the highest normal level), and elevated levels of creatinine, with renal dysfunction, dark urine, and myoglobinuria. However, there is still the possibility of increased levels of CPK to potentially serious stages without any muscle symptoms or, otherwise, muscle manifestations in the absence of elevated CPK. Thus, monitoring CPK is recommended during treatment with statins. [9,10]

The actual incidence of statin-induced myopathy is uncertain because it depends on multiple factors, including the criteria used for the characterization of statin-induced myopathy, the dose and type of statin, the drug interaction, as well as levels of physical activity. [11]

Thus, there is not a definitive consensus on the literature, that brings results from clinical trials suggesting that the incidence of muscle symptoms in the placebo group and the group treated with statin is the same [12-14] opposing to others large studies that show muscle symptoms occurring in about 10 to 20% in the treated groups. [15-17]

A large study that followed 7,924 patients treated with high doses of statins, found that 10.5% developed muscle symptoms, in approximately one month after beginning the statin therapy, 38% developed muscle pain, and while 4% was effectively confined to bed or unable to work. Moreover, fluvastatin was the drug that was associated with lower rate of muscle symptoms. [16]

A major problem in interpreting and comparing the results of large observational community-based studies has been the fact that many of them are supported by patient's self-report about muscle symptoms, without evaluation by experienced neuromuscular specialists. [18]

MECHANISMS UNDERLYING STATIN-INDUCED MUSCLE TOXICITY

The mechanisms by which statins cause muscle damage still require elucidation. The cases described in the literature suggest that statins cause depletion of intermediate metabolites of cholesterol synthesis, induce apoptosis and may lead to alterations in chloride conductance channels in the myocyte. [19].

As mentioned above, inhibition of HMG-CoA reductase induced by statin leads to depletion of intermediates metabolites resulting from the synthesis of cholesterol, with reduction of mevalonic acid (farnesol and geranygeraniol). It has been suggested that statins cause intracellular deficiency of ubiquinone (CoQ10) specifically because an intermediate needed for the CoQ10 synthesis (coenzyme Q10) – the farnesyl pyrophosphate – is blocked. The reduction of CoQ10 results in decreased oxidative phosphorylation, required for myocyte normal cellular respiration process. The reason is that ubiquinone is an isoprenoid compound which acts in the oxidation of nutrients to produce ATP, whose main function is to serve as electron transport to mitochondria. [20]

In this context, England et al. [21] observed that simvastatin is able to change the synthesis of ubiquinone. A study conducted by these researchers demonstrated mitochondrial abnormalities through electron microscopy in patients who developed myopathy. It is speculated whether these changes can foment and/or evoke in skeletal muscle the clinical expression of a pre-existing mitochondrial disorder.

Although Nakahara et al. [22] had found reduced ubiquinone levels in muscle of rabbits treated with pravastatin or simvastatin, the activities of mitochondrial enzymes were not affected by either drug. Thus, the authors concluded that skeletal myopathy was not prompted by a mitochondrial respiration disorder due to a low level of ubiquinone.

Corroboration evidence was provided by Schaefer et al. [23] The authors had emphasized that the mitochondrial damage does not seem to be the primary cause of skeletal myopathy induced by cerivastatin, because mitochondrial changes were limited to degenerative or necrotic myofibers. The predominance of normal mitochondria both in muscles of treated mice and in untreated controls, and the lack of a decrease in mitochondrial function in all highly damaged muscle tissue, argues that the ultrastructural perceived changes in mitochondria are possibly secondary to muscle degeneration or necrosis. In this case, rather than its cause, would be its effect.

Apoptosis, or programmed cell death, is a fundamental mechanism to maintenance and remodeling of tissue structures. However, when inappropriately activated, apoptosis can lead to pathological conditions. The atorvastatin, lovastatin and simvastatin increase apoptosis of vascular smooth muscle cells, in a dose-dependent effect. The mechanisms by which statins cause apoptosis are still unclear. Larger studies are needed to demonstrate whether the increased apoptosis could cause myotoxicity during the statins treatments. [24]

Another possible explanation for statin-induced muscle toxicity is associated with intracellular chloride channels. These structures in the muscle are responsible for hyperpolarization of the cell and, as a result, the muscle relaxation. Changes in cell membrane permeability can also blockage this phenomenon. Besides, modifications in cell membrane properties have been described with the use of these drugs. Thereby, the more lipophilic statins can easily cross the cell membrane due to these changes and generate a great potential for muscle injury. [24]

It has been reported that women are at higher risk, with 1.5 to 1.7 chances of clinically relevant drug adverse reactions greater than men. [25,26] Most drugs are metabolized by the hepatic enzyme cytochrome system. Lipophilic statins such as lovastatin, simvastatin, fluvastatin, atorvastatin and pivastatin undergo first-pass metabolism in the liver via reactions catalyzed by cytochrome P450 3A4 (CYP3A4). The women, however, have higher levels of CYP3A4. This may mean that they are theoretically more able to clear statins out of their bodies. Therefore, at first sight, it seems contradictory that women have a greater susceptibility to the adverse effects of statins. However, dosage factors and issues of weight and body fat can compensate for any differences in the concentrations of CYP3A4. [25,27] This is because although males weighing more than women, in general, the dosages of medications in elderly adults are rarely standardized through the weight. In some cases, this may expose elderly women at a dose which is higher than its organisms can efficiently metabolize and eliminate. Women also tend to have a higher percentage of body fat, which affects the volume of distribution of some drugs and can significantly increase the half-life of a variety of drugs, including more lipophilic statins. [25, 28]

Furthermore, physiological levels of CoQ10 significantly greater (1.11 x 0.86 mmol / L) were reported in men compared to women. Whether this factor predisposes myopathy in women related to men has not been well documented in the literature. Moreover, other processes lead to the depletion of CoQ10, such as diabetes and hypothyroidism, and can be consider risk factors for myopathy. [29] It is also possible that a behavioral aspect of pain perception may affect the likelihood of an individual complain of discomfort or associated with statin-related muscle pain disorder. [30] There is a tendency for women to be more sensitive to pain as well as to describe it as being more serious and recurring when compared with men. [31]

Association between Exercises and Statins

The favorable effects of exercise on the lipoprotein profile are well evidenced in dyslipidemic patients (usually pure hypertriglyceridemic or with associated hypercholesterolemia and low HDLc levels) with adequate dietary pattern. Thus, the treatment of dyslipidemia frequently associates the use of statins with a regular physical activity program.

Although physical training induces beneficial cardiovascular adaptations, it is known that muscle damage can be generally produced from the exercises performed with eccentric actions above the usual level of effort. [32] In this case, it can be evidenced by ultrastructural damage, rupture of the sarcolemma [33,34] and increased serum activity of muscle enzymes such as CPK and lactate dehydrogenase [35], as well as an increased number of macrophages, monocytes and neutrophils has also been observed in response to higher exercise intensity. [36]

The prolonged and strenuous exercise also induces increased CPK levels, which is highly dependent on the duration and intensity of exercise and also on the individual fitness level. Among these variables, the duration of exercise is the most important. Incidentally, the highest CPK levels measured post-exercise are found in runners and triatholon athletes, reaching levels as high as 50 times its reference value. Differently, short-term racing leads to a much smaller increases in CPK levels. Another important aspect is related to the type of exercise: while swimming or cycling tends to a minimal or no elevation of CPK levels, races in mountain and weight lifting tend to produce the highest elevations of these enzymes. Most of CPK released after exercise belongs to the MM fraction (that means a fraction founded in skeletal muscles and the heart – CK-MM), and among the causes of increased CPK after exercise are tissue hypoxia, muscle glycogen depletion, lipid peroxidation, accumulation of free radicals and direct mechanical damage to the contractile elements, especially the Z-disk of the sarcomere. [37]

Given the fact that muscle disorders induced by statins may lead to increased plasma levels of CPK, this parameter is used as a predictor for drug interruption when it reaches more than ten times its reference value [38]. Thus, it is important to consider the association between use of statins, regular practice of exercise and muscle symptoms to evaluate the causes of myopathy or to estimate the potentiality of this association to induce muscle injury.

Phillips et al. [39] were the first researchers to examine the association of statins and muscle strength in 4 subjects (2 men and 2 women elderly) with symptoms of myopathy and despite normal levels of CPK, they found 10-40% reductions in the strength of hip abduction.

Sinzinger and O'Grady [40] reported that 78% of professional athletes with a family history of hypercholesterolemia did not tolerate statin therapy due to muscle pain and cramps. However, most of them did not show increased levels of CPK.

Experimental study performed by Seachrist et al., [41] that administered cerivastatin at a dose of 1.0 mg / kg to Sprague-Dawley rats, found significantly higher levels of CPK in the control group, which was not associated with exercise. However, it was found greater severity of musculoskeletal degeneration in the exercised group, suggesting that the CPK level should not be the only parameter to evaluate muscle degeneration, highlighting that the muscular evaluation should also be important. In this case, exercise can trigger muscle damage induced by cerivastatin, allowing it to occur earlier and with greater magnitude than that is seen in the sedentary group.

In this context, Accioly et al. [42] conducted an experimental study in order to examine the effects of exercise on muscle function with or without the use of statins. Male dyslipidemic Wistar rats (*Rattus norvegicus*) were subjected to low-intensity exercise performed on a treadmill in 60 minutes daily sessions for eight weeks. Simvastatin and fluvastatin were the used statins, with the dosages determined by the allometric scaling method, which is based on metabolic rate of the animal. [43] After the training period, histological analysis of the soleus muscle was performed. Typical histological features of muscle injury were identified in 30% of animals subjected to the protocol of exercise, even without administration of statins. Moreover, the inactive rats treated with simvastatin or fluvastatin showed 80% and 30% of muscle damage, respectively. Exercised animals treated with simvastatin showed 90% of muscle damage and those treated with fluvastatin presented 70%. The authors also noted that the use of statins alone was able to generate muscle damage, but in a lower proportion compared to animals subjected to physical activity without statin treatment. However, the association between statins and exercise potentiated muscle damage. As fluvastatin caused minor injury, it can be inferred that possibly its hydroxy acid constituent may confer tissue selectivity, mainly hepatic, conferring to it a possibility to cause less severe muscle damage. [44] Other studies also supporting the fact that differences between lactone and acid forms can have an impact on the muscle injury potential. [4] It was demonstrated that, at least *in vitro*, a significantly higher potency of the lactone forms, than the respective acid forms, to induce myotoxicity is noted in human skeletal muscle cells. These results clearly indicate the need to differentiate between acid and lactone forms in investigation of statin myotoxicity. [4]

Bonfim et al. [45] also investigated the association of simvastatin and exercise in dyslipidemic animals. Gastrocnemius muscle was evaluated through histological and immunohistochemical analysis, showing that simvastatin was harmful to the gastrocnemius muscle in sedentary mice and the association of this medicine with exercise on a treadmill led to a greater severe muscle injury.

Other available relevant evidence is that type II fibers are known to be more injured in statin treatment. This is because these fibers are glycolytic, depending on glucose as substrate. For this reason, the depletion of carbohydrate during exercise may become particularly sensitive to injuries in type II fibers, what also explains the increased tendency of injury on the use of statins.

In an observational study conducted in France, investigating muscle symptoms in an unselected sample of 7,924 patients with dyslipidemia, in treatment with usual high doses of statin therapy, founded that muscle symptoms were reported by 832 patients (10.5%), about one month after initiation of statin therapy. In addition, 315 patients (38%) reported that muscle pain prevented daily activities while 31 (4%) were confined to bed or unable to work. The fluvastatin has also been associated with lower rates of muscle symptoms (5.1%) between the statin group. [46]

In order to check whether statin-induced muscle damage associated with exercise are dose-dependent, the CPK levels were analyzed in 79 men with LDLc> 100 mg / dL. They were instructed to discontinue statin treatment for 6 weeks and were randomly distributed into two groups: atorvastatin 10 mg (n = 42) or 80 mg (n = 37), during 5 weeks. The exercise was established as a walking on a treadmill for 45 minutes at an intensity of 65% of maximum heart rate. CPK in plasma were measured daily and also the reported muscle pain was checked daily as well as the same measurements were assessed 4 days after of the completion of exercise protocol. An increase in CPK levels and muscle pain related to the pre-exercise levels was found after the stablished exercise protocol without differences between the groups that received high or low doses of statins, suggesting that exercise increases levels of CPK, even with low dose of statin. It is possible, however, that the adopted exercise was not sensitive enough to detect dose-dependent differences in the effects of statin therapy and muscle damage. [47]

Further investigations about the muscle damage induced by statins also consider possible influences of these drugs on the physiological capacity of muscle repair. Pointing that the deleterious effects of statins are intimately linked to physical activity intensity, the resulting injury could be dependent on failures in muscle repair, mediated by cells responsible for this function – satellite cells. These cells, located between basal lamina of myofibers and the sarcolemma, participate in postnatal muscle growth as well as in the regeneration process of the injured muscle. Normally quiescent in adult skeletal muscle, satellite cells become activated when muscle is injured [48] as well as on mechanical muscle overload, starting to proliferate and, finally, to fuse either to injured muscle fibers or between those to form new muscle fibers [49]. *In vitro* studies demonstrated that the ability of proliferation and fusion of skeletal myotubes in culture is decreased with treatment with statins [50] and it has been suggested delaying the effect of simvastatin on myocytes derived from satellite cells differentiation. [48] Also it was showed that the resting intracellular calcium concentration was reduced in statin treated satellite cells and myotubes. [50]

Furthermore, it is known that HMG-CoA and its main end-products (eg prenyls, dolichol) are crucial for the myogenesis to occur. [48] However, the role-played by this enzyme in the differentiation and maturation of adult satellite cell derived myocytes responsible for muscle regeneration remains to be elucidated. [48]

One of the studies with this investigative purpose noted that the delayed myogenic process occurred *in vitro* and *in vivo* in the presence of simvastatin were prevented with mevalonate addition, demonstrating that the impaired processes was resulting from the inhibition of HMG-CoA activity rather than to an effect exerted by the drug per se, a finding that can highlight the pivotal role played by HMG-CoA in muscle regeneration. [48]

Moreover, polynuclear myotubes formed from the differentiation of satellite cells of healthy human donors that received simvastatin on day 5 of differentiation, showed, after 48 hours, a dose-dependent decrease in both glucose uptake and oxidation in mature myotubes. [51] In this context, the dysregulation of glucose metabolism by simvastatin shows another damaging effect of statins on skeletal muscle, that can contribute to the understanding of the myotoxicity followed statin treatment. [51]

Mechanisms of Muscle Toxicity That Associate Statins and Exercise

The mechanisms by which physical exercise combined with statin treatment contributes to muscle injury are still obscure [41] although several hypotheses explaining the statin-induced myotoxicity have been put forward. [51] Some theories are suggested in the literature:

- Plasma protein concentration enlarges during exercise due the loss of water from the plasma to the tissues, which is explained by an increase in osmolarity from the active tissues, increase in hydrostatic pressure, and loss of body fluids as sweat. Thus, the plasma protein concentration increases what may influence the drug concentration in plasma and tissues. Also, it is theorized that changes in the drug distribution may occur due to the blood redistribution for active muscles, causing some inability to achieve the intended drug effects on their sites of action. [52]
- Many drugs, including statins, are excreted in bile and urine. Renal excretion is the effect of glomerular filtration, tubular secretion and tubular reabsorption. Thus, the glomerular filtration rate depends on the amount of blood in the kidneys. [53] During exercise, a decrease in renal blood flow occurs, and this can represent a 30% rate decrease from the glomerular filtration. These pharmacokinetic changes during exercise are dose-dependent. It is also possible that, by reason of physical exercise, an increase in blood flow to the muscles is evoked, resulting in a greater concentration of drug in muscle tissue, with subsequent toxicity. [54]
- Muscle contraction lead to depletion of glycogen and also in a reduced availability of adenosine triphosphate (ATP), which together generate an increase membrane permeability and muscle fiber damage, with a consequent efflux of muscle enzymes,

that may be exacerbated by the use of statins. The membrane of skeletal muscle is predominantly composed by phospholipids, which certainly decrease with statin treatment and this may be the reason for the exacerbation of damage associated with exercise. [55].

- Another theory considers the intramuscular CoQ10 depletion, which leads to mitochondrial dysfunction with a subsequent abnormal energy metabolism and muscular symptoms. The hypothesis is that the reduction of CoQ10 is directly associated with the reduction of low-density lipoproteins, that are responsible for the coenzyme transport. [56]
- Mitochondrial dysfunction as a consequence from the increased reactive oxygen species (ROS) generated in higher levels in subjects receiving statins and performing physical activity. [57]
- Statins can reduce the expression of genes related to oxidative phosphorylation (an event required for ATP and phosphocreatine to release energy), such as genes related to ribosomal and mitochondrial proteins. [58].
- Statins increase apoptosis. The calpain activation pathway (which is a protease that stimulates apoptosis) is upregulated under treatment with simvastatin. Moreover, it was also showed that treatment with simvastatin suppresses anti-apoptotic genes and activates apoptotic genes. [59]
- The last hypothesis considers calcium, which could leave the mitochondria and disrupt the calcium cycle in the sarcoplasmic reticulum. Calpain is extremely dependent on calcium for its activation. As calpain is a protease which stimulates apoptosis, the mechanisms can be correlated, having calcium as the major problem. [60]

Conclusion

In light of the foregoing in this chapter, it can be noted that there is not a consensus in the literature about the muscle damage effects that are attributed to statins treatment, that are also exacerbated by exercise practice. Moreover, a possibility that may not be excluded, considers that multifactorial mechanisms can be involved with the muscular adverse effects. When considering exercise as one of the most effective and cheapest intervention in reducing morbidity and mortality from cardiovascular disease [61,62], the prohibition or contraindication of its practice among dyslipidemic individuals represents a counterintuitive situation in a realm of our expertise.

Thus, the literature demands studies that clearly elucidate the mechanisms that associate myopathy with statins, in attempt to promote drug manipulations aiming to reduce their adverse effect. On the other hand, from this knowledge, even more appropriate exercises can be prescribed to these individuals, since workload, level of energy depletion, and injury recovery time might be more properly adjusted from studies with this purpose.

REFERENCES

[1] Endo, A. A historical perspective on the discovery of statins, Proceedings of the Japan Academy - Series B:. *Physical and Biological Sciences*. 2010; 86(5): 484-493.
[2] Vaughan CJ, Gotto AM. Update on statins 2003. *Circulation*. 2004;110:886-92.
[3] Forti N, Diament J. *Fármacos hipolipemiantes*. Rev Soc Cardiol Estado de São Paulo 2005;15:25-30.
[4] Skottheim IB, Gedde-Dahl A, Hejazifar S, Hoel K, Asberg A. Statin induced myotoxicity: The lactone forms are more potent than the acid forms in human skeletal muscle cells in vitro. *Eur J Pharm Sci*. 2008;33(4-5):317-25.
[5] Albuquerque DC, Ferreira AG, Rocha RM, Albuquerque FN, Esporcatte R. Estatinas nas Síndromes Coronarianas Agudas: há evidências suficientes para a sua utilização? *Revista da SOCERJ*. 2004; 2:88-96.
[6] MRC/BHF Heart Protection Study of cholesterol lowering with simvastatin in 20 536 high-risk individuals: a randomised placebocontrolled trial. *The Lancet*. 2002; 360:7-22.
[7] Graham DJ, Staffa JA, Shatin D, Andrade SE, Schech SD, La Grenade L, et al. Incidence of hospitalized rhabdomyolysis in patients treated with lipid lowering drugs. *JAMA*. 2004; 292:2585-2590.
[8] Law M, Rudnicka AR. Statin Safety: a systematic review. *Am J Cardiol*. 2006; 97:52C-60C.
[9] Staffa JA, Chang J, Green L. Cerivastatin and reports of fatal rhabdomyolysis. *N Engl J Med*. 2002; 346(7):539–40.
[10] Sathasivam S. Statin induced myotoxicity. *Eur J Intern Med*. 2012; 23: 317–324.
[11] Armitage J. The safety of statins in clinical practice. *Lancet*. 2007; 370:1781–90.
[12] Newman CB, Palmer G, Silbershatz H, Szarek M. Safety of atorvastatin derived from analysis of 44 completed trials in 9416 patients. *Am J Cardiol*. 2003;92:670–6.
[13] Newman C, Tsai J, Szarek M, Luo D, Gibson E. Comparative safety of atorvastatin 80 mg versus 10 mg derived from analysis of 49 completed trials in 14,236 patients. *Am J Cardiol*. 2006;97:61–7.
[14] Ridker PM, Danielson E, Fonseca FAH, et al. Rosuvastatin to prevent vascular events in men and women with elevated C-reactive protein. *N Engl J Med*. 2008;359:2195–207.
[15] Nichols GA, Koro CE. Does statin therapy initiation increase the risk for myopathy? An observational study of 32,225 diabetic and nondiabetic patients. *Clin Ther*. 2007; 29:1761–70.
[16] Bruckert E, Hayem G, Dejager S, Yau C, Begaud B. Mild to moderate muscular symptoms with high-dosage statin therapy in hyperlipidemic patients–the PRIMO study. *Cardiovasc Drugs Ther*. 2005; 19:403–14.
[17] Cohen JD, Brinton EA, Ito MK, Jacobson TA. Understanding statin use in America and gaps in patient education (USAGE): an internet-based survey of 10,138 current and former statin users. *J Clin Lipidol*. 2012; 6:208–15.
[18] Needham M, Mastaglia FL. Statin myotoxicity: A review of genetic susceptibility factors. *Neuromuscular Disorders*. 2014; 24: 4–15.

[19] Christopher-Stine L. Statin myopathy: an update. *Curr Opin Rheumatol*. 2006; 18:647-653.
[20] Plosker GL, Wagstaff AJ. Fluvastatin: a review of its pharmacology and use in the management of hypercholesterolaemia. *Drugs*. 1996; 51:433-59.
[21] England JDF, Viles A, Walsh JC, Stewart PM. Muscle side effects associated with simvastatin therapy. *M Journal Aust*. 1990; 153:562-63.
[22] Nakahara K, Kuriyama M, Sonoda Y, Yoshidome H, Nakagawa H, Fujiyama J, Higuchi I et al. Myopathy induced by HMGCoA reductase inhibitors in rabbits: a pathological, electrophysiological, and biochemical study. *Toxicol. Appl. Pharmacol.* 1998; 152: 99–106.
[23] Schaefer WH, Lawrence JW, Loughlin AF, Stoffregen DA, Mixson LA, Dean DC, et al. Evaluation of ubiquinone concentration and mitochondrial function relative to cerivastatin-induced skeletal myopathy in rats. *Toxicology and Applied Pharmacology*. 2004; 194:10– 23.
[24] Knapp AC, Huang J, Starling G. Inhibition of HMGCoA reductase sensitize human smooth muscle cells to FAZ-ligand and cytokineinduced cell death. *Atherosclerosis*. 2000; 152:217-27.
[25] Anderson GD. Gender differences in pharmacological response. *Int Rev Neurobiol*. 2008; 83:1–10.
[26] Hofer-Dueckelmann C, Prinz E, Beindl W, Szymanski J, Fellhofer G, Pichler M et al. Adverse drug reactions (ADRs) associated with hospital admissions – elderly female patients are at highest risk. *Int J Clin Pharmacol Ther*. 2011; 49:577–586.
[27] Wolbold R, Klein K, Burk O, Nüssler AK, Neuhaus P, Eichelbaum M, et al. Sex is a major determinant of CYP3A4 expression in human liver. *Hepatology*. 2003. 38:978–988.
[28] Mangoni AA, Jackson SH. Age-related changes in pharmacokinetics and pharmacodynamics: basic principles and practical applications. *Br J Clin Pharmacol*. 2004; 57:6–14.
[29] Kaikkonen J, Nyyssönen K, Tuomainen TP, Ristonmaa U, Salonen JT. Determinants of plasma coenzyme Q10 in humans. *FEBS Lett*. 1999; 443:163–166.
[30] Racine M, Tousignant-Laflamme Y, Kloda LA, Dion D, Dupuis G, Choinière M. A systematic literature review of 10 years of research on sex/gender and pain perception – part 2: do biopsychosocial factors alter pain sensitivity differently in women and men? *Pain*. 2012;153:619–635.
[31] Goffaux P, Michaud K, Gaudreau J, Chalaye P, Rainville P, Marchand S. Sex differences in perceived pain are affected by an anxious brain. *Pain*. 2011; 152:2065–2073.
[32] Apple FSE, Rhodes M. Enzymatic estimation of skeletal muscle damage by analysis of changes in serum creatine kinase. *Journal of Applied Physiology*. 1988; 65:2598-600.
[33] Armstrong RB, Ogilvie RW, Schwane JA. Exccentric exercise-induced injury to rat skeletal muscle. *Journal of Applied Physiology*.1983; 54:80-93.
[34] Clarkson PM, Tremblay I. Exercise-induced muscle damage, repair, and adaptation in humans. *Journal of Applied Physiology*. 1988; 65:1-6.
[35] Lac G, Maso F. Biological markers for the follow-up of athletes troughout the training season. *Pathologie Biologie*. 2004; 52:43-49.

[36] Matsuura N, Kawamata S, Ozawa J, Kai S, Sakakima H, Abiko S. Injury and repair of the soleus muscle after electrical stimulation of the sciatic nerve in the rat. *Arch of Histology and Cytol.* 2001; 4:393-400.

[37] Katirji B, Al-jaberi MM. Creatine Kinase Revisited. Journal of Clinical Neuromuscular *Disease.* 2001; 2:158-163.

[38] Owczarek J, Jasinska M, Orszulak-Michalak. Drug-induced myophathies. An overview of the possible mechanisms. *Pharmacological reports.* 2005; 57:23-34.

[39] Phillips PS, Haas RH, Bannykh S, Hathaway S, Gray NL, Kimura BJ, Vladutiu GD, England JD. Statin-associated myopathy with normal creatine kinase levels. *Ann Intern Med.* 2002; 137(7): 581–5.

[40] Sinzinger II, O'Grady J. Professional atletes suffering from familial hypercholesterolemia rarely tolerate statin treatment because of muscular problems. *Bras J Clin Pharmacol.* 2004; 57:525-28.

[41] Seachrist JL, Loi CM, Evans MG, Criswell KA, Rothwell CE. Roles of exercise and pharmacokinetics in cerivastatin-induced skeletal muscle toxicity. *Toxicological Sciences.* 2005; 88:551-561.

[42] Accioly MF, Camargo Filho JCS, Padulla SAT, Lima ALZ, Bonfim MR, Pinhel MAS et al. Effect of physical exercise and statins on the muscle function in animals with dyslipidemia. *Rev Bras Med Esporte.* 2012; 18: 198-202.

[43] Pachaly JR, Brito HFV. Interspecifc Allometric Scaling. In: Fowler ME, Cubas PR. *Biology, Medicine and Surgery of South American Wild Animals,* Ames. Iowa University Press; 2001. p.475-481.

[44] Plosker GL, Wagstaff AJ. Fluvastatin: a review of its pharmacology and use in the management of hypercholesterolaemia. *Drugs.* 1996;51:433-59.

[45] Bonfim MR, Camargo Filho JCS, Vanderlei LCM, Padulla SAT, Accioly MF, Souza DRS et al. Muscle response to the association of statin and physical exercise in rats. *Int. J. Morphol.* 2009; 27:1155-1161.

[46] Bruckert E, Hayem G, Dejager S, Yau C, Begaud B. Mild to moderate muscular symptoms with high-dosage statin therapy in hyperlipidemic patients--the PRIMO study. *Cardiovasc Drugs Ther.* 2005; 19:403–14.

[47] Parker BA, Thompson PD. Effect of Statins on Skeletal Muscle: Exercise, Myopathy, and Muscle Outcomes. *Exerc Sport Sci Rev.* 2012; 40(4): 188–194.

[48] Trapani L, Segatto M, La Rosa P, Fanelli F, Moreno S, Marino M et al. 3-Hydroxy 3-Methylglutaryl Coenzyme A Reductase inhibition impairs muscle regeneration. *Journal of Cellular Biochemistry.* 2012;113:2057–2063.

[49] Sartorelli V, Fulco M.Molecular and cellular determinants of skeletal muscle atrophy and hypertrophy. *Sci STKE.* 2004; 2004(244):re11.

[50] Füzi M, Palicz Z, Vincze J, Cseri J, Szombathy Z, Kovács I, et al. Fluvastatin-induced alterations of skeletal muscle function in hypercholesterolaemic rats. *J Muscle Res Cell Motil.* 2012; 32:391–401.

[51] Smith R, Solberg R, Jacobsen LL, Voreland AL, Rustan AC, Thoresen GH, et al. Simvastatin inhibits glucose metabolism and legumain activity in human myotubes. *PLOS ONE,* 2014;9:1-9.

[52] Van Baak MA. Influence of exercise on the pharmacokinetics of drugs. *Clin P Pharmacokinet.* 1990; 19:32-43.

[53] DiPiro JT, Spruill WJ, Blouin RA, Prue DiPiromer JM. Concepts in clinica DiPirol pharmacokinetics. 3ª ed. Bethesa (MD): American Societu of Health Systems *Pharmacistis;* 2002

[54] Lenz TL, Lenz NJ, Faulkner MA. Potential interactions between exercise and drug therapy. *Sports Med.* 2004; 34:293-306.

[55] Urso ML, Clarkson PM, Hittel D, Hoffman EP, Thompson PD. Changes in ubiquitin proteasome pathway gene expression in skeletal muscle with exercise and statins. *Arterioscler Thromb Vasc Biol.* 2005; 25(12):2560–6.

[56] Marcoff L, Thompson PD. The role of coenzyme Q10 in statin-associated myopathy: a systematic review. *J Am Coll Cardiol.* 2007; 49(23):2231–7.

[57] Wu JS, Buettner C, Smithline H, Ngo LH, Greenman RL. Evaluation of skeletal muscle during calfexercise by 31-phosphorus magnetic resonance spectroscopy in patients on statin medications.*Muscle Nerve.* 2011; 43(1):76–81.

[58] Hubal MJ, Reich KA, De Biase A, Bilbie C, Clarkson PM, Hoffman EP et al. Transcriptional deficits in oxidative phosphorylation with statin myopathy. *Muscle Nerve.* 2011; 44(3):393–401.

[59] Yu JG, Sewright K, Hubal MJ, Liu JX, Schwartz LM, Hoffman EP et al. Investigation of gene expression in C(2)C(12) myotubes following simvastatin application and mechanical strain. *J Atheroscler Thromb.* 2009; 16(1):21–9.

[60] Liantonio A, Giannuzzi V, Cippone V, Camerino GM, Pierno S, Camerino DC. Fluvastatin and atorvastatin affect calcium homeostasis of rat skeletal muscle fibers in vivo and in vitro by impairing the sarcoplasmic reticulum/mitochondria Ca2+-release system. *J Pharmacol Exp Ther.* 2007; 321(2):626–34.

[61] Mann N, Rosenzweig A. Can exercise teach us how to treat heart disease? *Circulation.* 2012;126(22):2625–35.

[62] Booth FW, Gordon SE, Carlson CJ, Hamilton MT, Davis JC, Verhagen E, et al. Waging war on modern chronic diseases. *J Appl Physiol.* 2000; 88(2):774-87.

In: Statins
Editor: Eric R. Travers
ISBN: 978-1-63463-057-3

Chapter 10

STATINS: DIABETOGENICITY IS WEAK, BUT AN ANTIATHELOGENIC EFFECT IS MORE REAL

Shouji Shimoyama*
Gastrointestinal Unit, Settlement Clinic, Towa,
Adachi-ku, Tokyo, Japan

ABSTRACT

Hyperlipidemia is one of the major risk factors of cardiovascular disease (CVD). Hydroxymethylglutaryl coenzyme-A (HMG-CoA) reductase inhibitors, or statins, have now become the most commonly prescribed drugs to intended lower serum low-density lipoprotein cholesterol levels, which eventually prevent primary or secondary CVD events. However, it has also been argued that statin therapy may associate with new onset diabetes mellitus (DM) in clinical trials and metaanalyses. This association is universally observed across different statins –the homologous class effect– in some studies, while there could be varying levels of risk or gradient risk increases depending on the individual statins or their doses in some studies. Although the strength of association is weak and heterogeneous, the consistency cannot be denied. Therefore, it is critical that clinicians be aware of this presumed risk of developing DM because DM *per se* is a risk factor for CVD. This minireview presents current knowledge on the association between statins and developing DM and discusses the benefit-risk balance, i.e., the balance between numbers needed to treat and the numbers needed to harm, as well as potential confounding factors that could play a role in the statin-DM association. This comprehensive evaluation draws the conclusion that the benefits of statin therapy outweigh the new onset DM and reinforces the importance of continued statin therapy, – though the statin-DM association continues to be considered a risk among a certain segment of patients with specific characteristics. This motivates more further, more in-depth research to realize treatment optimization through identifying the most beneficial patient population while minimizing the risk of new onset DM.

Keywords*:* Statins, Diabetes Mellitus, Adverse events, Cardiovascular disease

* Tel.: +81-3-3605-7747, Fax: +81-3-3605-0244, E-mail: shimoyama@apost.plala.or.jp.

INTRODUCTION

Hyperlipidemia is one of the major risk factors of cardiovascular disease (CVD). Hydroxymethylglutaryl coenzyme-A (HMG-CoA) reductase inhibitors, or statins, act to decrease low-density lipoprotein cholesterol (LDL-C) and have been documented as beneficial drugs in the primary or secondary prevention of CVD events. Each 1.0mmol/L (39mg/dl) decrease in LDL-C proportionally reduces the rate of all causes of mortality by 9-13%, or major vascular events by 21% in patients both with and without diabetes mellitus (DM) [1]. Also, a 1.0mmol/L reduction of LDL-C reduced strokes by 20%, especially in patients with known vascular diseases [2]. These protective effects against cardiovascular events occur within the 1st year of statin use. Therefore, statins are now the most commonly prescribed drugs for lowering serum lipid levels to obtain cardiovascular health and survival benefits. However, with the increasing prescription of this drug, several adverse events have been expressed, and new onset DM has emerged as an unforeseen negative outcome.

The literature contains conflicting results regarding new onset DM with statins. Randomized controlled trials (RCTs) of rosuvastatin versus placebos demonstrated a significant association between rosuvastatin use and a higher incidence of newly physician-reported DM [3]. Similarly, a very recent retrospective cohort study has elucidated a significantly increased risk of DM development by rosuvastatin, atorvastatin, and simvastatin use, irrespective of the purpose for primary and secondary prevention [4]. In contrast, a West of Scotland Coronary Prevention (WOSCOPS) study demonstrated a 30% risk reduction of new onset DM [5] by pravastatin use.

In addition, some investigators [4, 6] observed that the risks of new onset DM were influenced by the doses or potency of statins, though others [7] did not. Given these inconsistencies, several metaanalyses have been conducted to explore possible associations between statin and new onset DM. They have yielded conflicting but possible evidence of a statin-DM association [8-14]. Against these backgrounds, the U.S. Food and Drug Administration has recognized the risk of developing DM and updated the labeling of all statins to warn the possibility of new onset DM.

On the other hand, type 2 DM per se confers a two-fold excess risk for CVD [15], and intensive glycemic control could significantly reduce coronary events [16]. In addition, besides CVD events, DM associates with a substantial risk of various types of diseases. For example, fifty-year-old patients with DM are associated with 6-year poorer expected survival rates than those without DM [17].

In this regard, there might be a dilemma that treating elevated LDL-C by statins for the purpose of CVD prevention would in turn increase new onset DM that might cancel the cardioprotective benefit of statins.

There exist multiple streams of inconsistent data pertaining to a statin-DM association. This minireview introduces current knowledge on the statin-DM association with its plausible mechanisms and risk-benefit balance, as well as potentially unresolved questions remaining to be elucidated on this matter.

Taking the available evidence into account, at present, the importance of continued statin therapy is reinforced. Given that current studies suffer, to different degrees, from methodological shortcomings, proposals for research directions are also addressed as future perspectives.

OVERVIEW OF METAANALYSES

The literature contains several metaanalyses examining the statin-DM association [8-14] (Table). The association between statin and new onset DM was neutral in the earlier metaanalyses while it appears consistently positive in the more recent ones. However, the incidence of new onset DM varied substantially among the RCTs included in these metaanalyses. In one metaanalysis [10], only two studies (JUPITER and PROSPER) showed a significantly positive DM risk while most studies exhibited nonsignificant trends towards decreased or increased DM risk. These seemingly inconsistent findings in individual RCTs suggest that the strength of the statin-DM association appears weak at best.

One metaanalysis compared a risk of new onset DM between intensive doses of statin and moderate doses [18]. Intensive doses of statin therapy resulted in a 12% increased risk of DM as compared with moderate doses of statin.

These currently available results suggest that the use of statins may cause a DM, although weak, and that they do so in a dose-dependent manner.

PLAUSIBLE MECHANISMS OF STATIN-DM ASSOCIATION

The mechanisms underlying the increased incidence of DM remain elusive. Several plausible mechanisms to explain the statin-DM association have been very recently reviewed [19]. Statins may impair pancreatic beta-cell function through lowering cholesterol levels, decrease glucose transporter-4 expression, alter insulin signaling substrates, and decrease adipocyte maturation. These metabolic effects on several factors that affect glucose tolerance are partly mediated by decreased products of the cholesterol biosynthesis pathway downstream to mevalonate [20].

Individual statins have different effects on glucose regulation [21] through different molecular mechanisms [22]. In the clinical field, one metaanalysis –including RCTs– investigating the influence of statins on insulin sensitivity demonstrated that insulin sensitivity was increased by pravastatin, decreased by simvastatin, and showed no change by atorvastatin and rosuvastatin. These results on the basis of molecular and clinical research suggest that statins do not appear to demonstrate a class effect on insulin sensitivity [23].

RISK BENEFIT BALANCE

These above results of metaanalyses raised clinically important dilemma, where statin use for the purpose of cardiovascular protection in turn enhances cardiovascular harm through DM development. To provide one answer to this dilemma, it is important to estimate the risk-benefit balance, i.e., the balance between cardioprotective benefit and risks of new onset DM. Calculation of numbers needed to treat (NNT) and numbers needed to harm (NNH) reassures one that statins' benefit exceeds their DM risk [10, 11, 24]. NNT (59-125) [11, 24] is generally smaller than NNH (256) [10], and NNH/NNT is roughly around 2~4, suggesting that developing DM in one patient correspond to 2~4 patients enjoying the benefits of cardiovascular health.

Table. Metaanalyses investigating statin-DM association

Author	Number of participants	Follow-up length (year)	Control arm	Statins	Number of included trials	Number of trials		Relative risk (RR) or odds ratio (OR) of new onset DM (95% confidence interval)	Methods of DM diagnosis	Remarks
						Primary prevention	Secondary prevention			
Coleman [8]	39791	2.7-6.0	PBO	Overall	7	3	4	RR: 1.03 (0.89-1.19)	WHO criteria, 2mmol/L increase in fasting blood glucose, prescribing DM medication, physician or patient-report DM.	
				Ato	1	1	0	RR: 1.14 (0.91-1.42)		
				Pra	3	2	1	RR: 0.84 (0.86-1.49)		
				Ros	1	0	1	RR: 1.13 (0.86-1.49)		
				Sim	2	0	2	RR: 1.14 (0.98-1.33)		
				Excluding Pra	4	1	3	RR: 1.14 (1.02-1.28)		
Rajpathak [9]	57593	3.9 (mean)	PBO	Overall	6	3	3	RR: 1.06 (0.93-1.22)	Elevated fasting glucose, initiation of pharmacotherapy, physician-report DM.	Increasing age or female gender is a significant risk for DM.
				Excluding Pra	5	2	3	RR:1.13 (1.03-1.23)		
Sattar [10]	91140	4 (mean)	PBO or Standard care	Overall	13	5	8	OR: 1.09 (1.02-1.17)	WHO criteria, elevated fasting blood glucose, prescribing DM medication, physician-report DM.	Increasing age was a significant risk for DM. No difference found between lipophilic and hydrophilic statins.
				Ato	1	1	0	OR: 1.14 (0.89-1.46)		
				Lov	1	1	0	OR: 0.98 (0.7-1.38)		
				Pra	6	2	4	OR: 1.03 (0.90-1.19)		
				Ros	3	1	2	OR: 1.18 (1.04-1.33)		
				Sim	2	0	2	OR: 1.11 (0.97-1.26)		

Author	Number of participants	Follow-up length (year)	Control arm	Statins	Number of included trials	Number of trials		Relative risk (RR) or odds ratio (OR) of new onset DM (95% confidence interval)	Methods of DM diagnosis	Remarks
						Primary prevention	Secondary prevention			
Mills [11]	111003	0.5-6.1	PBO or usual care	Overall (Ato, Lov, Pra, Ros, Sim)	17	8	8	RR:1.09 (1.02-1.16)	NA	
Naci [12]	113698	NA	PBO	Overall (Ato, Lov, Pra, Ros, Sim)	NA	NA	NA	OR:1.09 (1.02-1.16)	NA	
				Ros	NA	NA	NA	OR: 1.16 (1.02-1.31)		
Tayler [13]	24407	NA	PBO	Overall (Lov, Ros)	2	2	0	RR:1.18 (1.01-1.39)	NA	
Navarese [14]	64137	1.9-6.0	PBO or no treatment	Overall	13	4	9	NA	Starting medication, elevated plasma glucose level.	
		4.9 (mean)	PBO	Ato(80mg)	1	0	1	OR: 1.15 (0.90-1.50)		
		3.2-6.0 (mean)	PBO or no treatment	Pra(40mg)	4	1	3	OR: 1.07 (0.86-1.30)		
		1.9-2.7 (median)	PBO	Ros(20mg)	2	1	1	OR: 1.25 (0.82-1.90)		
		5.0 (mean), 5.4 (median)	PBO	Sim(40mg)	2	0	2	OR: 1.21 (0.94-1.56)		
		3.3 (median)	PBO	Ato(10mg)	1	1	0	OR: 1.04 (0.75-1.46)		
		2.0 (median), 5.3 (mean)	no treatment	Pra(20mg)	2	1	1	OR: 0.90 (0.71-1.36)		
		3.9 (median)	PBO	Ros(10mg)	1	0	1	OR: 1.11 (0.81-1.52)		

PBO; Placebo, Ato; Atorvastatin, Lov; Lovastatin, Pra; Pravastatin, Ros; Rosuvastatin, Sim; Simvastatin, RR; Relative risk, NS; Not significant, NA; Not available
RR; relative risk, OR; odds ratio

Advantages of statins over their disadvantages have been also expressed in an alternative way. Cannon et al. estimated the benefit of preventing cardiovascular events being 9-fold higher than the risk of DM development [25]. Similarly, intensive statin therapy for 1 year resulted in one fewer CVD event in every 155 patients at the expense of one additional new onset DM in every 498 patients [18]. In this study, as compared with moderate dose statin, intensive dose statin documented a 16% absolute reduction in cardiovascular events with only a 12% absolute increase in DM risk. These estimates suggest that net cardiovascular benefits could remain and outweigh any diabetogenic harm of statin.

It must be noted that such a risk-benefit balance alters according to the potential confounders as described later. In fact, a previous metaanalysis [10], in which the majority of participants were elderly or middle-aged men, described the occurrence of one new onset DM in every 1000 statin-treated patients, an incidence which contrasts sharply with those by JUPITER subanalysis in which 5 additional cases of new onset DM occurred in every 1000 women [26], or those by PROSPER in which an additional 4.7 new onset DM cases occurred for every 1000 elderly patients [10].

In consideration of NNT and NNH, the two populations with distinct CVD risk, i.e., statin use for primary or secondary CVD prevention, should be separately investigated. The NNT is larger among patients with a low risk of major CVD events for primary prevention than those among patients with secondary CVD prevention [27]. These comparisons could be translated into an estimation that the cardiovascular benefit seen among the patients in primary prevention trials seem to be less as compared with that in the secondary prevention trials. Furthermore, the NNT and NNH were respectively 250 and 351 in primary prevention trials, while they were respectively 98 and 202 in secondary ones [10, 27]. Taking the ratios of NNH/NNT into account, these figures suggest that higher CVD risk individuals will still strongly favor statin therapy because of the net statin benefit, while such benefit becomes less evident for lower CVD risk patients. Therefore, the risk benefit balance may differ according to levels of background CVD risks.

Potential Confounders

Assuming that the statin-DM association is real, however, several potential confounders or limitations should always be taken into account when interpreting the current publications.

a) Statin-Induced DM and Naturally-Occurring DM: Possessing Common Background Metabolic Disorders

Many patients who should be suitable for statin therapy are likely to have several concurrent metabolic disorders which are also potential risk factors for the development of DM. Baseline elevated fasting blood glucose and triglyceride, a higher body mass index, and hypertension are independent predictors of statin-induced new onset DM, and the risk of statin-induced new onset DM is further increased along with an accumulation of these [28]. Considering that such risk factors are often seen in patients with DM who do not take statin, it is plausible that statins may push predisposing individuals toward the development of DM or simply hasten the DM that would have developed anyway by these risk factors regardless of whether or not the person took statin. In this regard, the Cambridge Diabetes Risk Score may be one of the simple tools which can help identify patients who are at risk of developing DM [29].

This possibility is supported by several investigations. The participants in the WOSCOPS study, as a group, were considered as a population without insulin resistance because the overall triglyceride/high density lipoprotein cholesterol ratio was 1.7, but those who developed DM even among the WOSCOPS participants manifested features of insulin resistance such as a higher baseline body mass index, higher baseline glucose, and higher baseline triglyceride levels [30]. Similar findings were reported by subanalyses of the PROSPER [31] and JUPITER [32] studies. In the PROSPER study [31], individuals with new onset DM carried features of metabolic syndrome more prominently than those without new onset DM. In the JUPITER trial [32], rosuvastatin treatment resulted in an increase of new onset DM by 28% in subjects with one or more risk factors for DM (but a 39% reduction of primary endpoint), which contrasted sharply with the absence of any increase in new onset DM in the case of individuals with no risk factors for DM (but a 52% reduction in primary endpoint) [32]. Furthermore, the only 5.4 week difference in duration from the start of the study to DM detection between rosuvastatin and placebo groups can be interpreted as DM development at nearly the same acceleration rate between the two groups [32]. These findings further suggest that factors other than rosuvastatin use may be at least partly responsible for new onset DM.

b) Other Confounders

First, older age [9, 10], female gender [9, 26, 33], and Asian ethnic groups [34] are significantly more susceptible to develop DM by statins. Why the WOSCOPS study, unlike other trials, resulted in a 30% reduction of DM risk by pravastatin could be partly explained by its study design in which only men were participants in that study. Second, different diagnostic criteria of new onset DM among studies included in the metaanalyses cause inevitable heterogeneity. Excluding trials in which DM diagnosis is based on the physician-report attenuates the DM risk, which was no longer significant [10]. Third, studies reporting a statin-DM association –even if suggestive– were not prospectively designed to address this question. Strictly speaking, clinical trials designed to assess new onset DM as a prespecified endpoint with a systematic surveillance program are required; otherwise, a subgroup post-hoc analysis may introduce bias. Fourth, whether the statin-DM association is due to class effect or differs among individual statins, potency, or doses is not definitively determined. With regard to the potency of LDL-C reduction, rosuvastatin and atorvastatin are the most effective, yielding an average degree of LDL-C reductions that approaches 50% for atorvastatin and exceeds 50% for rosuvastatin [35], followed by simvastatin, lovastatin, pravastatin, and fluvastatin [36]. When looking at such statin potency or doses, the results of a metaanalysis [10] or observational study [6] indicate that statin-induced DM risk presumably depends on the statins' potency, while head-to-head comparisons between individual statins on developing DM prove nonsignificant [12]. In addition, the rate of new onset DM did not differ between intensive and moderate doses of statins [7]. Furthermore, the association of lipophilic statins with an increased risk of DM demonstrated in one observational study [37] was not confirmed by a metaanalysis [10]. Fifth, interpretation of the statin-DM association reported especially in cohort or retrospective analyses requires caution due to "detection bias" because patients taking statin may have more health concerns, are more likely to seek medical surveillance, and have more chances to be advised to undergo clinical examinations; thus, they are likely to have a greater likelihood for a DM diagnosis. For example, the disparity that an association between body mass index and statin-induced DM was positive in some studies [28, 31, 32] while inverse in one study [34] may be attributable to study design (RCT vs. observational). Both patients taking statins and those not on statin therapy must undergo the same routine assessment for the screening of new-onset DM to avoid detection bias. Sixth, "survival bias" may also occur by improved survival through the cardioprotective effect of statin, which may allow patients to be exposed to greater risk of developing DM and to render more chances to diagnose it. Seventh, in the reported metaanalyses, the follow-up duration was relatively short and did not allow sufficient time to determine the "true" cases of statin-induced DM. Since glucose intolerance or insulin resistance starts many years before clinically overt DM, participants should be screened at the start of the study whether or not they have DM or are even in its preclinical stage, and those in a prediabetic stage should be excluded from the clinical study to evaluate strictly the "actual" effect of statin on the development of DM.

Considering these several confounders or methodological shortcomings, RCTs should be conducted to investigate new onset DM as a primary endpoint, using a well-designed and identical screening frequency in both statin and placebo groups –excluding participants who show preexisting hyperinsulinemia or insulin resistance– as well as under the uniform diagnostic criteria of new onset DM.

Supposing that Statin Has a Risk of New Onset DM, What Should Clinicians Consider Next?

At present, it is difficult to refute the statin-DM association. These facts cause alarm and raise one important question: does statin-induced DM accelerate CVD events akin to "pure" DM? CVD risks in statin-induced DM patients may not always be the same as those in the "pure" DM patients. A combined analysis of three atorvastatin trials [28] documented that the occurrence of major CVD events was 11.3% in patients who developed atorvastatin-induced DM, which was even lower than that (17.5%) in the already-known DM while equivalent to that (10.8%) in those who did not experience atorvastatin-induced DM. These observations imply that the causal mechanisms underlying CVD events differ between statin-induced DM and "pure" DM. The risks of major CVD events in patients taking 80mg atorvastatin were equivalent regardless of whether DM was newly developed, suggesting that the CVD risk was not appreciably magnified in the new onset DM patients even by higher doses of atorvastatin.

Conclusion and Future Perspectives

Adverse events inevitably accompany medical drugs. Since adverse events cannot be avoided, the potential health benefit should be balanced against the potential risk for any prescription drugs. Given the undeniable statin-DM association, the populations of statin-induced DM cannot be negligible even if the absolute DM risk is small because of the widespread use of statins and rapid increase in DM patients globally [38]. However, it is still uncertain whether statins may causatively implicated in the development of DM because studies which assert a causal association suffer from methodological shortcomings including incomplete outcome validation and inadequate confounding control. Until these questions are completely resolved, the assumption that the benefits of statin outweigh the risk seems to be vindicated.

Such uncertainty leads future research in several directions. First, the risk-benefit balance may differ between populations with lower and higher risks of CVD events (i.e., no history or a past history of CVD), so that the currently available benefit may not be applicable to populations at a lower risk of CVD events. There is clinically meaningful evidence that statin reduces all cause mortality in secondary prevention [4], while metaanalyses concerning statins' benefit in reducing total mortality in primary prevention have provided conflicting results [4, 39].

This means that balancing the treatment benefit of CVD event reduction with the risk of new onset DM should be separately considered by stratifying the CVD risk. Unfortunately, data from observational studies are unavoidably vulnerable to biases and susceptible to confounding by variations in the health care afforded to those prescribed statins. Perhaps these biases can inflate or deflate true associations or erroneously suggest effects even in cases where none exists. In this regard, RCTs that use new onset DM as a primary prespecified endpoint should be separately conducted with each statin or for each cohort with distinct CVD risks, with the assumption that the potential risk-benefit profile of statin use is different between primary and secondary prevention. This research direction aims to identify populations who are most benefitted by statin therapy while minimizing the risk of new onset DM, with a selection of the most appropriate statin drugs. This stance will ultimately realize individualized statin therapy under considerations of patient-oriented management based on the statins' cardioprotective vs. diabetogenic balance. A second issue of concern to be clarified in the future is the ascertainment of the true CVD risks in patients with statin-induced DM as "specific" DM. Whether statin-induced DM is a transient or established disease remains to be elucidated.

Finally, the mechanisms underlying the statin-DM association and determination of the time it takes to develop DM under these mechanisms have not been fully elucidated. Additional studies are warranted to confirm when, why, how, and to whom statins cause DM as well as what happens next once statin-induced DM occurs. These issues deserve research focus and should be investigated in parallel. A thorough understanding of statin biology is essential for a better management of patients taking statins.

Although the totality of the data currently available provides reassurance that the benefits of statin outweigh the risk, new onset DM will continue to be a risk associated with statins. Until definite conclusions concerning the evidence and mechanisms of statin-induced DM as well as DM-induced future complications are elucidated and drawn, clinicians should comprehensively manage hyperlipidemic patients by prescribing statins, along with monitoring blood glucose closely during statin use on one hand, and on the other, by fundamental approaches such as advising a healthy lifestyle and diet, endurance exercise, and body weight control with a reduction of total calorie intake and avoidance of sugary drinks, rather than eliminating statins.

REFERENCES

[1] Cholesterol Treatment Trialists' (CTT) Collaborators, Kearney P. M., Blackwell L., Collins R., Keech A., Simes J., Peto R., Armitage J., Baigent C. Efficacy of cholesterol *Lancet,* 2008, 371, 117-125.

[2] Law M. R., Wald N. J., Rudnicka A. R. Quantifying effect of statins on low density lipoprotein cholesterol *BMJ,* 2003, 326, 1423.

[3] Ridker P. M., Danielson E., Fonseca F. A., Genest J., Gotto A. M. Jr., Kastelein J. J., Koenig W., Libby P., Lorenzatti A. J., MacFadyen J. G., Nordestgaard B. G., Shepherd J., Willerson J. T., Glynn R. J.; JUPITER Study Group. Rosuvastatin to prevent vascular events in men and women with elevated C-reactive protein. *N. Engl. J. Med.,* 2008, 359, 2195-2207.

[4] Carter A. A., Gomes T., Camacho X., Juurlink D. N., Shah B. R., Mamdani M. M. Risk of incident diabetes among patients treated with statins: population based study. *BMJ,* 2013, 346, f2610.

[5] Freeman D. J., Norrie J., Sattar N., Neely R. D., Cobbe S. M., Ford I., Isles C., Lorimer A. R., Macfarlane P. W., McKillop J. H., Packard C. J., Shepherd J., Gaw A. Pravastatin and the development of diabetes *Circulation,* 2001, 103, 357-362.

[6] Dormuth C. R., Filion K. B., Paterson J. M., James M. T., Teare G. F., Raymond C. B., Rahme E., Tamim H., Lipscombe L.; Canadian Network for Observational Drug Effect Studies Investigators. Higher potency statins and the risk of new diabetes: multicentre, observational study of administrative databases. *BMJ,* 2014, 348, g3244.

[7] Ko D. T., Wijeysundera H. C., Jackevicius C. A., Yousef A., Wang J., Tu J. V. Diabetes mellitus *Circ. Cardiovasc. Qual. Outcomes*, 2013, 6, 315-322.

[8] Coleman C. I., Reinhart K., Kluger J., White C. M. The effect of statins on the development of new-onset type 2 diabetes *Curr. Med. Res. Opin.*, 2008, 24, 1359-1362.

[9] Rajpathak S. N., Kumbhani D. J., Crandall J., Barzilai N., Alderman M., Ridker P. M. Statin therapy and risk of developing type 2 diabetes: a meta-analysis. *Diabetes Care,* 2009, 32, 1924-1929.

[10] Sattar N., Preiss D., Murray H. M., Welsh P., Buckley B. M., de Craen A. J., Seshasai S. R., McMurray J. J., Freeman D. J., Jukema J. W., Macfarlane P. W., Packard C. J., Stott D. J., Westendorp R. G., Shepherd J., Davis B. R., Pressel S. L., Marchioli R., Marfisi R. M., Maggioni A. P., Tavazzi L., Tognoni G., Kjekshus J., Pedersen T. R., Cook T. J., Gotto A. M., Clearfield M. B., Downs J. R., Nakamura H., Ohashi Y., Mizuno K., Ray K. K., Ford I. Statins and risk *Lancet,* 2010, 375, 735-742.

[11] Mills E. J., Wu P., Chong G., Ghement I., Singh S., Akl E. A., Eyawo O., Guyatt G., Berwanger O., Briel M. Efficacy and safety of statin treatment for cardiovascular disease: a network meta-analysis of 170,255 patients from 76 randomized trials. *QJM,* 2011, 104, 109-124.

[12] Naci H., Brugts J., Ades T. Comparative tolerability and harms of individual statins: a study-level network meta-analysis of 246 955 participants from 135 randomized, controlled trials. *Circ. Cardiovasc. Qual. Outcomes,* 2013, 6, 390-399.

[13] Taylor F., Huffman M. D., Macedo A. F., Moore T. H., Burke M., Davey Smith G., Ward K., Ebrahim S. Statins for the primary prevention of cardiovascular disease. *Cochrane Database Syst. Rev.*, 2013, 1, CD004816.

[14] Navarese E. P. 1., Buffon A., Andreotti F., Kozinski M., Welton N., Fabiszak T., Caputo S., Grzesk G., Kubica A., Swiatkiewicz I., Sukiennik A., Kelm M., De Servi S., Kubica J. Meta-analysis of impact of different types and doses of statins on new-onset diabetes mellitus. *Am. J. Cardiol.*, 2013, 111, 1123-1130.

[15] Emerging Risk Factors Collaboration, Sarwar N., Gao P., Seshasai S. R., Gobin R., Kaptoge S., Di Angelantonio E., Ingelsson E., Lawlor D. A., Selvin E., Stampfer M., Stehouwer C. D., Lewington S., Pennells L., Thompson A., Sattar N., White I. R., Ray K. K., Danesh J. Diabetes mellitus, fasting *Lancet,* 2010, 375, 2215-2222.

[16] Ray K. K., Seshasai S. R., Wijesuriya S., Sivakumaran R., Nethercott S., Preiss D., Erqou S., Sattar N. Effect of intensive control of glucose *Lancet,* 2009, 373, 1765-1772.

[17] Emerging Risk Factors Collaboration, Seshasai S. R., Kaptoge S., Thompson A., Di Angelantonio E., Gao P., Sarwar N., Whincup P. H., Mukamal K. J., Gillum R. F., Holme I., Njølstad I., Fletcher A., Nilsson P., Lewington S., Collins R., Gudnason V., Thompson S. G., Sattar N., Selvin E., Hu F. B., Danesh J. Diabetes mellitus, fasting *N. Engl. J. Med.*, 2011, 364, 829-841.

[18] Preiss D., Seshasai S. R., Welsh P., Murphy S. A., Ho J. E., Waters D. D., DeMicco D. A., Barter P., Cannon C. P., Sabatine M. S., Braunwald E., Kastelein J. J., de Lemos J. A., Blazing M. A., Pedersen T. R., Tikkanen M. J., Sattar N., Ray K. K. Risk of incident diabetes with intensive-dose compared with moderate-dose statin therapy: a meta-analysis. *JAMA,* 2011, 305, 2556-2264.

[19] Brault M., Ray J., Gomez Y. H., Mantzoros C. S., Daskalopoulou S. S. Statin treatment and new-onset diabetes: A review of proposed mechanisms. *Metabolism,* 2014, 63, 735-745.

[20] Xia F., Xie L., Mihic A., Gao X., Chen Y., Gaisano H. Y., Tsushima R. G. Inhibition of cholesterol biosynthesis impairs insulin secretion and voltage-gated calcium channel function in pancreatic beta-cells. *Endocrinology,* 2008, 149, 5136-5145.

[21] Koh K. K., Sakuma I., Quon M. J. Differential metabolic effects of distinct statins. *Atherosclerosis,* 2011, 215, 1-8.

[22] Navarese E. P., Szczesniak A., Kolodziejczak M., Gorny B., Kubica J., Suryapranata H. Statins and risk *Am. J. Cardiovasc. Drugs*, 2014, 14, 79-87.

[23] Baker W. L., Talati R., White C. M., Coleman C. I. Differing effect of statins on insulin *Diabetes Res. Clin. Pract.*, 2010, 87, 98-107.

[24] Cholesterol Treatment Trialists' (CTT) Collaboration, Baigent C., Blackwell L., Emberson J., Holland L. E., Reith C., Bhala N., Peto R., Barnes E. H., Keech A., Simes J., Collins R. Efficacy and safety *Lancet,* 2010, 376, 1670-1681.

[25] Cannon C. P. Balancing the benefits *Lancet*, 2010, 375, 700-701.

[26] Mora S., Glynn R. J., Hsia J., MacFadyen J. G., Genest J., Ridker P. M. Statins for the primary prevention of cardiovascular events in women with elevated high-sensitivity C-reactive protein or dyslipidemia: results from the Justification for the Use of Statins in Prevention: An Intervention Trial Evaluating Rosuvastatin (JUPITER) and meta-analysis of women from primary prevention trials. *Circulation,* 2010, 121, 1069-1077.

[27] Cholesterol Treatment Trialists' (CTT) Collaborators, Mihaylova B., Emberson J., Blackwell L., Keech A., Simes J., Barnes E. H., Voysey M., Gray A., Collins R., Baigent C. The effects of lowering LDL *Lancet,* 2012, 380, 581-590.

[28] Waters D. D., Ho J. E., DeMicco D. A., Breazna A., Arsenault B. J., Wun C. C., Kastelein J. J., Colhoun H., Barter P. Predictors of new-onset diabetes *J. Am. Coll. Cardiol.*, 2011, 57, 1535-1545.

[29] Rahman M., Simmons R. K., Harding A. H., Wareham N. J., Griffin S. J. A simple risk *Fam. Pract.*, 2008, 25, 191-196.

[30] McLaughlin T., Abbasi F., Cheal K., Chu J., Lamendola C., Reaven G. Use of metabolic markers to identify overweight *Ann. Intern. Med.*, 2003, 139, 802-809.

[31] Sattar N., McConnachie A., Shaper A. G., Blauw G. J., Buckley B. M., de Craen A. J., Ford., Forouhi N. G., Freeman D. J., Jukema J. W., Lennon L., Macfarlane P. W., Murphy M. B., Packard C. J., Stott D. J., Westendorp R. G., Whincup P. H., Shepherd J., Wannamethee S. G. Can metabolic syndrome usefully predict cardiovascular disease and diabetes? Outcome data from two prospective studies. *Lancet,* 2008, 371, 1927-1935.

[32] Ridker P. M., Pradhan A., MacFadyen J. G., Libby P., Glynn R. J. Cardiovascular benefits *Lancet,* 2012, 380, 565-571.

[33] Goodarzi M. O., Li X., Krauss R. M., Rotter J. I., Chen Y. D. Relationship of sex *Diabetes Care*, 2013, 36, e100-101.

[34] Culver A. L., Ockene I. S., Balasubramanian R., Olendzki B. C., Sepavich D. M., Wactawski-Wende J., Manson J. E., Qiao Y., Liu S., Merriam P. A., Rahilly-Tierny C., Thomas F., Berger J. S., Ockene J. K., Curb J. D., Ma Y. Statin use and risk *Arch. Intern. Med.,* 2012, 172, 144-152.

[35] Nicholls S. J., Ballantyne C. M., Barter P. J., Chapman M. J., Erbel R. M., Libby P., Raichlen J. S., Uno K., Borgman M., Wolski K., Nissen S. E. Effect of two intensive statin *N. Engl. J. Med.*, 2011, 365, 2078-2087.

[36] Jones P., Kafonek S., Laurora I., Hunninghake D. Comparative dose efficacy study of atorvastatin versus simvastatin, pravastatin, lovastatin, and fluvastatin in patients with hypercholesterolemia (the CURVES study) *Am. J. Cardiol.*, 1998, 81, 582-587.

[37] Danaei G., García Rodríguez L. A., Fernandez Cantero O., Hernán M. A. Statins and risk *Diabetes Care*, 2013, 36, 1236-1240.

[38] Nolan C. J., Damm P., Prentki M. Type 2 diabetes *Lancet,* 2011, 378, 169-181.

[39] Ray K. K., Seshasai S. R., Erqou S., Sever P., Jukema J. W., Ford I., Sattar N. Statins and all-cause mortality *Arch. Intern. Med.*, 2010, 170, 1024-1031.

INDEX

D

G

H

I

N

O

P

R

S

T

U

V

W

Y